Primary Care Procedures in Women's Health

Sandra M. Sulik • Cathryn B. Heath
Editors

Primary Care Procedures in Women's Health

An International Guide for the Primary Care Setting

Third Edition

Springer

Editors
Sandra M. Sulik
Family Medicine
St Joseph's Health
Syracuse, NY, USA

Cathryn B. Heath
Medical Director
Rutgers University Student Health
New Brunswick, NJ, USA

ISBN 978-3-032-07060-9 ISBN 978-3-032-07061-6 (eBook)
https://doi.org/10.1007/978-3-032-07061-6

This Springer imprint is published by the registered company Springer Nature Switzerland AG
The registered company address is: Gewerbestrasse 11, 6330 Cham, Switzerland

In memory of my mom, who provided constant faithful support and encouragement; and to my family, Jeff, Maryann, Julie, Read, Tammy, Abbie, Joe, Lydia, and Lisa, who have always believed in me. Special thanks to Julie for her help with photos and formatting, to my nurses Jill and Patti and my many patients who graciously allowed picture taking during their procedures. My thanks to Cathy for her friendship, support, and energy throughout this process. Thanks to all our contributing authors for sharing their expertise and wisdom.

SMS

Special thanks to my wonderful husband John and my dear friend Sandy. To my family, friends, colleagues, staff, and patients: How lucky I am to be surrounded by such wonderful people! To Brendan, Austin, and Claire who have provided strength, encouragement, wisdom, and patience. Thank you to all who contributed their time writing and rewriting chapters and to our colleagues at Springer Nature for assisting us with this journey.

CBH

Preface

There are many reasons for primary care providers to offer women's health procedures in an outpatient setting. Patients feel more comfortable having procedures done by clinicians whom they already know and trust. Continuity of care is still valued by patients, who trust their primary care providers to work with them as collaborators in the decision-making process. Patients have found that their options for care have become limited, not by their own decision but by the lack of training of their provider. In rural areas, the barriers of time, expense, and travel often prevent many women from obtaining necessary care; yet many of the procedures that these patients are requesting are relatively easy to learn.

This book is designed to assist not only the clinician performing the procedures covered but also the office staff with setting up the equipment tray prior to performing the procedure and with preparing office documents and coding information needed to complete the procedure. Most procedures covered can be done with a minimum investment in equipment and require minimal training. Some of the procedures either require or are best performed after a training course; however, even in these cases, this book will serve as a solid aid and review to the practitioner in performing the procedures within the office setting. The book can be used as a quick reference guide to re-familiarize the practitioner with the steps to a given procedure.

The book begins with basic chapters that are applicable to all procedures. Each chapter thereafter outlines one women's health procedure and contains an overview of background information, indications, contraindications, complications, equipment needed, procedure steps, an office note, patient instructions, and a patient handout. Case studies serve as illustrations of typical patients found in practices who have needed the procedure. The "tricks and helpful hints" section draws on the years of experience of providers who have performed each procedure many times and have overcome common difficulties often encountered by newcomers to the procedure. A setup picture of equipment is included to assist office staff in gathering the appropriate materials prior to starting the procedure. Algorithms assisting the provider with the steps to take at decision points of each procedure are also included to serve as a quick guide. References and additional resources are provided for further education, learning, and equipment needs. Illustrations, images, and photos further enrich the chapters.

We have elected to start our procedure book with the most common of procedures found in women's health—these include pelvic examinations and Pap smear collection—and its content extends to some of the more complicated office procedures, such as manual vacuum abortions and loop electrical excision procedure (LEEP). There are sections on basic women's health, contraceptive, diagnostic, and therapeutic procedures. Primary care physicians experienced with performing the procedure have written the chapter content. Also included are specific chapters on coding and billing, authored by a physician who oversees a large student health center. A separate chapter is included on the medico-legal aspects of performing women's health procedures in an office setting. This chapter outlines the necessary legal and regulatory considerations to address before adding many of these procedures to an office practice. We have also included a chapter on population health in this edition, which emphasizes process improvement in an outpatient clinical setting.

Many procedures have become a "lost art." A number of these common women's health procedures are not routinely taught in residency or training programs, and, hence, many practitioners do not offer them in their offices. Some are trained during residency but have not performed the procedure for some time and need a review prior to performing the procedure. This book will serve as a quick refresher for those procedures for which the clinician may have had previous training but may not have performed for a while.

The old standard of "see one, teach one, do one" gets more difficult as procedures become more complex and require more training before they can be performed. A number of excellent procedure courses are offered by the American Academy of Family Physicians, American College of Obstetrics and Gynecology, and the American Society of Colposcopy and Cervical Pathology. Suppliers of medical equipment also offer training courses. A training package is often offered as part of the purchase of more expensive pieces of equipment or may be mandated by the manufacturer prior to being able to place an order for the device. Finding a local experienced physician to precept and mentor a less experienced clinician in the initial few procedures is another way to become skilled in performing most of these procedures. Proctoring or precepted experience is crucial, especially for complex procedures, not only to reduce medico-legal liability but also to ensure patient safety.

Having the patient schedule a separate appointment to have a procedure performed allows the patient time to read the information provided about the upcoming procedure, ask appropriate questions, and prepare herself for the actual procedure. This allows for the proper amount of time to be scheduled for the procedure to be done; for the inexperienced clinician, additional time should be scheduled. Scheduling new procedures at the end of an office session allows more time. As the practitioner's confidence grows, scheduling times can be adjusted. Scheduling an office session dedicated to just procedures can also be helpful.

A well-trained staff is the clinician's best asset. A lunchtime training session can be very helpful for teaching the staff proper sterilization of instruments, sterile and nonsterile equipment setup, and how best to assist with the procedure itself. Appropriate equipment setups can greatly ease the procedure. Proper Occupational Safety and Health Administration (OSHA) guidelines must also be followed. For most women's health procedures, it is wise to have an assistant in the room with the provider to assist as well as to comfort and chaperone the patient. A written consent should be completed prior to most procedures.

It is important to understand the appropriate billing of your services in order to be properly compensated for your work. Both CPT® codes developed by the American Medical Association and the ICD10 (International Classification of Diseases, 10th Revision, Center for Disease Control and Prevention) codes are provided as suggested codes for each procedure. There may be other more appropriate codes; therefore, each procedure should be coded based on the procedures done or services rendered. Some minor procedures, such as cervical polyp removal, do not have a specific CPT® code. In those circumstances, the CPT® manual recommends that the clinician code the appropriate-level office visit. As covered in our billing and coding chapter, certain insurance plans reimburse differently for some of the contraception devices, and insurance reimbursement varies across the county. It is important that the provider be aware of these differences as these procedures are offered to the patient in the office. Prior authorization is sometimes necessary as well. Some devices (levonorgestrel intrauterine system or etonorgestrel implantables) may need to be ordered through the patient's insurance company and delivered to the office before insertion.

We also wish to acknowledge that there is a changing landscape regarding gender, and that not all women necessarily have female reproductive organs consistent with their gender. We have opted to choose the word "patient" in place of "women" since some of the people who desperately need empathic care and need these procedures are not women. We will use terminology specifically related to "women" when citing scientific studies who have used this terminology within their work.

It is our hope that this book will act as a manual for women's health procedures for all providers and their staff, including family physicians, gynecologists, general internists, residents, nurse practitioners, nurse midwives, and physician's assistants. There are presently no other texts specifically written for providers and staff of women's health services. It is our hope that this book will allow the clinician to become competent, efficient, and comfortable in performing each procedure in the office on a regular basis.

Syracuse, NY, USA — Sandra M. Sulik
New Brunswick, NJ, USA — Cathryn B. Heath

Contents

Contributors

Rhina Acevedo, MD Department of Family Medicine and Community Health, Rutgers School of Biomedical Health Sciences, New Brunswick, NJ, USA

Jennifer Amico, MD, MPH Department of Family Medicine and Community Health, Rutgers Robert Wood Johnson Medical School, New Brunswick, NJ, USA

Melissa Arthur, PhD Faculty, St. Joseph's Family Medicine Residency, Professor, Department of Psychiatry, Upstate Medical University, Syracuse, NY, USA

Meghan E. Boshart, MD PGY2, Boston Medical Center Family Medicine Residency, Boston, MA, USA

H Reeve Bright, MD, MPH Department of Family Medicine, Hoboken University Medical Center, CarePoint Health, Hoboken, NJ, USA

Dawn Brink-Cymerman, MD Faculty, St. Joseph's Family Medicine Residency, Syracuse, NY, USA

Anthony L. Ciricillo, MD Liberty Resources, Syracuse, NY, USA

DeAnn Cummings, MD Faculty, St. Joseph's Family Medicine Residency, Syracuse, NY, USA

Sara-Ann Fox, MD Faculty, St. Joseph's Family Medicine Residency, Syracuse, NY, USA

Roshan Ghimire, MD Faculty, St. Joseph's Family Medicine Residency, Syracuse, NY, USA

Cathryn B. Heath, MD Medical Director, Rutgers University Student Health, New Brunswick, NJ, USA

Stephen D. Hoag, MD St. Joseph's Family Medicine Residency, Syracuse, NY, USA

Catherine I. Keating, MD Berkshire Family Practice Associates, North Adams, MA, USA

Nadine Khouzam, MD Faculty, St. Joseph's Family Medicine Residency, Syracuse, NY, USA

David E. Kolva, MD Retired Faculty, St. Joseph's Family Medicine Residency, Syracuse, NY, USA

Jeffrey P. Levine, MD Department of Family Medicine and Community Health, Rutgers Robert Wood Johnson Medical School, New Brunswick, NJ, USA

Kenya M. Lyons, MD California Central Coast, Planned Parenthood, Santa Monica, California, USA

Barbara Jo McGarry, MD Department of Family Medicine and Community Health, Rutgers Robert Wood Johnson Medical School, New Brunswick, NJ, USA

Kristen McNamara, MD Faculty, St. Joseph's Family Medicine Residency, Syracuse, NY, USA

Elizabeth H. McNany, MD Faculty, St. Joseph's Family Medicine Residency, Syracuse, NY, USA

Joshua A. Mleczko, DO Capital Health Primary Care – Bordentown, Bordentown, NJ, USA

Matthew L. Picone, MD Faculty, St. Joseph's Family Medicine Residency, Syracuse, NY, USA

Ryan Planer, MD Faculty, St. Joseph's Family Medicine Residency, Syracuse, NY, USA

Anna Sliwowska, MD Department of Family Medicine and Community Health, Rutgers Robert Wood Johnson Medical School, New Brunswick, NJ, USA

Sandra M. Sulik, MD St. Joseph's Health; Professor Emeritus, Upstate Medical Center, Syracuse, NY, USA

Laurie Turenne-Kolpan, MD Faculty, Department of Family Practice, Hunterdon Medical Center, Flemington, NJ, USA

Chapter 1
Introduction: The Case for Procedures in Primary Care

Cathryn B. Heath and Sandra M. Sulik

Case Studies

A patient came to the office requesting an intrauterine device (IUD) placement, a procedure that the author had not done in several years. She told the patient that she had not done this procedure in quite some time and offered to send her to another physician. The patient's response was that she preferred her own primary care physician do the procedure, and the patient suggested that the author "just read the book and then go ahead." The procedure was successful and was the first of many IUD placements within this physician's practice in New Jersey.

A patient came into the office in Student Health due to a strange bump she noticed on her vulva. She tried to do a computer search to find out what it could be and was now worried she could have cancer of the vulva or perhaps a sexually transmitted disease. Upon seeing the family physician at Health Services, she was diagnosed with a Bartholin Gland cyst and, after discussing her options by shared decision making, opted to have it drained. She was relieved that she didn't have to find another provider and could have the procedure done at the health center by someone she knew and trusted.

A patient came in to see their physician with symptoms of pressure in her vagina which worsened upon standing. With many health problems, the patient was considered at high risk for major morbidity and mortality from surgery. She came to the office for a pessary fitting, as there were few physicians in town who fit pessaries.

C. B. Heath (✉)
Rutgers University Student Health, New Brunswick, NJ, USA
e-mail: heathcb@scarletmail.rutgers.edu

S. M. Sulik
St. Joseph's Health; Professor Emeritus, Upstate Medical Center, Syracuse, NY, USA
e-mail: Sandra.sulik@sjhsyr.org

S. M. Sulik, C. B. Heath (eds.), *Primary Care Procedures in Women's Health*,
https://doi.org/10.1007/978-3-032-07061-6_1

The patient was successfully treated with a pessary, which avoided major surgery and relieved her urinary incontinence. The grateful woman used the pessary successfully for many years.

Location of Practice

These cases exemplify the necessity for women's health procedures being performed by primary care physicians, such as family physicians, pediatricians, and obstetricians/gynecologists, and internists and by primary care providers such as midwives, advanced nurse practitioners, and physician's assistants. Currently, a significant healthcare disparity exists for women who reside in rural areas. Over 20% of the population of the United States resides in rural areas with rates as low as 26.5 primary care providers/100,000 patients in Mississippi and the rates in Georgia and Texas being only slightly higher (31/100,000 and 33.61/100,000, respectively) [1]. Primary care providers in this study included physicians, physician assistants, and advanced practice nurses. While rates of internal medicine providers and specialist providers were higher in the United States in urban and suburban areas, family physicians and nurse practitioners were in higher preponderance in rural areas, particularly in the US Midwest [2].

The scope of practice of rural physicians has by necessity been broad, although the rate of surgical procedures reported by rural physicians in Canada was similar to those who practice in a more urban setting [3]. Female physicians performed more women's health procedures than other procedures in any setting.

In many instances, access to a specialist for routine procedures is difficult, and, thus, many generalist providers are doing procedures that in more suburban and urban regions are considered reserved for specialists. In a study of colonoscopy in rural communities, family physicians performed colonoscopies on patients with symptoms as well as on patients for screening. Family physicians successfully reached the cecum in 96% of the cases, with an average time of 15.9 min, finding neoplastic polyps in 22% of the patients and cancer in 2.5% of the patients [4].

Continuity of Care: "The Medical Home"

Patients prefer seeing the same provider and consider seeing the same provider every time they have a health problem as very important [5]. Patients prefer, in many cases, to have procedures done by a practitioner whom they know and trust. For instance, in a study conducted at an inner-city clinic, 70% of patients thought it appropriate for their family physicians to do medical abortions. Forty-seven percent thought it appropriate for their family physicians to do first-trimester surgical abortions. Of the women who would personally consider an abortion, 73% preferred to have it done by their family physician, 22% preferred to go to a freestanding abortion clinic, and 5% had no preference [6]. In a survey done by the Kaiser Family Foundation, 54% of obstetricians/gynecologists stated that they would be very or somewhat likely to prescribe mifepristone for medication abortions. Fifty percent of family physicians, nurse practitioners, and physician's assistants reported interest in prescribing mifepristone. At the time of the survey, only 5% of family physicians currently performed surgical abortions [7]. As of 2020, there are only 3% of family physicians performing either medical or surgical abortions [8].

In 2017, the rate of clinical procedures performed by family physicians at their practice revealed that 31% performed endometrial sampling, 74% performed skin procedures including biopsy and cryotherapy, and 12% performed colposcopy, among a variety of other procedures [9].

Many patients expect their generalist providers to perform common procedures, especially those done in an outpatient setting. Most patients appreciate continuity and find that receiving care (including procedures) from one provider improved the physician–patient relationship [9].

Procedure Training

A number of procedures have become a lost art, making it difficult for patients to access providers who feel comfortable performing these procedures. Physicians in the past have relied on learning procedures in medical school or residency, yet newer, more advanced procedures can only be offered in a postgraduate setting for most practicing physicians.

In medical school, family medicine clerkships provide some basis for learning common women's health procedures, such as obtaining a Pap smear. In a procedure knowledge survey, Pap smear was the only women's health procedure that students felt competent at being able to perform independently [10]. In Canada, 91% of physicians reported learning procedures in medical school or in a family medicine residency, whereas only 12.6% learned procedures in clinical practice settings, followed by 6.4% who reported learning procedures in formal skills training. Those in rural practice learned a relatively greater proportion of procedural skills through formal skills training [11].

While the general guidelines for women's health procedure skills within a family medicine residency have mandatory procedures (Pap smears, wet mount, and KOH prep, vulvar biopsy, Bartholin cyst management, intrauterine device insertion/removal), some less common procedures are considered something that a resident should be exposed to but not necessary become proficient with doing (colposcopy, cervical cryotherapy). There are some significant barriers to teaching and performing office-based procedures which need to be overcome by residency practices, including assuring adequate volume to be able to teach the procedure, that the appropriate faculty are available, and that there is enough given time in the schedule to be able to perform the procedure [12]. This is particularly difficult for procedures like vulvar biopsy or Bartholin cyst management.

Insurance Coverage

The good news is that many insurance plans across the United States are covering contraceptive procedures more commonly than ever before. Due to the Patient Protection and Affordable Care Act, the United States now mandates that insurance cover the cost of preventive care and contraceptives. However, there are still many women who do not currently have healthcare coverage.

Conclusion

Whatever the rationale, women's health procedures are in demand, especially in a primary care setting, and are rewarding for both physician and patient alike. No matter where the location of the practice or what type of patient or provider may be involved, generalist providers can offer these procedures as part of their daily practice. All of these procedures are easy to learn, most require minimal equipment, and they offer services that improve women's health and the range of options for the care that all patients wish to receive from their provider.

References

1. Hing E, Hsiao C. State variability in supply of office-based primary care providers: United States 2012. NCHS data brief, no 151. Hyattsville: National Center for Health Statistics; 2014.
2. Naylor KB, Tootoo J, Yakusheva O, Shipman SA, Bynum JPW, Davis MA. Geographic variation in spatial accessibility of U.S. healthcare providers. PLoS One. 2019;14(4):e0215016. https://doi.org/10.1371/journal.pone.0215016. Published 2019 Apr 9.
3. Jaakkimainen R, Schultz S, Sood P. Office-based procedures among urban and rural family physicians in Ontario. Can Fam Physician. 2012;58(10):E578–E5874.
4. Edwards JK, Norris TE. Colonoscopy in rural communities: can family physicians perform the procedure with safe and efficacious results? J Am Board Fam Pract. 2004;17:353–8.
5. Baker R, Mainous AG, Gray DP, Love MM. Exploration of the relationship between continuity, trust in regular doctors and patient satisfaction with consultations with family doctors. Scand J Prim Health Care. 2003;21(1):27–32.
6. Rubin SE, Godfrey E, Gold M. Patient attitudes toward early abortion services in the family medicine clinic. J Am Board Fam Med. 2008;21(2):162–4.
7. Koenig JD, Tapias MP, Hoff T. Are US health professionals likely to prescribe mifepristone or methotrexate? J Am Med Womens Assoc. 2000;55:155–60.
8. Patel P, Narayana S, Summit A, et al. Abortion provision among recently graduated family physicians. Fam Med. 2020;52(10):724–9. https://doi.org/10.22454/FamMed.2020.300682. Accessed 2 Feb 2025.

9. Haggerty JL, Pineault R, Beaulieu MD, Brunelle Y, Gauthier J, Goulet F, Rodriguez J. Practice features associated with patient-reported accessibility, continuity, and coordination of primary health care. Ann Fam Med. 2008;6:116–23.
10. Garcia-Rodriguez JA, Dickinson JA, Perez G, Ross D, Au L, Ross S, Babenko O, Johnston I. Procedural knowledge and skills of residents entering Canadian Family Medicine Programs in Alberta. Fam Med. 2018;50(1):10–21.
11. Crutcher RA, Szafran O, Woloschuk W, Chaytors RG, Topps DA, Humphries PW, Norton PG. Where Canadian family physicians learn procedural skills. Fam Med. 2005;37(7):491–5.
12. Langner S, Deffenbacher B, Nagle J, Khodeaee M. Barriers and methods to improve office-based procedural training in a family medicine residency. J Med Educ. 2016;7:158–9.

Chapter 2
Coding, Billing, and Reimbursement for Procedures

Cathryn B. Heath

Introduction

Coding, billing, and reimbursement are an integral part of the procedures performed in today's modern medical office. Performing the procedure is only part of the process. Providers and their business managers must establish a system to ensure that the device (i.e., pessary, intrauterine device, etc.) and the performance of the procedure are reimbursed prior to initiating the procedure within a medical practice. Since some devices are very expensive, it can be a costly mistake not to be reimbursed. Appropriate billing with concomitant reimbursement can gradually change the emphasis and tenor of a clinician's practice improving satisfaction for patients and clinicians alike. Once the billing process has been established, it can then be modified to add additional procedures.

Procedure Coding

To ease coding and billing processes, we have included within each chapter appropriate codes for the device (if applicable) and the procedures described.

We suggest that, if possible, a discussion of risks and benefits, side effects, cost, other choices beyond the recommended procedure, and other providers who can perform this procedure, and answering any questions that a patient may have occur at a separate office visit. The rationale for doing so is that it allows the patient to decide with all the information given whether they wish to proceed. It also allows patients to premedicate with a nonsteroidal anti-inflammatory if necessary. This

---

C. B. Heath (✉)
Rutgers University Student Health, New Brunswick, NJ, USA
e-mail: heathcb@scarletmail.rutgers.edu

S. M. Sulik, C. B. Heath (eds.), *Primary Care Procedures in Women's Health*,
https://doi.org/10.1007/978-3-032-07061-6_2

discussion can also give your staff sufficient time to contact insurance regarding reimbursement. However, it may not be possible for the patient to return considering that they may need to take time away from work or travel far to get to the clinician's office, so communication between the patient, the clinician, and the business office is important.

Most procedures have global codes. This means that all visits regarding the procedure are coded based on the procedure alone. Thus, if a procedure such as a Bartholin's gland excision requires a second visit for a recheck, the recheck is considered part of the original global procedure code and would not be billed as a second office visit. Similarly, if there are sutures being removed for a procedure done in the office, the suture removal should be covered in the global fee. If suturing or the procedure has been done elsewhere and the patient is only coming in for a recheck or suture removal, the clinician can bill for this task. If the follow-up office visit is related to reviewing pathology, one can bill separately for a visit to review and discuss the treatment options of colposcopy pathology.

If a clinician is seeing a patient for reasons other than just the procedure, the office visit and procedure need to be coded separately. For instance, if a patient is being seen for a gynecologic exam and requests that her intrauterine device (IUD) be removed, the clinician would code for a well-woman exam, use a -25 modifier, and then code for the IUD removal. If the patient prefers to return another day for the IUD removal, one would only code for the actual procedure on the IUD removal visit.

Coding compatibility with the procedure is essential to ensure payment. For those practicing in the United States, Medicare's website (http://www.cms.gov) is an excellent place to start [1]. Healthcare Common Procedure Coding System ("HCPCS" or "hick pics") has two levels. Level I coding is used to code for the procedure itself, associated with the appropriate Current Procedural Technology (CPT®, AMA, Chicago, IL) code. Level II HCPCS allows for coding for products, devices, and supplies. Within the United States, there are stipulations for which CPT® codes will be approved by private payers and/or Medicare and Medicaid for a procedure, and it depends on whether the specific insurance will reimburse a clinical provider for the procedure and/or device. Insurance approval of procedures varies by the medical insurance product purchased by the insured's place of work in the US, insurances purchased in an open market by the patient, or on state-specific Medicaid programs. Other countries with universal health coverage may not have the same experience.

Documentation and Billing of Procedures

Documentation needs to start with a consent prior to the procedure that the provider reviewed risks, benefits, side effects, other possible providers of this procedure, and follow-up. If anesthesia of any type is used, elicit any past reactions to anesthesia, and describe risks and benefits and possible side effects of the use of the anesthesia use as well. The consent should be signed by both the provider and the patient prior to the procedure. After the procedure is finished, the procedure steps need to be documented. Many clinicians use a pre-formatted template for consents and the procedure note. Samples of such notes are included in each chapter. If a provider is supervising a learner, the provider needs to be present for the entire procedure. Documentation needs to reflect this arrangement. Follow-up instructions on post-procedure care and possible aftereffects, contact information in case of an adverse event within the discharge instructions, and the appointment for follow-up if needed should be given to the patient prior to leaving.

Size and location of excised lesions should be documented, as reimbursement is determined by size, location, number of lesions removed, and the pathology of the lesion (benign versus malignant). Billing for excision of lesions should be submitted based not only on the size of the lesion but also on the size of the margins. For instance, if a 1 cm lesion is removed using a margin of 0.2 cm on each side, the size would be considered 1.4 cm [2]. Follow-up should be clearly stated in order to document whether a subsequent visit should be considered part of the procedure.

Coding and billing for skin procedures or colposcopy biopsies is further complicated by the specific pathologic diagnosis of the lesion itself. For instance, coding for removal of a benign versus malignant lesion may be difficult until the biopsy results have returned to the office, which may be anywhere from 10 to 14 days after the date the actual procedure is performed. However, removal of a malignancy is generally reimbursed at an average of two to three times the amount of the removal of a benign lesion. Thus, in some instances in which the CPT® code may be dramatically changed by the pathology results, it may be advisable to hold billing the procedure until the pathology report returns and is reviewed.

One can also attempt to bill for an unsuccessful procedure, though the likelihood of being reimbursed for the procedure is much less [3]. Coding needs to be specific; for instance, if a procedure fails due to anatomic reasons, use a -52 code. If the procedure fails due to concern over a patient's well-being (e.g., she had severe pain or vasovagal symptoms), it is considered a discontinued procedure and is coded as a -53. The payer will need to know the extent of what was done; attaching a copy of the office note to the claim will usually suffice.

Durable Medical Goods

Devices such as IUDs may be stocked by an office if the procedure is performed on a frequent basis. If the office is providing the device, the clinician needs to bill the specific HCPCS or "J code" associated with the device as well as bill the code for the procedure itself. Alternatively, some offices order the device after the patient comes in for a consultative visit prior to the procedure. In this case, the staff can arrange with the patient's insurance company to assist with the provision of a device. The IUD is then sent to the office in the patient's name; when it is received, the patient is called so that insertion can be scheduled. In this case, the provider will bill the procedure code but not bill for the device.

Pharmaceutical companies will frequently send a replacement for a device used in an unsuccessful procedure. This process can be started either online or through the pharmaceutical representative for that device. The pharmaceutical company will request the lot number of the device, the reason for the unsuccessful procedure, any adverse events that occurred due to the device, and other information to replace the device. They may also request the device itself for process improvement purposes. Keeping the device and the packaging until otherwise instructed differently by the pharmaceutical respresentative involved is best practice.

Insurance Company Coverage

Within the United States, medical procedures are highly scrutinized by insurance companies due to the expense of the procedure itself. Some insurances require prior authorization for procedures, which may include submitting prior office notes, labs, or radiology reports to substantiate the need for the actual procedure. This varies nationally by region and by the policy negotiated by the patient's employer. There are organizations that will assist women advocating with their insurance to obtain women's health procedures, such as the National Women's Law Center "Cover her" project (Center 2024) [4].

In the United States, it is imperative to have knowledgeable staff in your business office who are prepared to obtain authorization for the device or procedure, bill with appropriate coding, review and revise, and resubmit any rejected claims. It is important to have the patient sign an Advance Beneficiary Notice ("ABN") stating that she is willing to pay for the procedure and the device prior to performing the procedure for any costs not covered by her insurance.

As billing improves, rejected claims decrease in number. It is a common mistake to presume all patients of a particular insurance carrier cover a particular outpatient procedure. In the United States, the subtypes of a particular insurance vary, so it is best to check with the insurance carrier on each specific patient's insurance product.

Coding also can be improved and facilitated by using specific coding software, websites, or standardized forms, some of which may even be accessed by either an electronic medical record or a handheld electronic device.

Charity Care Procedures

Charity care services also may be available for procedures such as IUD insertion or implantable devices. For instance, the Arch Foundation was established as a not-for-profit institution to help low-income women who have no insurance coverage for the levonorgestrel intrauterine systems manufactured by Bayer. Primary Care residencies who participate in charity care programs for teaching learners how to insert or implant contraceptive devices may in some cases be able to access devices from manufacturers at low or no cost. Planned Parenthood or Family Planning may offer a lower cost option for those who are underinsured or not insured as well.

Summary

Appropriate coding and billing improve women's access to important health procedures. Due to the coding specificity, tracking payment and improving the process of payment are relatively easy tasks for any clinician's practice. Familiarizing oneself and one's billing staff with coding for procedures by type of procedure and by type of payment by specific insurance company will increase the likelihood of payment, thus rewarding the clinician for providing services that are requested by the patient or necessary for good clinical care.

References

1. HCPCS coding questions. Baltimore: Centers for Medicare and Medicaid Services. https://www.cms.gov/medicare/coding-billing/healthcare-common-procedure-system. https://www.cms.gov/Medicare/Coding/MedHCPCSGenInfo/index.html. Accessed 17 Feb 2024.
2. Fox G, McCann L. Twelve errors to avoid in coding skin procedures. Fam Pract Manag. 2013;20(1):11–6.
3. LARC coding. Long acting reversible contraceptives. University of California in San Francisco. https://larcprogram.ucsf.edu/coding. Accessed 17 Feb 2024.
4. Cover her. Washington, DC: National Women's Law Center. https://nwlc.org/coverher/. Accessed 17 Feb 2024.

Additional Resource

Websites

The Arch Foundation: http://www.archfoundation.com.

Chapter 3
Legal Aspects of Office-Based Women's Health Procedures

Sandra M. Sulik and David E. Kolva

Introduction

As primary care practitioners face increasing liability risk in this litigious society, careful planning and timely consultation with your competent legal advisor are critically important to reduce your exposure to lawsuits or misconduct sanctions.

The United States Supreme Court overturned the Roe vs Wade and Planned Parenthood vs Casey precedents with the ruling on June 24, 2022 in the Dobbs vs Jackson Women's Health Organization decision. This decision that there is no constitutional protection for abortion and allowed states to restrict or ban abortion with preexisting laws or new legislation has led to a public health crisis for many people. This decision has impacted the care of patients across the United States needing reproductive care. It also has forced clinicians practicing in states that have banned abortion to reconcile the law with their clinical recommendations for conditions such as molar pregnancy, ectopic pregnancy, miscarriage, previable rupture of membranes, and other such conditions [1].

The most common reasons primary care clinicians are sued are failure to diagnose in a timely manner, failure to consult in a timely manner, negligent procedures, and failure to provide informed consent. It is crucial to follow patient complaints to a full diagnosis, prepare them mentally for the procedure through informed consent, and know when it is time to consult a colleague or refer to a specialist. Ensuring well-documented notes highlighting key components is important as well.

S. M. Sulik (✉)
St. Joseph's Health; Professor Emeritus, Upstate Medical Center, Syracuse, NY, USA
e-mail: Sandra.Sulik@sjhsyr.org

D. E. Kolva
St Joseph's Family Medicine Residency, Syracuse, NY, USA

S. M. Sulik, C. B. Heath (eds.), *Primary Care Procedures in Women's Health*,
https://doi.org/10.1007/978-3-032-07061-6_3

Since the US regulation of medical practice is largely an individual state activity, and laws vary widely by locality, this chapter is not intended to provide personal legal advice. When your practice makes decisions about new policies or procedures, they should be clearly recorded in a practice policy and procedure manual. A user-friendly manual, in print and/or electronic form, will standardize policy and procedure throughout a medical practice and facilitate training of new employees. The clinician leader of the practice must be the role model for establishing a safe culture to protect and respect every patient and ensure the practice maintains and audits the consent process.

Office Physical Plant Zoning

Local zoning laws regulate the use of the office building premises for the provision of medical services. If your existing practice location is in complete compliance with local zoning law requirements, none of the procedures described in this book should require additional special permits or variances since they fall into the category of usual medical diagnostic and therapeutic services for licensed physicians.

If you are adding loop electrosurgical excision procedures (LEEP) or electrosurgery services to your practice, you should consult with an electrician to evaluate your electrical service requirements. Equipment manufacturers will provide the detailed specifications to ensure safe operation.

OSHA Concerns

In 2001, the federal Occupational Safety and Health Administration (OSHA) substantially revised the 1991 compliance standards for employers to prevent employees' exposure to bloodborne pathogens [2]. Your practice must have an exposure control plan to reflect these standards, and it must be reviewed and updated at least once a year. The employer is responsible for staff training and compliance as well as proper documentation of these activities. Practitioners and assistants who perform any procedure which could involve a possible blood exposure should have serological documented immunity to hepatitis B. The practice must have a written protocol that clearly outlines proper handling, storage, and disposal of "sharps" (needles and blades), toxic chemicals (acetic acid and Lugol's and Monsel's solutions), and regulated medical waste. Personal protective equipment and emergency eyewash stations must be provided by the employer.

The practice must create engineering controls that allow for the proper ventilation of waste nitrous oxide gas from certain cryosurgical instruments if this equipment is used for cryosurgery of cervical or vulvar lesions. Similarly, a smoke evacuation system should be available for electrosurgical procedures to minimize aerosolized tissue inhalation. Appropriate cautions on look-alike sound-alike medications administered in the practice and cautions to avoid use of chemical sprays with cautery instruments remind staff to be mindful to avoid practice errors.

Promotion of Services

If the practitioner is providing outpatient women's health procedures for patients within the United States outside of the practice's enrolled panel on a referral basis from other practitioners, then state and federal "anti-kickback" laws prevail. These laws, the Anti-Kickback Statute (42 U.S.C. §1320a-7b(b)) and the Physician Self-Referral Law (Stark) (42 U.S.C. § 1395nn), prohibit self-referrals, fee-splitting arrangements, and other types of activity between business entities [3]. You must consult an attorney who is knowledgeable in this technical area of the law before promoting or advertising your services to patients or clinicians outside of your group practice.

Individual States in the United States regulate the scope and content of advertisements of physicians' services. Fraudulent or misleading advertisement is considered professional misconduct in most states and may negate your malpractice insurance coverage for these services if results are guaranteed or falsely solicited [4].

Credentialing Concerns

While surgery performed in facilities licensed under state Public Health Laws (such as hospitals or ambulatory surgery centers) is subject to regulatory standards established under such law, procedures performed by primary care clinicians in private offices are not subjected to the same standards. The practitioner's authority to perform office-based procedures is derived from the license to practice medicine issued by the state in which the practitioner is licensed. States are increasingly establishing clinical guidelines for office-based surgery [5]. The practitioner should become familiar with their state's guidelines for definitions of standards of care and quality (see http://lawatlas.org/datasets/office-based-surgery-laws accessed February 2, 2025). These guidelines can serve as a good resource template for creating your office policy concerning staff education and training for individual procedures. Procedures done by learners should be done in the presence of the billing clinician.

One of the most important rules of risk management is that the practitioner must be able to prove competency in the performance of these outpatient procedures. Procedure-specific competence should include education, training, experience, and evaluations of performance. Proof of competence should include documentation of procedures performed during postgraduate residency programs and/or proof of satisfactory completion of approved didactic courses offered as continuing medical education (CME). For example, the American Academy of Family Physicians offers a Continuing Medical Education syllabus in colposcopy and outlines methods to facilitate credentialing [6]. Insertion of subdermal implants requires a training course provided by the pharmaceutical company (FDA required) prior to being authorized to provide the implants in the office. Your practice should have a system to record the ongoing number of procedures performed by each practitioner and have a formal "re-evaluation of competency" policy in place.

The practitioner must research the terms of coverage of the practice's professional malpractice policy to make sure that the planned procedures are covered under the existing policy. Unlicensed personnel should not be assigned duties or responsibilities that require professional licensure [5]. The practice should have a formal "in-service" instruction program for office personnel involved in these procedures and document successful completion in the personnel record. This program should also address the knowledge needs of telephone-triage or advice nurses who are most likely to receive telephone calls for postoperative care concerns from patients.

Informed Consent

Informed consent is a process of communication with a competent patient about the planned procedure in sufficient detail to allow a decision whether to proceed with the intervention [7]. The key legal components of informed consent have evolved over the last 50 years in the United States. Not only is this process an ethical obligation, but it also is now a legal duty of professional conduct as described in statutes and case law in all 50 states, the District of Columbia, and all US territories. Informed consent is also a key component of the shared decision-making process [8].

For the procedures described in this book, informed consent must include the following components:

1. Information on the patient's pathology or current medical condition
2. Other scientifically valid treatment options
3. Rationale for the chosen procedure
4. Anticipated beneficial outcomes of the procedure
5. Potential harmful complications or consequences of the procedure, including major and minor side effects
6. Consequences of *not* having the procedure (informed refusal)

There can be no deliberate or willful misrepresentation of facts in these discussions with patients. In addition, the discussion must be in a language that is understandable to the patient in terms of education level and native tongue. Certified medical interpreters should be provided for patients whose native language is discordant with the practitioner. Many studies have shown a higher medicolegal risk when using family members as "ad hoc" interpreters [9].

The Americans with Disabilities Act requires the provider of medical services to provide appropriate means for hearing-impaired patients to function in the medical environment. Because informed consent discussions are of the highest importance, only medically certified interpreters should be hired by the practice to serve in this function with hearing-impaired patients. The cost of this service must be absorbed by the practice and not billed to the patient.

The informed consent discussion should be performed by the practitioner in the office setting prior to the procedure. This discussion should be recorded in the patient's medical record, with care to mention the use of any drawings or audiovisual aids [10]. Many practices have preprinted informational brochures that are part of the informed consent discussion. The patient's signature authorizes the procedure *only at the successful conclusion of the informed consent process.* If the patient refuses to have the intervention after this discussion, this refusal should be documented with a discussion of the repercussions fully acknowledged by the patient. Documentation within the medical records that consent was obtained prior to the procedure is considered best practice.

The increasingly popular usage of electronic medical records (EMR) has allowed groups to create standardized electronic consent systems and forms. The use of these new standardized systems has improved the documentation accuracy of the informed consent process [11]. New practice models for primary care introduce more complex rules concerning informed consent and release of information procedures, treatment and warm hand-off protocols, documentation and electronic record keeping, agreements with other providers, and billing [12].

Rights of Minors

While primary care physicians provide the majority of health care to adolescents, there is "significant evidence that both physicians and adolescents are uninformed of adolescent's legal rights to confidential reproductive health care" [13]. The Guttmacher Institute (https://www.guttmacher.org/state-policy/explore/overview-minors-consent-law) sponsors an online reference source that is updated monthly to provide information on key issues affecting these rights indexed by each individual state within the US [14]. The practitioner AND the office staff must be knowledgeable about their own state's law concerning consent and confidentiality when treating minors. In general, the law recognizes special conditions where the minor child may consent to diagnostic and treatment activities without parental approval or knowledge in matters concerning sexually transmitted infections (STIs), contraception, and reproductive (pregnancy) health including abortion [15]. When the practitioner consents to perform these gynecological procedures on minors, there are practical clinical concerns that may arise in the office with regard to billing, scheduling, telephone calls, and medical records privacy. The practice's policy and procedure manual should anticipate these potential breaches and detail the proper method of handling each issue. If your practice participates in the federal Title X Family Planning Program or the State Children Health Insurance Program (SCHIP), you must be knowledgeable about the confidentiality and consent rules for these programs. The major specialty organizations have all published policy statements regarding health care for adolescents [16]. Practice leadership should require all clinicians who perform gynecological procedures be aware of a minor's rights to medical care. In the United States, minors become adults at age 18 and should be treated as such; clinicians need to be careful to avoid breaking the confidentiality of their patients.

Use of Chaperones

There is no *uniform* national legal requirement mandating the use of a chaperone during female pelvic examinations or procedures. Even though all medicolegal risk managers recommend the routine use of chaperones, there is wide variation in this practice between American physicians [17] and their European counterparts [18]. The American Medical Association has addressed this in their code of ethics recommending practices that provide appropriate gowns, private facilities for undressing, use of draping, and clear explanations of the different components of the exams. Patients should be made aware of the chaperone policy of the practice, and offered a chaperone for any sensitive exam even if the patient has a trusted companion with them. Chaperones should be an authorized member of the healthcare team. There should be time for a private conversation to discuss any sensitive issues prior to the presence of the chaperone [19]. The "Me Too" movement has allowed more individuals to speak up about improper sexual behavior within and out of medicine. Physicians too are aware that they can become targets of unethical or unwell patients who may allege misconduct that never happened but is difficult to disprove without a chaperone present [20]. One study showed that the characteristics of physicians convicted of sexual misconduct involved a combination of five factors: male physicians (100%), older than the age of 39 (92%), who were not board certified (70%), and practicing in non-academic settings (94%) where they always examined patients alone (85%) [21].

In April 2006, the Federation of State Medical Boards adopted a policy that defines physician sexual misconduct and provides recommendations for physician education [22]. When reviewing the definitions of sexual impropriety and sexual violation in this publication, it is clear that most false accusations or misunderstandings can be avoided with the proper use of a *medically trained* chaperone *always* when performing these women's health procedures or any procedure involving touching a patient's genitals. The practice policy and procedure manual should state this clearly. It is also a good investment to avoid the emotionally wrenching experience of a false sexual misconduct charge. For most of the procedures described in this book, a chaperone is the beneficial "second pair" of hands to assist the operator in the completion of the procedure. Most experts recommend that the chaperone be the same sex as the patient; thus, a male physician should have a female chaperone for a female patient. Presence of a chaperone should be documented in the medical record.

Patient Pre-procedure Preparation Concerns

Solutions to prevent healthcare errors were unveiled in May 2007 by the World Health Organization's (WHO) Collaborating Centre for Patient Safety Solutions. Two of the solutions deal with office-based procedures: patient identification and performance of the correct procedure at the correct body site. Your practice should adopt the "Universal Protocol for Preventing Wrong Site, Wrong Procedure, Wrong Person Surgery" as standard office policy [23]. It is the responsibility of the practitioner to verify the adequacy of the informed consent process and double-check the patient's identity and planned procedure. The office should have an adequate privacy area to allow for patient disrobing and gowning.

Procedure-Specific Legal Concerns: Cervical Cytology and Pap Smears

Your office should have an established policy for the review of all laboratory reports before the reports are filed into the medical record [24]. The primary care provider must review and acknowledge ALL Pap smear cytology reports. Your office notification system must be fool-proof and have built-in reminders for follow-up of patients with abnormal Pap smear results until diagnostic resolution. Patient risk factors contributing to inadequate follow-up include low-income group, ethnic minority, and low health literacy [25]. Clinical errors occurring that led to Pap smear litigation include failure to notify patients of their abnormal test result, missing or inconsistent follow-up patterns, failure to investigate persistent bleeding following a Pap smear, and failure to biopsy an abnormal cervix given a normal Pap smear result [26]. The practitioner *must* be knowledgeable about the positive and negative predictive values of the Pap smear results to give adequate informed consent.

Recent publications contain excellent consensus statements that summarize the 2019 American Society for Colposcopy and Cervical Pathology (ASCCP) Guidelines for evidence-based management of abnormal cervical cytology [27]. These protocol algorithms should be referenced in your informed consent discussion and documentation.

Procedure-Specific Legal Concerns: Pessary

New self-positioning pessaries are effective, easy to use, and have few complications [28]. The most serious complications from pessary use are attributable to neglected devices in patients lost to follow-up [29]. These rare complications include urosepsis, impaction, vesicovaginal fistulae, and incarceration of the cervix and small bowel.

Procedure-Specific Legal Concerns: Contraceptives

When the practitioner discusses the contraceptive needs of the patient, the six key components of the previously discussed informed consent process must be addressed. Elements of the patient's current medical condition that are important in shared decision making regarding the proper contraceptive method for a patient include age, emotional maturity, health literacy, parity, number of sexual partners, cardiac risk profile including hypertension and diabetes, migraines with auras, coagulopathy, history of cancers, history of pelvic inflammatory disease or sexually transmitted infections, HIV and hepatitis B status, tobacco use, street drug or alcohol use, access to medical care follow-up, family history, and latex allergy. The practitioner must also have published information available to compare the relative effectiveness rates of each method [30]. This information should be included in table form on the practice's informed consent forms. It is important to document in the patient chart the risks and benefits and potential complications of the method chosen and prescribed.

Procedure-Specific Legal Concerns: Long-Acting Reversible Contraception (LARC)-IUDs, and Implants

The *intrauterine device (IUD)* and the *birth control implant* are long-acting reversible contraception methods. The thought process of a generation of physicians was forever changed by the Dalkon Shield litigation history during the 1970s. It was the largest "defective product" tort case in history and had reduced IUD usage in the United States to the lowest level of any industrialized nation in the world [31]. The IUDs approved for current use in the United States have eliminated the design flaws that plagued the Dalkon Shield. Use of LARCs has increased over the years with approximately 14% of women choosing a LARC as their preferred method [32]. Proper patient selection and post-insertion education and follow-up are important factors to reduce complications and to enhance effectiveness [33]. Contraindications and adverse effects should be included on the informed consent forms. Documentation of the absence of pregnancy before insertion is legally critical. The most serious complication of the IUD insertion procedure is uterine perforation with a reported rate of 1 per 1000 insertions for copper IUDs and 2.2 per 1000 insertions for hormone-releasing IUD [34]. Complications of the subdermal implant occur with improper insertion, difficult removal, or migration of the implant. Proper training and insertion techniques will avoid many of these complications [35].

Procedure-Specific Legal Concerns: Colposcopy and Loop Electrocautery Excision Procedure (LEEP)

The process of informed consent is of the utmost importance when discussing abnormal Pap smear results with patients and determining who should undergo further procedures. Some patients consider an abnormal Pap smear to automatically indicate cancer and wonder why they are not being managed more aggressively. The majority of college-educated women do not know the role of human papillomavirus (HPV) in cervical neoplasia [36]. An overlooked communication problem is the confusion between the abbreviations "HPV" and "HIV" and "HSV" when talking with patients. Please be careful!

The highest medicolegal risk in the performance of a colposcopy is an inadequate examination with inappropriate follow-up. With the advent of the Pap Guidelines with less frequent screening, the decreased number of abnormal results, and the introduction of the HPV vaccine, the volume of colposcopic procedures has decreased. The ASCCP has developed a set of quality recommendations for colposcopic practice. These include documentation guidelines including such aspects as visualization of the squamocolumnar junction, presence of acetowhite lesions, full visualization of the cervix, taking several biopsies, and a timeline for contacting patients with high-grade and invasive disease [37].

Your office notification system must be foolproof and have built-in reminders for follow-up of patients with abnormal colposcopic findings until diagnostic resolution. A telephone call to a patient before a scheduled recheck appointment has been shown to improve compliance with follow-up. Text reminders with reply message capability can also be useful in reminding patients about followup appointments. Mail reminders have NOT been found to be helpful to improve compliance but are legally important for documentation purposes.

Even though colposcopy is regarded as a core procedural technique for family physicians, the skill and comfort level of the individual practitioner must be assessed with a verifiable credentialing process and an ongoing quality assurance process. The practice should set its own standards for the number of procedures that should be performed to maintain credentials. Ideally, clinicians who will perform colposcopy in the office will maintain their skills by participating in the ASCCP society and updating their skills at advanced CME courses. The practice should also consider the clinical and pathologic situations where referral to a gynecology specialist is required since "failure to diagnose cancer" is still a leading cause of malpractice actions against primary care practitioners [38].

Loop electrosurgical excision procedure (LEEP) of the cervix has been shown to be an effective office technique that may obviate the need for cold knife conization surgery in the treatment of CIN 2 and CIN 3 [39]. The informed consent discussion must include the reason for selection of the cervical ablation procedure, including risks of incomplete excision, cervical stenosis, and incompetent cervix in subsequent pregnancy [40]. Your practice must have an adequate reminder system for post-procedure follow-up of pathology reports and patient recall.

Procedure-Specific Legal Concerns: Endometrial Biopsy

The endometrial biopsy has virtually replaced dilatation and curettage (D&C) for the workup of abnormal uterine bleeding. It is performed in the office, is cost-effective, and is 90% sensitive for endometrial cancer and 82% sensitive for atypical hyperplasia in postmenopausal bleeding [41]. When coupled with transvaginal ultrasound, saline sonohysterography, and/or hysteroscopy in patients with a low risk for endometrial cancer, the combined results had accuracy rates comparable to formal D&C [42]. During your informed consent discussion with patients with unexplained uterine bleeding, the risk assessment for uterine cancer must be categorized based on age, menopause status, nulliparity, body mass index, insulin resistance syndromes (such as polycystic ovary syndrome), family history, hormone replacement therapy, and tamoxifen use. Documentation of the absence of pregnancy before endometrial biopsy is legally critical. A nondiagnostic tissue sample in patients with persistent bleeding requires referral for further workup. Again, remember that "failure to diagnose cancer" is still a leading cause of malpractice actions against primary care practitioners.

The main complication of endometrial biopsy is uterine perforation, although the reported rates are extremely rare [41].

Procedure-Specific Legal Concerns: Elective Termination of Pregnancy in the United States

There is probably no other medical procedure that provokes as much worldwide divisive emotional and ethical debate as the elective termination of pregnancy. With the overturning of Roe vs Wade by the US Supreme Court, it is imperative for women's healthcare practitioners to know their own state's laws and terminology regarding the elective termination of pregnancy. Two excellent Internet sites contain up-to-date information on the status of state laws governing elective termination of pregnancy: the Guttmacher Institute [43] (www.guttmacher.org) and the National Abortion Federation (https://prochoice.org/health-care-professionals/educational-resources/). These sites contain information on Medicaid abortion funding, mandatory counseling and waiting periods, parental involvement in minors' abortions, and mandatory reporting to state health department requirements.

"Pregnancy termination and miscarriage treatment use overlapping sets of skills and procedures" [44]. It is critical for the practitioner to perform a thorough history, physical examination, and determination of gestational age for all pregnant patients. All the elements of the informed consent process need to be well documented. The risk of the planned procedure on future fertility must be discussed and documented. Post-procedure contraception needs should also be answered. The practitioner's office staff and after-hours call groups should be comfortable providing advice and care for any post-procedure complications to avoid any charge of patient abandonment. Quality standards produced by the National Abortion Federation should be adopted, and policies and procedures for care should be clear. These include that abortions must be provided by trained providers working within their scope of practice, ancillary services for ultrasound, laboratory, pain relief, and infection control must be provided by trained individuals; follow up care must be provided.

Telemedicine has been safely used to provide abortion services for medical abortion, informed consent, and follow-up. Complications of elective termination include pain, hemorrhage and (rarely) retained products; in surgical procedures in addition to the above, infection and (rarely) uterine perforations can occur.

References

1. Kirchner E. Legal challenges for family physicians in the Post-Roe v Wade Era. Am Fam Physician. 2023;107(4):344–7.
2. http://www.osha.gov/dcsp/osp/index.html. Accessed 4 June 2018.
3. Satiani B. Exceptions to the stark law: practical considerations for surgeons. Plast Reconstr Surg. 2006;117(3):1012–22, discussion 1023.
4. All professional liability policies have “intentional acts exclusions” where coverage may be reserved or denied. Some companies provide a more exhaustive list of acts that would trigger denial of coverage.
5. Clinical guidelines for Office-Based Surgery. Committee on Quality Assurance in Office-Based Surgery. A report to: New York State Public Health Council and New York State Department of Health. 2000. Accessed 29 May 2007 at: www.health.state.ny.us/nysdoh/obs/purpose.html.
6. American Academy of Family Physicians. Position paper: colposcopy. https://www.aafp.org/about/policies/all/colposcopy.html. Accessed 4 June 2018.
7. Updated 7 May 2007. http://www.ama-assn.org/ama/pub/category/4608.html. Accessed 29 Sept 2007.
8. Woolf SH, Krist A. The liability of giving patients a choice: shared decision making and prostate cancer. Am Fam Physician. 2005;71(10):1871–2.
9. Betancourt JR, Jacobs EA. Language barriers to informed consent and confidentiality: the impact on women's health. J Am Med Womens Assoc. 2000;55(5):294–5.
10. Issa MM, Setzer E, Charaf C, et al. Informed versus uninformed consent for prostate surgery: the value of electronic consents. J Urol. 2006;176(2):694–9.
11. Moseley TH, Wiggins MN, O'Sullivan P. Effects of presentation method on the understanding of informed consent. Br J Ophthalmol. 2006;90(8):990–3.
12. Hudgins C, Rose S, Fifield PY, Arnault S. Navigating the legal and ethical foundations of informed consent and confidentiality in integrated primary care. Fam Syst Health. 2013;31(1):9–19.
13. Lieberman D, Feierman J. Legal issues in the reproductive health care of adolescents. J Am Med Womens Assoc. 1999;54(3):109–14.
14. Guttmacher Institute. Overview of minor's consent law. https://www.guttmacher.org/state-policy/explore/overview-minors-consent-la. Accessed 4 June 2018.
15. Ford C, English A, Sigman G. Confidential health care for adolescents: position paper of the Society for Adolescent Medicine. J Adolesc Health. 2004;35(2):160–7.
16. Diaz A, Neal WP, Nucci AT, et al. Legal and ethical issues facing adolescent health care professionals. Mt Sinai J Med. 2004;71(3):181–5.
17. Rockwell P, Steyer TE, Ruffin MT 4th. Chaperone use by family physicians during the collection of a Pap smear. Ann Fam Med. 2003;1:218–20.

18. Rymer J, Durbaba S, Rosenthal J, et al. Use of chaperones by obstetricians and gynaecologists: a cross-sectional survey. J Obstet Gynaecol. 2007;27(1):8–11.
19. American Medical Association. Code of Medical Ethics. Opinion 1.2.4. Use of chaperones. 2016. https://www.ama-assn.org/delivering-care/use-chaperones. Accessed 20 Apr 2024.
20. Pimienta AL, Giblon R. The case for medical chaperones. Fam Pract Manag. 2018;25(5):6–8.
21. DuBois JM, Walsh HA, Chibnall JT, et al. Sexual violation of patients by physicians: a mixed-methods, exploratory analysis of 101 cases. Sex Abus. 2019;31(5):503–23.
22. Federation of State Medical Boards Policy Statement. Addressing sexual boundaries: guidelines for State Medical Boards. Adapted April 2006. http://www.fsmb.org/grpol_policydocs.html. Accessed 4 June 2018.
23. https://www.jointcommission.org/standards_information/up.aspx. Accessed 4 June 2018.
24. White B. Four principles for better test-result tracking. Fam Pract Manag. 2002;9(7):41–4.
25. Engelstad LP, Stewart LS, Nguyen BH, et al. Abnormal Pap smear follow-up in a high-risk population. Cancer Epidemiol Biomarkers Prev. 2001;10:1015–20.
26. Frable WJ. Litigation in gynecologic cytology. Path Case Rev. 2005;10(3):106–14.
27. 2019 ASCCP Risk-based management consensus guidelines for abnormal cervical cancer screening tests and cancer precursors: erratum. J Low Genit Tract Dis. 2020;24(4):427. https://doi.org/10.1097/LGT.0000000000000056.
28. Farrell SA, Baydock S, Amir B, et al. Effectiveness of a new self-positioning pessary for the management of urinary incontinence in women. Am J Obstet Gynecol. 2007;196(474):e1–474.e8.
29. Trowbridge ER, Fenner DE. Conservative management of pelvic organ prolapse. Clin Obstet Gynecol. 2005;48(3):668–81.
30. Trussell J. Contraceptive failure in the United States. Contraception. 2004;70:89–96.
31. Hubacher D. The checkered history and bright future of intrauterine contraception in the United States. Perspect Sex Reprod Health. 2002;34(2):98–102.
32. Lanzola EL, Ketvertis K. Intrauterine device. 26 June 2023. In: StatPearls [Internet]. Treasure Island (FL): StatPearls Publishing; 2024. PMID: 32491335.
33. Johnson BA. Insertion and removal of intrauterine devices. Am Fam Physician. 2005;71(1):95–102.
34. Penney G, Brechin S, de Souza A, Bankowska U, Belfield T, Gormley M, Olliver M, Hampton N, Howlett-Shipley R, Hughes S, Mack N, O'Brien P, Rowlands S, Trewinnard K, Faculty of Family Planning and Reproductive Health Care Clinical Effectiveness Unit. FFPRHC Guidance. The copper intrauterine device as long-term contraception. J Fam Plann Reprod Health Care. 2004;30(1):29–41. 34. Le T, Hicks W, Menard C, et al. Human papillomavirus testing knowledge and attitudes among women attending colposcopy clinic with ASCUS/LGSIL pap smears. J Obstet Gynaecol Can. 2004;26(9):788–92.
35. Irgens-Moller N, Baum C. Complications of long-acting reversible contraceptive modalities. Pediatr Emerg Care. 2023;39(6):443–9. https://doi.org/10.1097/PEC.0000000000002970.
36. Le T, Hicks W, Menard C, et al. Human papillomavirus testing knowledge and attitudes among women attending colposcopy clinic with ASCUS/LGSIL pap smears. J Obstet Gynaecol Can. 2004;26(9):788–92.
37. Mayeaux E Jr, et al. ASCCP colposcopy standards: colposcopy quality improvement recommendations for the United States. J Low Genit Tract Dis. 2017;21(4):242–8. https://doi.org/10.1097/LGT.0000000000000342.
38. Callaway P. Does a family physician who offers colposcopy and LEEP need to refer patients to a gynecologist? J Fam Pract. 2000;49:534–6.
39. Lyman DJ, Morris B. LEEP in the family practice setting. J Am Board Fam Pract. 2003;16(3):204–8.
40. Mathevet P, Chemali E, Roy M, et al. Long-term outcome of a randomized study comparing three techniques of conization: cold knife, laser and LEEP. Eur J Obstet Gynecol Reprod Biol. 2003;106(2):214–8.
41. Williams PM, Gaddey HL. Endometrial biopsy: tips and pitfalls. Am Fam Physician. 2020;101(9):551–6. PMID: 32352730.

42. Vitale SG, Buzzaccarini G, Riemma G, Pacheco LA, Di Spiezio SA, Carugno J, Chiantera V, Török P, Noventa M, Haimovich S, De Franciscis P, Perez-Medina T, Angioni S, Laganà AS. Endometrial biopsy: indications, techniques and recommendations. An evidence-based guideline for clinical practice. J Gynecol Obstet Hum Reprod. 2023;52(6):102588. https://doi.org/10.1016/j.jogoh.2023.102588. Epub 2023 Apr 13. PMID: 37061093.
43. Guttmacher Institute. https://www.guttmacher.org/united-states/abortion. Accessed 30 Apr 2024.
44. 2024 clinical policy guidelines for abortion care. National Abortion Federation. Quality/Standards – National Abortion Federation (prochoice.org). Accessed 30 Apr 2024.

Chapter 4
Population Health in Women's Healthcare

Cathryn B. Heath

Introduction

Population health is defined as the health outcomes of a group of individuals, including the distribution of such outcomes within the group [1]. Groups of individuals can include geographic regions such as communities, ethnic groups, age of the patients, or socioeconomic classes. The determinants include medical care systems, the social environment, and the physical environment, all of which have a biological impact on individuals within the group. It also includes the resource allocations involved in linking determinants to outcomes. There are three major components to population health, namely, health outcomes, policies and interventions, and patterns of health determinants. Population management utilizes interventions on individuals and organizations to improve morbidity patterns.

Health Outcomes

Determining health outcomes requires a collection of data to support the study of an office. The electronic medical record (EMR) can be a particularly rich source of data, although it is not a necessity for data collection. One of the important tasks related to population health is creating registries; this is particularly applicable for procedures that are done with lengthy time intervals, such as the current recommendations for cervical cancer screening. A registry is a list of patients who by their age, sex, or disease are eligible for screening. Registries track patients eligible for a particular procedure due to their age, sex, and/or disease ("denominator") and those

C. B. Heath (✉)
Rutgers University Student Health, New Brunswick, NJ, USA
e-mail: heathcb@scarletmail.rutgers.edu

S. M. Sulik, C. B. Heath (eds.), *Primary Care Procedures in Women's Health*,
https://doi.org/10.1007/978-3-032-07061-6_4

who have had the procedure ("numerator"), thus creating a percentage of patients who have had the intervention. Many insurance companies who request these reports also require reporting on those patients who would be eligible for a procedure by age and gender but are ineligible for the procedure ("exclusion") due to mitigating factors. For example, breast cancer survivors would be excluded from breast cancer *screening* as they will have breast cancer *surveillance*. Breast cancer survivors are excluded from breast cancer screening rates. Criteria for numerators, denominators, and exclusions are available in a variety of sources, including the National Quality Forum (NQF) and the Centers for Medicare and Medicaid Services (CMS). All measures which a practice report are required to be consistent with the standards set for each measure by the Centers for Medicare and Medicaid Services (CMS) or by the standards set nationally by organizations such as the National Quality Forum. National percentiles for each quality measure then allow a practice to compare their rate of screening to similar practices nationwide.

Advanced registries track additional information, such as the date when a patient is due for a screening or procedure, which provider is associated with the patient, and the results of the procedure. Many components of a registry can be automated within an electronic health record and can create a percentage rate of a screening measure that is reportable to the practice and to outside interested parties. Practices then use these registries to create policies and interventions which improve the healthcare of the patient.

One of the major obstacles to creating registries within an EMR is making sure that the data that is being followed is present within extractable data fields for aggregation purposes. For many EMRs, if the data is present in free text by having been typed into a blank field, it may not be extractable. Making sure that the data is "in observation terms," i.e., in extractable data fields (as opposed to free text), is important. The more automated the process, the more likely the data will reflect true results as opposed to results that reflect poor data collection.

Registries can be kept on paper or in electronic spreadsheets, if a practice does not use an EMR or their EMR is not capable of creating registry reports. A "tickler" file is a common reminder system that creates a "next due" date that is then reviewed on a regular basis by office staff. Common tickler files have been created on index cards, or even postcards which are then mailed as reminders to patients to return for a given test. Text messages can also be sent by some medical EMRs to remind the patient to schedule an appointment for a specific screening test. Documentation that a reminder was sent should be kept within a registry or the patient's chart. Registries can track patients with specific diseases (abnormal pap smears), patients who are due for routine screening (Pap smear), or patients who may be due for review of their contraceptives, particularly those with long-acting reversible contraceptives (LARCs), such as intrauterine devices or subdermal implants. In addition, tracking whether the clinician viewed and acted upon a result from a procedure is essential. This is particularly relevant for any Pap smear or biopsy (e.g., a colposcopy biopsy or genital skin biopsy). Analysis of data from registries helps drive the improvement process by measuring changes in outcomes due to a change in policies within an office setting or on a national basis. Wu reports on the low use rate of highly effective contraceptives such as LARCs where she noted that although still half of all pregnancies in the United States were unintended, the rate of LARC use was still comparatively low at

14% [2]. A process improvement project regarding unintended pregnancies may then set as their goal improving rates of LARCs within a community or a practice.

Policies and Interventions

Policies within an office can create structure and accountability for staff and providers alike. Agreement on the given guidelines is a first step to developing office policies for clinical practice. Once determined, assigning responsibility for tasks outlined within the policy lessens confusion of who is responsible for the tasks, improves efficiency, and allows all staff work to the "top of their license," a term meaning tasks can be allotted by levels of expertise. Creating an efficient workflow centered on a specific preventive service can then lead to a discussion on how to create an atmosphere for shared workload. Shared workload improves health outcomes by sharing responsibility for the care of the patient to the entire office. This is considered the essence of the Quadruple Aim in Medicine—improve quality, decrease cost, improve patient satisfaction, and decrease office burnout [3].

Reviewing data then creates opportunities to improve office procedures. There are many ways that this is done; common methodologies for this are "plan-do-study-act" (PDSA) or "Define-Measure-Analyze-Improve-Control" (DMAIC) to use data to create process improvement. Processes are then changed and restudied to ascertain whether the outcomes are better. Small changes can gradually improve health outcomes of the patients over time. For instance, a team at West Virginia State University studied their rate of patients who came for a colonoscopy and were found to have a high "poor prep" for the study. After reviewing the workflow and making changes within their EMR to create standard instructions which were reviewed with the patient, they decreased their rate of poor preps from 19% to 4% [4].

Similarly, for outpatient procedures, analyzing the actual specific procedure steps can then optimize how that procedure is performed. Studying the rate of outcomes (successful procedures without incident and with incidents of poor outcomes) can lead toward an improved procedure process. When there is a negative outcome to a procedure, a "root cause analysis" (RCA) is a process of collaborating among all parties to review the occurrence and take steps to avoid the occurrences in the future. RCAs review the process instead of placing blame on specific people involved. Corrective action may involve changing some methodology regarding the procedure's process which will benefit the patient population of the entire practice.

Patterns of Social Determinants

Social determinants of health include all the conditions under which people are born, grow, live, work, and age. Factors that influence health outcomes include access to medical care, access to nutritious foods, access to clean water and functioning utilities, education and health literacy, ethnicity and cultural orientation, family and other social supports, gender, housing and transportation, linguistic and communication capabilities, neighborhood safety, occupation and job security, exposure to violence and adverse factors in the home environment, sexual identification, social status, socioeconomic status, and spiritual/religious values. The clinician needs to be able to address social determinants of health to promote good health outcomes for individuals and populations.

Assessing social determinants of health and breaking down barriers, when possible, help meet the needs of individual patients and also help improve the health of a population. Using population-based cancer registries to examine incidence and mortality data helps identify disparities based on race and ethnicity. Cote et al. found that while the overall cancer incidence rates have been declining in the United States, endometrial cancer rates have continued to increase. While the incidence rates have increased for all racial/ethnic groups, non-Hispanic black women have a significantly higher incidence of aggressive endometrial cancers as well as higher mortality rates [5]. Population health requires attention to an entire population. In this manner, we are tasked with optimizing medicine and healthcare resources for the benefit of all. As national guidelines change for preventive screening, it is important to neither over- nor under-screen for preventive services. Analysis of screening data can identify current utilization rates, identify discrepancies from the norms, and help address changes in policies to improve screening rates. Some factors which may determine rates of screening procedures include variance by socioeconomic status of the patient, race of the patient, and even the gender of the provider. A study by Ince-Cushman found that the rate of cervical cancer screening done by women physicians was much higher than the rate of those done by male physicians, although the rate of mammography screening was similar for both male and female physicians [6]. Current rates then need to be analyzed with proposals on how to increase the rates for patients in need. For instance, a simple reminder that a patient may have a Pap smear done in a family medicine office may improve the rate of that specific procedure, as many women may not understand that they can receive such services there. Other factors that may make it difficult for women to receive services are the requirement for a woman to make two appointments for preventive healthcare, one for a preventive health examination and another for cervical cancer screening. This may be difficult for women who are not paid if they take time off work; combining the visit into one service would improve compliance. Or evaluate the frequency in which the preventive screening should be performed. The "yearly Pap smear" now only applies to a small group of patients. If a woman does not have insurance, an office needs to be able to give a patient the current rate for the procedure if done in the office and other low or no-cost alternatives, such as planned parenthood or family planning. Language can be a barrier as well; providing translation services is a requirement of ambulatory practices within the United States.

Another overlooked social determinant is the patient's weight; many providers are reluctant to do cervical cancer screening on patients who are morbidly obese with a body mass index (BMI) of 40–49.9 or the super morbidly obese (BMI greater than 50). Similarly, biases regarding cervical cancer or sexually transmitted infection screening in patients who are having sex with women, patients who have specific occupations, or are members of a religious order may impact current rates of screening.

Discussions of specific procedures and patients' reluctance or avoidance to have them might reveal prior undisclosed incidences of sexual assault, which need to be addressed in an empathic manner. Certain populations such as the developmentally disabled patient might need special accommodations to accomplish needed screening procedures. Developmentally disabled adult patients who require anesthesia to have simple dental work done would benefit from arranging a cervical cancer screening while they are under anesthesia if they cannot tolerate an examination otherwise.

Summary

Population health as a methodology for improving the health of patients has great relevance to procedural training. It is rewarding for patients and clinicians alike to improve the actual procedures as well as to improve the processes by which we care for the health of patients both individually and collectively.

References

1. Silberberg M, Martinez-Bianchi V, Lyn MJ. What is population health? Prim Care. 2019;46(4):475–84. https://doi.org/10.1016/j.pop.2019.07.001. Epub 2019 Jul 31. PMID: 31655744. Accessed 3 May 2024.
2. Wu JP, Moniz MH, Ursu AN. Long-acting reversible contraception—highly efficacious, safe, and underutilized. JAMA. 2018;6:397. https://doi.org/10.1001/jama.2018.8877.
3. Anandarajah A, Quill T, Privitera M. Adopting the quadruple aim: the University of Rochester Medical Center experience: moving from physician burnout to physician resilience: moving from physician burnout to physician resilience. Am J Med. 2018;131:979. https://doi.org/10.1016/j.amjmed.2018.04.034.
4. Shah-Khan SM, Cumerledge J, Reynolds GJ. Using the plan-do-study-act approach to improve inpatient colonoscopy preparation. BMJ Open Qual. 2017;6(2):e000230. https://doi.org/10.1136/bmjoq-2017-000230. eCollection 2017.
5. Cote M, Ruterbusch J, Olson H, et al. The growing burden of endometrial cancer: a major racial disparity affecting black women. Cancer Epidemiol Biomarkers Prev. 2015;24(9):1407. https://doi.org/10.1158/1055-9965.EPI-15-0316.
6. Ince-Cushman D, Correa JA, Shuldiner J, Segouin J. Association of primary care physician sex with cervical cancer and mammography screening. Can Fam Physician. 2013;59(1):e11.

Additional Resources

Greenberg RS. Medical epidemiology: population health and effective health care. 5th ed. New York: McGraw-Hill.

Nash DB, Fabius R, Skoufalos A, Clarke J, Horowitz M. Population health; creating a culture of wellness: with Navigate 2 eBook Access. 3rd ed. Burlington: Jones and Bartlett Learning.

Chapter 5
Empathic Pelvic Examination

Rhina Acevedo

Introduction

The pelvic examination is an important and basic procedure for primary care providers. It is an integral part of the evaluation of common gynecologic and abdominal complaints including but not limited to lower abdominal pain, pelvic pain, vaginal discharge, vaginal bleeding, and irregular menses. The American College of Obstetricians and Gynecologists (ACOG) recommends a routine annual health assessment visit starting at age 13–15 but states that unless the patient has symptoms that it is not necessary to perform a pelvic examination [1]. The United States Preventive Services Task Force (USPSTF), the American College of Physicians, and the American Academy of Family Physicians state there is insufficient evidence to recommend screening pelvic examinations in asymptomatic women except for those needing cervical cancer testing [2, 3]. The American Cancer Society (ACS) recommends that women begin cervical cancer testing at age 25. Those aged 25 to 65 should have a primary human papillomavirus (HPV) test every 5 years. If primary HPV testing is not available, screening may be done with either a co-test that combines an HPV test with a Papanicolaou (Pap) test every 5 years or a Pap test alone every 3 years [4]. USPSTF recommends cervical cancer screening to begin at age 21 [5]. For more information, see Chap. 8.

R. Acevedo (✉)
Department of Family Medicine and Community Health, Rutgers School of Biomedical Health Sciences, New Brunswick, NJ, USA
e-mail: acevedra@rwjms.rutgers.edu

S. M. Sulik, C. B. Heath (eds.), *Primary Care Procedures in Women's Health*,
https://doi.org/10.1007/978-3-032-07061-6_5

Patients with risk factors such as a past history of abnormal Pap smears (depending on the length of time since abnormality was diagnosed) or having symptoms of sexually transmitted infections may need pelvic examinations. There is currently no evidence to continue yearly pelvic examinations or Pap smears after the age of 65 years. Patients over 65 years of age with normal Pap test results in the previous 10 years should discontinue screening. Consideration needs to be made for personal history, including recent changes in male sexual partner or multiple male sexual partners. The US Preventive Services Task Force found insufficient evidence to suggest routine screening examinations past the age of 65 years [5]. Medicare presently does not pay for yearly routine screening pelvic examinations. Patients under the age of 21 years need pelvic examinations only if symptomatic with vaginal discharge or pelvic pain. Screening for sexually transmitted infections may be done by the patient by self-inserting vaginal swabs or with a urine specimen.

Although the Pap smear has been a mainstay for the evaluation of cancer of the cervix, there is no recommended screening for ovarian cancer. Three cohort studies assessed the diagnostic accuracy of the pelvic examination for detecting ovarian cancer in asymptomatic women. The studies together found that 96.7%–100% of pelvic examinations on asymptomatic women did not identify ovarian cancer [2]. Thus, many clinicians do not perform the bimanual examination on asymptomatic women. Clinicians may elect to perform a recto-vaginal examination on patients with deep pelvic and rectal pain.

See Algorithm 5.1 for the decision tree on the necessity of performing a pelvic exam.

Case Study

A 26-year-old G0P0 patient presents to your office for her first gynecological evaluation and cervical cancer screening. She had two HPV vaccinations prior to her 15th birthday. She has become sexually active with a male partner in the last 2 years. They are currently using condoms every time for contraception. She denies any current complaints. She reports that her menses are regular. She is not currently using any other contraceptive method. She is very nervous about her gynecologic examination.

Diagnosis (Algorithm 5.1)

Gynecologic women's health examination.

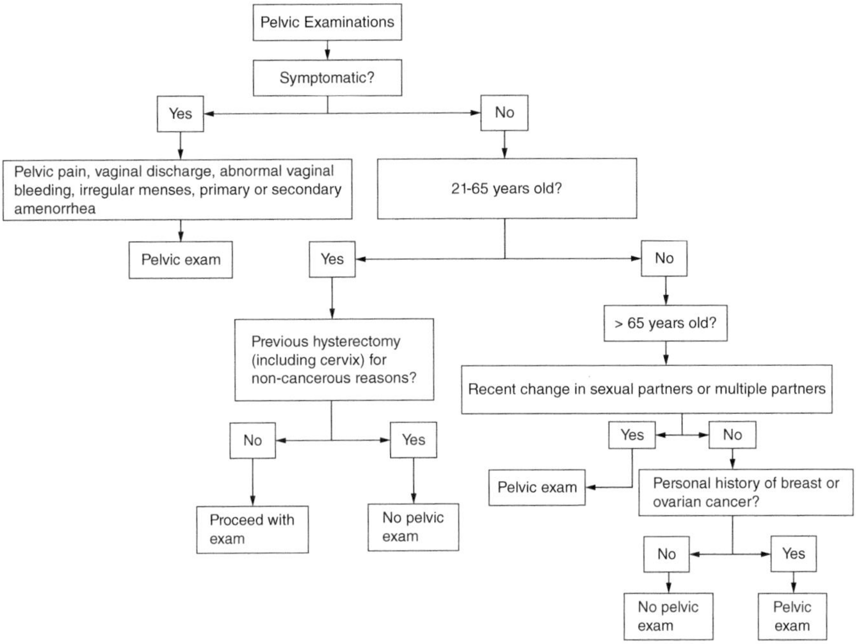

Algorithm 5.1 Decision tree on the necessity of performing a pelvic exam

Indications (Algorithm 5.1)

- Lower abdominal or pelvic pain
- Menstrual irregularities including
  - Primary amenorrhea (no menses by age 16)
  - Secondary amenorrhea
  - Menorrhagia (heavy bleeding)
  - Menometrorrhagia (irregular heavy bleeding)
- Vaginal discharge
- Postcoital bleeding
- Dyspareunia
- Dysmenorrhea
- Pregnancy
- Vaginal bleeding in pregnancy
- Postmenopausal bleeding
- Sexual assault
- Vaginal warts

Contraindications

- Patient refusal
- Placenta previa (contraindication to digital vaginal exam)

Equipment (Fig. 5.1)

- Appropriate-sized gown
- Sheet
- Light source
- Nonsterile latex-free gloves
- Water-based lubricating gel
- Large vaginal swabs
- Speculum: come in different sizes and forms, from metal to plastic, Pedersen and Graves
- If clinically appropriate
  - Pap smear (Fig. 5.3a)
    - (a) For fixed glass slide specimens—glass slide, wooden cervical spatula, and endocervical brush; or endocervical broom, cell fixation spray
    - (b) For liquid Pap—plastic spatula and endocervical brush or endocervical broom, liquid Pap smear jar (preferred)

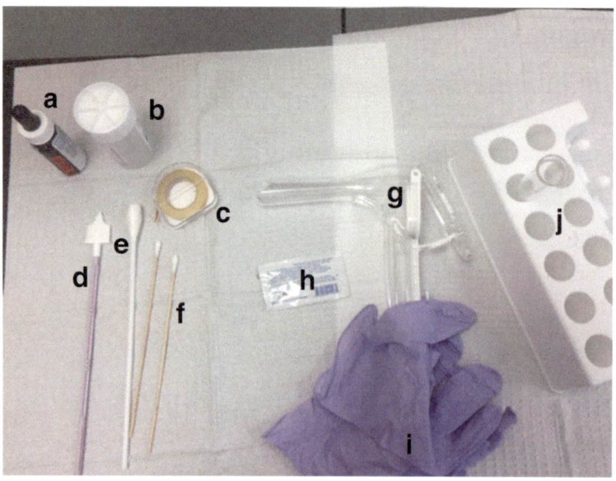

Fig. 5.1 Setup for pelvic examination: (**a**) saline for vaginitis specimens, (**b**) Liquid cytology jar for Pap specimen, (**c**) pH paper, (**d**) endocervical broom, (**e**) large vaginal swabs, (**f**) cotton-tipped applicators for pH and saline specimen for vaginitis, (**g**) small disposable Pederson speculum, (**h**) water-based lubricant, (**i**) nonsterile latex-free gloves, and (**j**) plastic test tube for vaginitis specimen. Light source is not shown in the photo

- Wet mount
  (a) Cotton swab, small test tube, saline, pH paper, glass slide
- Additional testing (if appropriate)—for gonorrhea and chlamydia, HPV, bacterial vaginosis, or Group B Streptococcus

Procedure

1. Take history before the patient changes into the gown. Using appropriate language and/or drawings, describe the pelvic examination to the patient. Answer any questions the patient may have regarding the upcoming procedure. Let the patient know that although the exam may be uncomfortable, it should not be painful and that every effort will be made to minimize her discomfort.
2. Offer a chaperone: ask if the patient wishes to have another person present in the room at the time of the examination. Chaperones may be a requirement in some states and should be of the same sex as the patient and should be personnel from the health center. If the patient requests a chaperone brought with them their presence should be confirmed with only the patient and the provider in the room. This would be in addition to the clinical chaperone, not in substitution.
3. Step out of the room so that the patient may change into a gown, instructing her to take off her clothing, including underwear.
4. Ask the patient to lie down on the table. Do the rest of the examination, leaving the pelvic examination for last. Have her lie down on the table, placing the stirrups in the appropriate positions, extending and externally rotating the stirrups. Consider elevating the head of the examination table slightly for patient comfort.
5. Ask the patient to place her heels in the stirrups and to slide down so that her perineum reaches the edge of the examination table. Be sure to use the drape or sheet across her abdomen and pelvic area.
6. Put on nonsterile gloves on both hands after washing your hands per CDC guidelines.
7. Ask the patient to let her knees fall to the sides as much as possible (Fig. 5.2). Describe to the patient each part of the procedure that you are about to perform.
8. Examine the labia for the presence of any lesions (warts, ulcerations, or abnormal moles). Also, examine the patient for the presence of a cystocele or rectocele.
9. If you are using a self-lit speculum, place the light source in the appropriate segment of the handle. If you are using a gooseneck lamp as a light source, position to provide appropriate lighting for visualization inside the vagina without burning the patient's thigh.
10. Apply warm water and/or a small amount of warm lubricant gel to the blades of the speculum. Introduce the tip of the speculum at a 45- to 90-degree angle to the introitus, and apply downward and posterior pressure until approximately three-fourths of the speculum's blades have been introduced. Introducing the

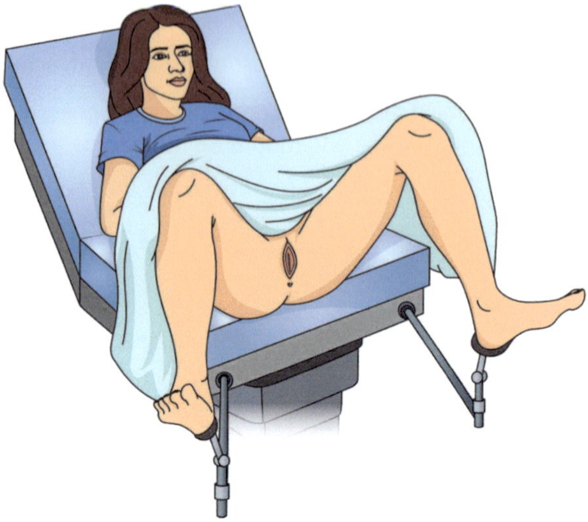

Fig. 5.2 Dorsal lithotomy position and pelvic exam position

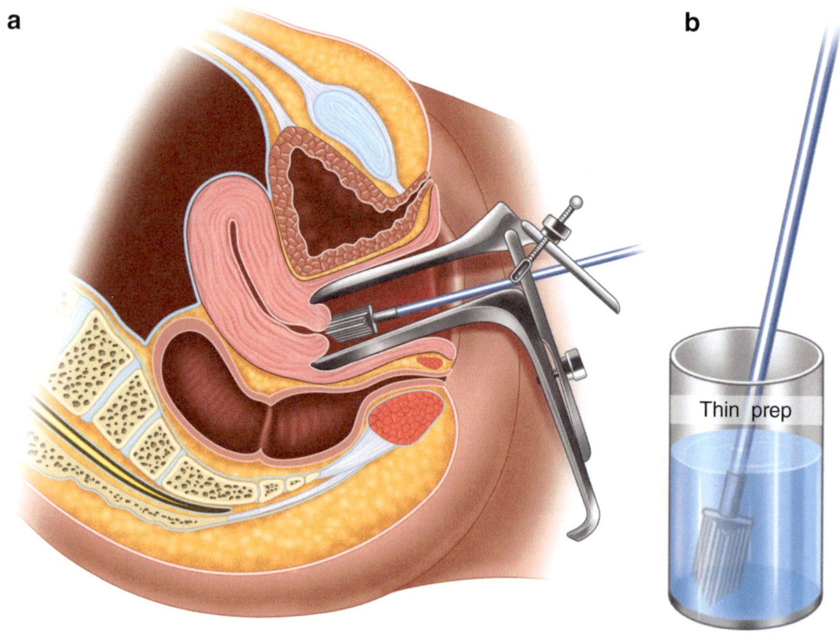

Fig. 5.3 (**a**) Speculum examination. (**b**) Liquid Pap smear

speculum slowly allows the tissue to accommodate the speculum. (Some labs caution against using gel as it may obscure the samples taken for a pap smear.)

11. Rotate the speculum so that the blades are at a perpendicular position in relation to the vaginal canal, and open the blades (Fig. 5.3a).
12. Reposition as needed in order to bring the cervix into full visualization between the blades of the speculum.

13. Inspect the vaginal walls for the presence of any lesions (i.e., warts and ulcers). Also note for presence or lack of moisture or rugae indicating atrophy.
14. Clean any cervical mucus from the cervix with the large cotton-tipped swab prior to obtaining either Pap smear or gonorrhea and chlamydia DNA probes.
15. Obtain clinically appropriate vaginal/cervical/endocervical/rectal samples and Pap smear, if indicated (Fig. 5.3b). Obtain culture specimens prior to obtaining Pap smear specimens. (The use of the endocervical brush to obtain an endocervical sample can produce some bleeding which could affect the evaluation of other samples such as a wet mount or gonorrhea/chlamydia DNA probes.)
16. Withdraw the speculum from the vaginal canal, being careful not to release the cervix quickly (do not "pop" the cervix).
17. If appropriate, perform a bimanual examination by introducing the index and middle finger of the dominant hand into the vaginal canal. The examiner then places the nondominant hand over the patient's lower abdomen. With the finger located inside the vagina, locate the cervix and apply upward pressure to the body of the uterus. Sweep the external hand down the midline of the lower abdomen to palpate the size of the uterus in order to measure uterine size.
18. Move internally placed fingers laterally to the adnexae on each side by applying upward pressure while applying downward pressure on the external hand to locate the ovaries.
19. If indicated by symptoms, perform a rectovaginal examination, withdrawing the internal vaginal fingers, changing gloves, and relubricating and then placing one finger inside the vaginal canal and one finger of the same hand into the rectum. Palpate the rectovaginal wall for thickening or herniations, and or deep pelvic and rectal pain.
20. Help the patient into a seated position by sliding back up the table first, and then removing the feet from the stirrups. Offer tissues for cleaning the lubricant and sanitary pads for any bleeding. Allow her to change prior to going over any results. Let her know when and how she can expect to be contacted about her results.

Complications and Risks

Although there is a small risk of trauma to the adjacent tissue, it is usually not necessary to obtain a written consent form for the performance of a pelvic examination.

Tricks and Helpful Hints

- Be aware of your patient's cultural needs. Different ethnic groups may hold to different beliefs and health practices than those of the provider. When appropriate, ask the patient about any other health beliefs or health maintenance practices

in which she may participate. Be respectful, listen with an open mind, and welcome the opportunity to learn about these differences. Being judgmental may be detrimental toward building trust between the patient and the clinician. If the clinician is concerned that a belief may be harmful, present the reservations in an open dialog and negotiate a solution that is acceptable to all.
- Specula come in various sizes and configurations:
  - Pedersen: It has narrow blades and is considered the speculum of choice. A medium-sized Pedersen speculum will usually suffice for women of any size.
  - Graves: It has wider blades, which are more useful in multiparous women or women with redundant vaginal walls.
  - Smaller-sized specula are more appropriate for women who have never been sexually active. Consider using a pediatric speculum; have one available for use if necessary.
  - Larger specula may be useful in patients with a cystocele or rectocele. It may be necessary to use vaginal wall retractors (see Chap. 5).
  - It is best to start with the smallest speculum that will allow full visualization of the cervix and to change to a larger size if needed.
- Have the patient take a deep breath to relax the perineal muscles while you are inserting the speculum.
- If you are having difficulty finding the cervix, withdraw the speculum from the vaginal canal and perform a digital examination to identify the presence and location of the cervix. Alternatively, withdraw the speculum approximately halfway down the vagina, being careful not to pinch the patient as the blades close slightly. Apply downward pressure on the entire speculum toward the rectum. Open the speculum blades partially to view the vaginal tissue. If more tissue is found superiorly, aim the speculum tip downward. Conversely, if more tissue is found inferiorly, aim the speculum tip upward.
- Inserting the speculum slowly allows the woman's perineal tissues to accommodate the speculum blades. This is especially important in women who are postmenopausal or nulliparous or women with vaginal infections.
- Some patients may find it more comfortable to have a "stirrup-free" pelvic examination. To use this technique, have the patient slide down to the edge of the exam table, placing her feet on the corners of the withdrawn extension of the table. She then externally rotates her knees. This technique was found to decrease both physical discomfort and the sense of vulnerability [6].
- Avoid prolonged conversations while the patient is lying on the table in stirrups. It is easier for a patient to absorb information while they are seated after the examination is over.
- If the patient's partner insists on being present, make sure that there is some time during the examination that the clinician and the patient are alone. Be sure to ask the patient if they have been harmed in any way. Posting discrete notices about safe houses for abuse in discrete places (usually restrooms) may be helpful.

Procedure Note

(*Provider to fill in blanks/circle applicable choice when given multiple choices and customize as necessary.*)

Patient placed in a dorsal lithotomy position. External genitalia examined without lesions or abnormalities. Speculum inserted without difficulty; cervix visualized; Pap smear (done/not done due to __________). Bimanual examination performed with uterus noted to be in ____________ (anteverted, retroverted) position. Approximately ___________ cm in size. Adnexae without masses or tenderness. Rectal examination (performed, not performed) with no noted lesions.

Coding

99385 New Patient Preventive Medicine Services, age 18–39
99386 New Patient Preventive Medicine Services age 40–64
99395 Established Patient Preventive Medicine Services, age 18–39
99396 Established Patient Preventive Medicine Services, age 40–64
Use problem-based coding for all visits related to specific concerns/complaints.

CPT® Codes (Current Procedural Terminology, AMA, Chicago, IL)
99385 New Patient Preventive Medicine Services, age 18–39
99395 Established Patient Preventive Medicine Services, age 18–39

ICD 10-CM-Diagnostic Codes (International Classification of Diseases, 10th Revision, Clinical Modification, Centers for Disease Control and Prevention)
Z01.419 Encounter for gynecological examination (general) (routine) without abnormal findings.
Z01.411 Encounter for gynecological examination (general) (routine) with abnormal findings
Use appropriate ICD 10 for specific concerns or complaints as appropriate

Post-procedure Patient Instructions

The patient may experience some vaginal spotting and is to be instructed to call if it does not resolve spontaneously within 2 days. The patient should be told to call the office with heavy vaginal bleeding (more than one pad per hour), vaginal discharge, or pain. She needs to be told how to expect the results of any Pap smears or cultures and how soon to expect the results.

Case Study Outcome

Pelvic examination was performed. A Pap smear and gonorrhea/chlamydia cultures were obtained and sent to the laboratory. Contraception options were discussed with the patient and prescribed. One week later, results revealed normal cytology and cultures. The patient was advised to return to the office for a wellness check in 1 year and told their own suggested interval for pelvic examination and Pap smear.

Post-procedure Patient Handout

(*Provider to customize as necessary.*)

You have had a pelvic examination today and may experience some vaginal spotting for 1 or 2 days, which will resolve spontaneously. Please call the office if you have heavy bleeding, vaginal discharge, or abdominal or pelvic pain. You will be notified of the results of your Pap smear and/or cultures within the next 2 weeks. If you have not heard from this office by then, please call us.

References

1. ACOG Committee Opinion No. 811 "The initial reproductive health visit". Obstet Gynecol. 2020;136:e70–80. Accessed 4 Feb 2025.
2. US Preventive Services Task Force. Screening for cervical cancer: US Preventive Services Task Force recommendation statement. JAMA. 2018;320(7):674–86. https://doi.org/10.1001/jama.2018.10897.
3. American Academy of Family Physicians. Clinical practice guidelines: screening pelvic exam. Accessed at: Screening for Gynecologic Conditions with Pelvic Examination: Recommendation Statement | AAFP on 4 Feb 2025.
4. The American Cancer Society. The American Cancer Society Guidelines for the prevention and early detection of cervical cancer. Accessed at: https://www.cancer.org/cancer/types/cervical-cancer/detection-diagnosis-staging/cervical-cancer-screening-guidelines.html. Last revised April 22, 2021 on 4 Feb 2024.
5. USPSTF: final recommendation statement cervical cancer: screening. Accessed at: https://www.uspreventiveservicestaskforce.org/uspstf/recommendation/cervical-cancer-screening (August 21, 2018) on 4 Feb 2024.
6. Seehusen DA, Johnson DR, Earwood JS, Sethuraman SN, Cornali J, Gillespie K, Doria M, Farnell E IV, Lanham J. Improving women's experience during speculum examinations at routine gynaecological visits: randomised clinical trial. BMJ. 2006;333(7560):171.

Additional Resources

Articles

Edelman A, Anderson J, Lai S, Braner DA, Tegtmeyer K. Pelvic examination. In videos in clinical medicine. N Engl J Med. 2007;356(26):e26.

Websites

https://www.asccp.org/screening-guidelines.
https://www.acog.org.

Video

https://www.youtube.com/watch?v=RwkKXCCA_0k.

Chapter 6
Difficult Exams: Cystocele, Rectocele, Stenotic Cervix/Cervical Dilatation, Nonsexually Active Women, and Elderly Women

Rhina Acevedo

Introduction

There are various anatomical conditions that can affect the performance of the pelvic exam and may lead to modifications of your pelvic examination techniques. These conditions include examinations of patients who are not sexually active, patients with cystoceles, rectoceles, atrophic vaginitis, or cervical stenosis.

Patients who have never been sexually active may have greater anxiety about their first pelvic examination; they would benefit from more time, explanation, and support during their examinations. Indications for examination of patients who have never had vaginal intercourse are limited to those with pelvic pain, discharge, or age above 21 [1]. Most examinations are possible; however, if the examination becomes too painful, the provider should discontinue the examination and consider referral for an examination under anesthesia or, alternatively, using a pelvic ultrasound. For non-emergent situations (i.e., Pap smear), a patient without prior sexual contact may benefit from first using tampons during menses prior to their first pelvic examination as tampon use has the patient experience the physical sensation of having something placed inside the vagina. Using the smallest speculum will also improve their comfort during the exam, as well as using lubricant liberally. Patients with vaginismus (involuntary vaginal muscle spasm), with dyspareunia (pain during intercourse), or who have been sexually violated may have symptoms of pain during an examination and may need to have additional time.

There are acquired and congenital changes of the pelvic structures that may also add difficulty in performing the pelvic exam. These include cystoceles, rectoceles, atrophic vaginitis, and cervical stenosis.

R. Acevedo (✉)
Department of Family Medicine and Community Health, Rutgers School of Biomedical Health Sciences, New Brunswick, NJ, USA
e-mail: acevedra@rwjms.rutgers.edu

S. M. Sulik, C. B. Heath (eds.), *Primary Care Procedures in Women's Health*,
https://doi.org/10.1007/978-3-032-07061-6_6

Rectoceles and cystoceles result from weakened pelvic support structures. Weakness can occur due to childbirth, pelvic trauma, and the aging process. A rectocele is produced when the weakened pelvic structure allows the rectum to bulge into the vaginal canal. The patient may report the presence of a sensation of heaviness in the vagina and constipation and may need to splint the vagina with her fingers in order to evacuate stool during a bowel movement [2].

Cystoceles occur when the pubovesical cervical fascia is weakened, allowing the descent of the bladder into the vaginal canal. Patients often have a sensation of fullness or pressure, stress incontinence, urinary urgency, or a feeling of incomplete voiding. A cystocele is best observed with the patient in the dorsal lithotomy position. With the posterior wall of the vagina depressed (manually or with the use of a retractor), the patient is then asked to Valsalva or cough to visualize the degree of cystocele that is present [2]. A cystocele that presents only on Valsalva or upright posture is considered grade 1. A grade 2 cystocele occurs when the cystocele is present at the introitus. Grade 3 is a cystocele that protrudes halfway beyond the introitus, and if it occurs with an everted vaginal cuff or cervix, it is called a "procidentia," complete pelvic floor collapse, or grade 4 cystocele. Alternatively, pelvic organ prolapse quantification (POPQ) measures nine sites in centimeters between the vagina and perineal body to the hymen [2].

Cervical stenosis can be either acquired or congenital. It commonly occurs in the region of the internal os. Acquired cervical stenosis can result from radiation therapy, previous infection, cancer, atrophic changes, and surgical interventions. Cone biopsy and cautery of the cervix, electrocautery, loop electrosurgical excisional procedure (LEEP), and cryotherapy can all lead to cervical stenosis [3]. Presenting symptoms vary depending on the patient's hormonal status (pre- or postmenopausal) and the degree of obstruction present. Premenopausal women with cervical stenosis may present with complaints of dysmenorrhea, pelvic pain, abnormal uterine bleeding, amenorrhea, or infertility. Postmenopausal women are predominantly asymptomatic but eventually may develop hydrometra (collection of clear fluid in the uterine cavity), hematometra (collection of blood in the uterine cavity), or pyometra (collection of exudate within the uterine cavity). The diagnosis of cervical stenosis is based on the inability to pass a 1- to 2-mm cervical dilator through the cervical os into the endocervical canal. The treatment for complete cervical stenosis is cervical dilatation (can be performed under ultrasound guidance). It is important to rule out the presence of endometrial carcinoma and endocervical carcinoma in patients with complete cervical stenosis [4].

Vaginal atrophy is the result of estrogen deficiency. This commonly occurs in postmenopausal women, but it may also occur in premenopausal women who have a relative estrogen deficiency. Premenopausal atrophy due to estrogen deficiency can occur in the immediate postpartum period, during lactation, or with the use of low-dose estrogen contraceptives, progesterone-only contraceptives, and estrogen blockers such as Danazol (Sanofi-Synthelabo, Barceloneta, Puerto Rico (Danocrine®) and tamoxifen. Patients with atrophic vaginitis may present with complaints of vaginal itching, vaginal soreness, spotting, urinary incontinence, dysuria, or dyspareunia [3]. On exam, the vaginal tissues appear pale and dry and have decreased distensibility and decreased vaginal rugae. The tissue may be friable and have areas of stenosis. Patients may also have adhesions of the vaginal wall, either externally or internally.

Case Study

A 64-year-old patient, G5P5005, presents to your office for a gynecologic well-woman examination and Pap smear. Her last pap smear with HPV co-testing was 5 years ago. There is no history of prior abnormal pap. The patient has had no vaginal bleeding since her last menses 12 years ago. She also reports some vaginal dryness and itching. As you introduce the speculum into the vaginal canal, the patient reports discomfort. As you examine the vagina, you notice that her vaginal walls are devoid of rugae and appear thin. When attempting to obtain an endocervical sample, it is impossible to insert the brush into the tightly closed cervical os.

Diagnosis (Algorithms 6.1 and 6.2)

- Atrophic vaginitis
- Cervical stenosis

Differential Diagnosis (Algorithms 6.1 and 6.2)

- Female sexual dysfunction
- Infectious vaginitis
- Vaginal neoplasia (most commonly squamous cell)
- Status post cervical cone or cryotherapy (differential for cervical stenosis)
- Estrogen deficiency due to postmenopausal state

Indications (Algorithms 6.1 and 6.2)

- Routine screening pelvic examination
- Lower abdominal and/or pelvic pain
- Irregular menses
- Postcoital bleeding
- Dyspareunia
- Pregnancy
- Postmenopausal bleeding
- Sexual assault

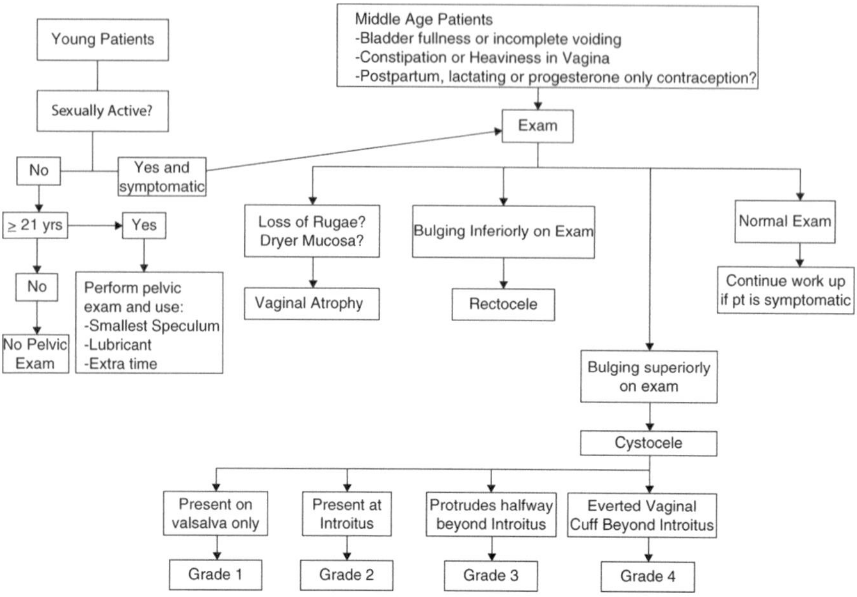

Algorithm 6.1 Decision tree for pelvic examinations of adolescent and middle-aged women

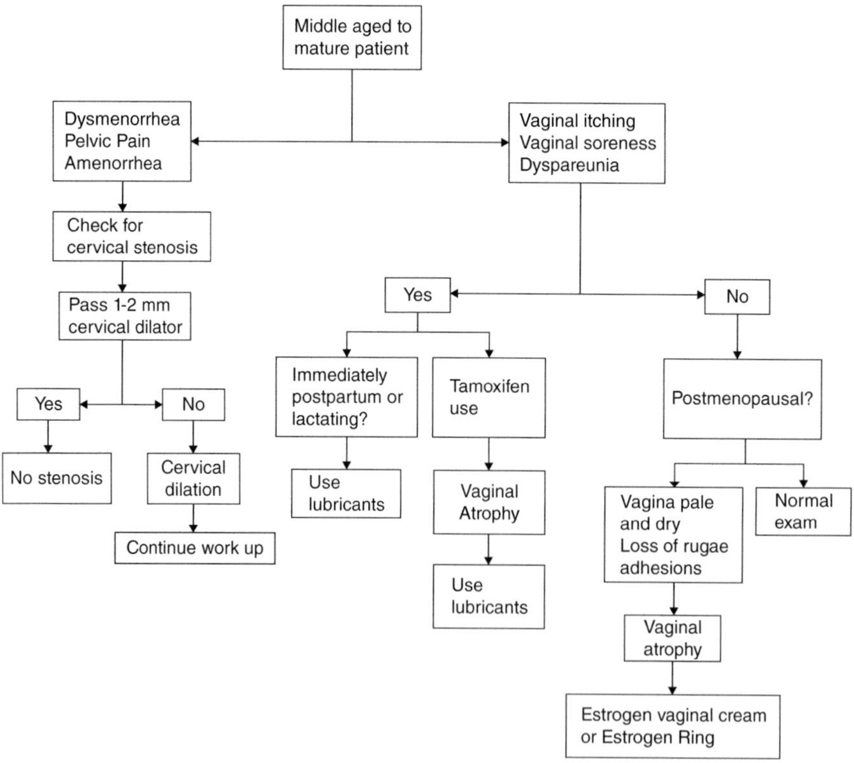

Algorithm 6.2 Decision tree for abnormal pelvic exams of middle-aged to mature women. *SERM-Selective Estrogen Receptor Modulator

Contraindications

- Patient refusal
- Placenta previa (contraindication to digital vaginal examination) (Fig. 6.1)

Equipment (Fig. 6.1)

- Gown (appropriately sized for patient)
- Sheet
- Light source
- Vaginal cotton swabs
- Nonsterile latex-free gloves
- Lubricating gel
- Speculum (Fig. 6.2): Metal or plastic—various sizes and shapes available, including Graves ("duck-billed") or Pederson ("straight"); each speculum comes in small (pediatric), medium, large, and extra-large sizes.
- Vaginal wall retractors: May be separate from the speculum or incorporated into the speculum

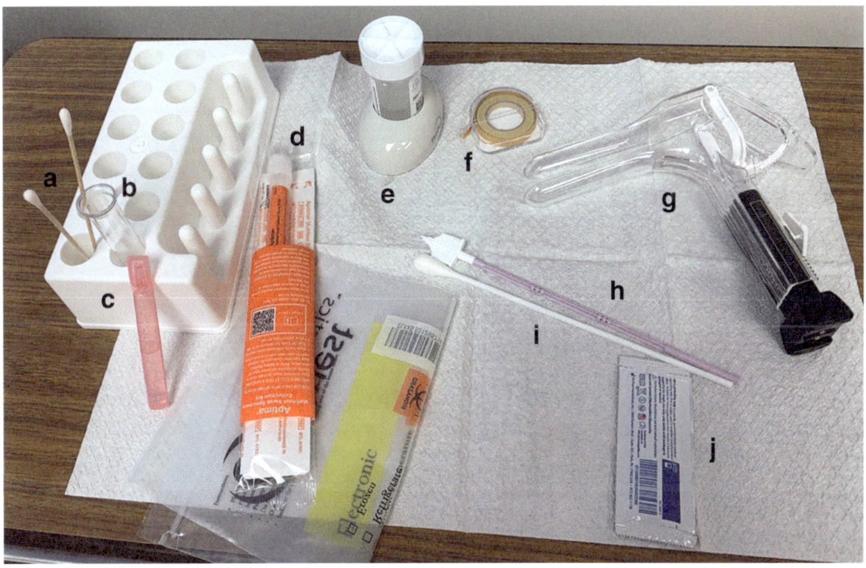

Fig. 6.1 Setup for pelvic examination: (**a**) cotton-tipped applicators for pH and saline specimen for vaginitis, (**b**) plastic test tube for vaginitis specimen, (**c**) saline, (**d**) culture swabs, (**e**) Pap smear jar for pap specimen, (**f**) pH paper, (**g**) disposable Pederson plastic speculum with light source, (**h**) endocervical broom, (**i**) large cotton tip swab, and (**j**)water-based lubricant

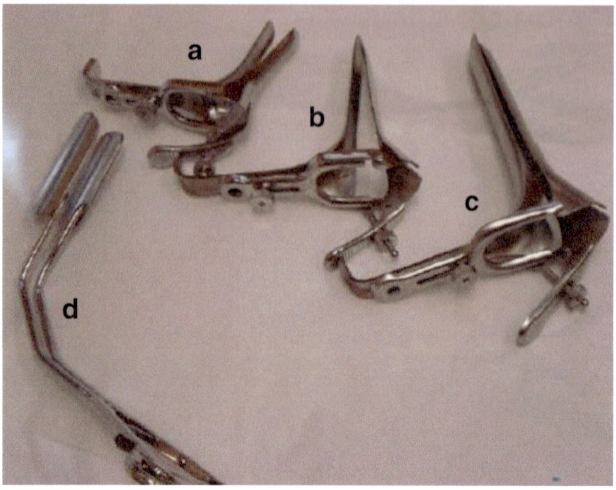

Fig. 6.2 Small Pederson speculum (**a**), medium Pederson speculum (**b**), large Graves speculum (**c**), with separate vaginal wall retractor/spreader (**d**)

- Wet mount specimen
  - Cotton swab
  - KOH
  - Small test tube with saline
  - pH paper
  - Glass slide with cover
  - Microscope
- Additional cultures as necessary
  - Gonorrhea and chlamydia
  - HSV (herpes virus)
- Pap smear equipment
  - Glass slide method (rarely used)
    (a) One glass slide
    (b) Fixation spray or jar with alcohol
    (c) Wooden cervical spatula and endocervical brush OR
    (d) Cervical broom
  - Liquid cell medium
    (a) Plastic cervical spatula and endocervical brush OR
    (b) Cervical broom

Procedure

Proceed with the steps described in Chap. 5 in the "Procedure" section, with the following variations:

1. Examine the labia for the presence of any lesions (warts, ulcerations).
2. Separate the labia and inspect the introitus for any masses or bulges.
3. Ask the patient to Valsalva and watch the area for any bulges on the superior (cystocele) (Fig. 6.3) or inferior (rectocele) (Fig. 6.4) aspect of the vaginal canal.
4. Place the index finger into the vaginal canal and apply downward pressure to displace the introitus, which will allow the examiner to visualize a cystocele or a rectocele.
5. Position the light source in order to optimize visualization of the vaginal canal.
6. Apply a small amount of warm lubricant gel to the blades of the speculum or wet the metal speculum with warm water. Use the smallest speculum available that will permit visualization of the vaginal walls and cervix.
7. Introduce the tip of the speculum at an angle to the vaginal canal entry and apply slow downward and posterior pressure until approximately three-fourths of the speculum blades have been introduced. Allow time to have the patient's vaginal tissue to accommodate the procedure.
8. Rotate the speculum so that the blades are perpendicular to the vaginal canal and open the blades. Reposition as needed in order to bring the cervix into full visualization between the blades of the speculum.
9. Inspect the vaginal walls for the presence of any lesions. Also note the presence or absence of rugae and vaginal moisture.
10. Obtain clinically appropriate vaginal/cervical/endocervical samples.
11. Carefully withdraw the speculum from the vaginal canal.

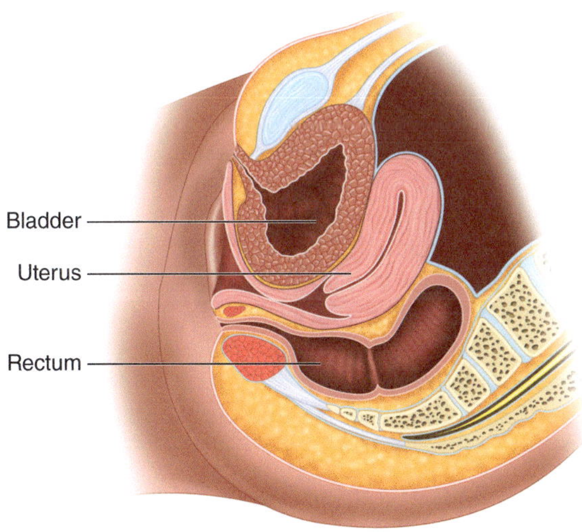

Fig. 6.3 Visualization of cystocele with patient in dorsal lithotomy position

Fig. 6.4 Rectocele with patient in dorsal lithotomy position

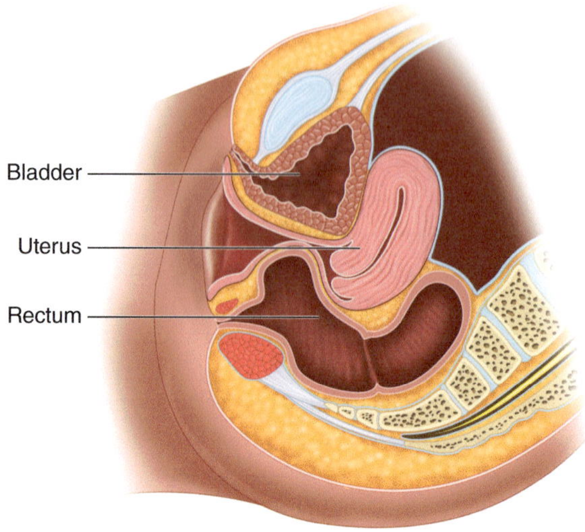

12. Perform a bimanual examination if necessary. For patients with a small introitus, one finger may be all that is necessary for the intravaginal portion of the bimanual examination.
13. Perform a rectovaginal examination if necessary, with the middle finger being introduced into the rectum and the index finger into the vagina.

Complications and Risks

There is a small risk of trauma to the adjacent tissue.

Tricks and Helpful Hints

- Do not assume that postmenopausal patients are not sexually active.
- Use a well-lubricated speculum when performing an examination of a patient with possible atrophic vaginitis. Consider using a Pedersen instead of a Graves speculum.
- A speculum with a wider blade (such as a medium- or large-sized Graves) will provide better support of superior and posterior structures if necessary due to mildly collapsing vaginal walls.
- For vaginal walls that persistently protrude into the field of vision, consider the following:
  - Use vaginal wall retractors with the speculum (must use medium or large Graves with retractors).

  - If vaginal wall retractors are unavailable, make a retractor out of a clean latex glove by cutting the thumb portion from the glove and then cutting the tip off the thumb portion of the glove (Fig. 6.5). Introduce the speculum blades into the rubber cylinder created (Fig. 6.6), and lubricate both the speculum and the cylinder prior to introducing it into the vagina.
  - Use a condom in the same fashion as the latex glove.

- For cervical stenosis:

  - Use an endometrial cell sampler to relieve mild cervical strictures. Then retry using the endocervical brush or broom.
  - Use cervical dilators.
  - Use intravaginal estrogen cream, one applicatorful, to the vagina nightly for 2–4 weeks and then obtain the specimen.
  - Use laminaria.
  - Use misoprostol 200 mg orally or intravaginally 4 h prior to the exam. (intravaginal preferred)

- In women who have never been sexually active, the clinician may opt to insert only one finger intravaginally during the bimanual examination.
- In extreme cases of tenderness or pain with examination, discontinue the exam and consider doing it under general anesthesia.
- In extreme cases of tenderness or pain, consider gently questioning women about previous sexual abuse. In some cases, pelvic examinations may need to be done after desensitization programs such as pelvic floor therapy or under general anesthesia.
- Be sure to question women alone about their needs for a chaperone. Chaperones in general should be health professionals, but they can be family members or partners if that is the preference of the patient. However, be sure to discuss this in private with the patient prior to agreeing to any nonprofessional chaperone, as abusive partners may insist on being present.

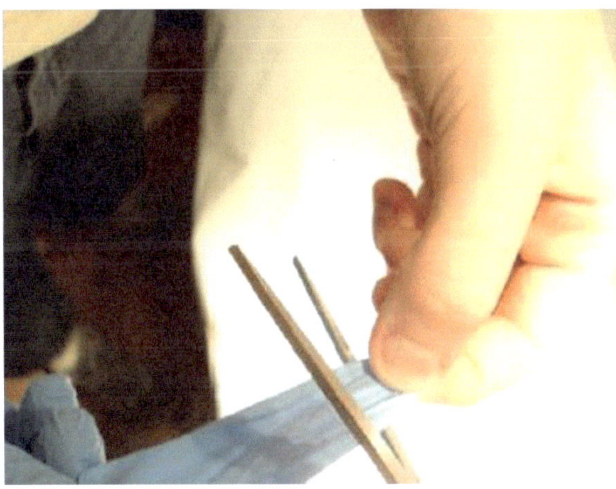

Fig. 6.5 Cutting a latex glove finger for a vaginal retractor

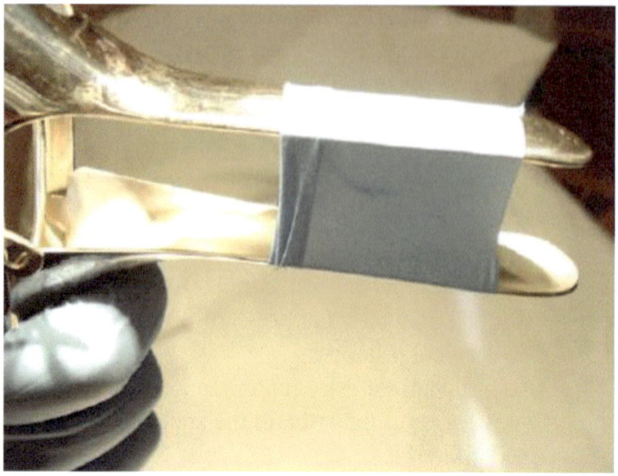

Fig. 6.6 Glove finger used as a vaginal retractor

Procedure Note

(Provider to fill in blanks/circle applicable choice when given multiple choices and customize as necessary.)

Patient was placed in the dorsal lithotomy position. Upon examination, __________ (cystocele, rectocele, vaginal atrophy, cervical stenosis) was noted. Careful speculum examination (with, without) vaginal retractors occurred; cervix was visualized, and Pap smear was obtained. Patient tolerated the procedure well and a note will be mailed or securely messaged with the results.

Coding

CPT® Codes (Current Procedural Terminology, AMA, Chicago, IL)

99384–99387 New Patient Preventive Medicine Services

99394–99397 Established Patient Preventive Medicine Service Use illness coding for patients presenting with symptoms

ICD 10-CM-Diagnostic Codes (International Classification of Diseases, 10th Revision, Clinical Modification, Centers for Disease Control and Prevention)

Z01.49 Encounter for gynecological examination (general) (routine) without abnormal findings

Z01.411 Encounter for gynecological examination (general) (routine) with abnormal findings

N81.1 Cystocele

N81.10 Cystocele, unspecified

N81.11 Cystocele, midline

N81.12 Cystocele, lateral

N81.6 Rectocele
N88.2 Stricture and stenosis of cervix uteri
N95.2 Postmenopausal atrophic vaginitis

Postprocedure Patient Instructions

The patient should be advised of any findings on the exam and how she will be notified of the results. She should also be advised that she may experience some scant vaginal spotting which is usually self-limited. If the patient begins to experience significant vaginal symptoms of heavy bleeding, discharge, or pelvic pain, she should return to the office for evaluation.

Case Study Outcomes

Vaginal examination revealed the presence of a cystocele and atrophic vaginitis. The patient was treated with estrogen vaginal cream. Upon re-evaluation 1 month later, the patient reported significant improvement of symptoms.

Postprocedure Patient Handout

(*Provider to fill in blanks/circle applicable choice when given multiple choices and customize as necessary.*)

You have just had a pelvic examination. This examination showed that you have (provider to circle diagnosis):

- A cystocele is a protrusion of the bladder into the vagina that happens due to the relaxation of the pelvic structures. Many women who have cystoceles have no symptoms at all. Some will notice urgency of urination, stress incontinence (losing urine with laughing, coughing, or sneezing), or a sense that their bladder is just not emptying. Some patients also experience only a vague sense of fullness of the bladder. If these symptoms are becoming bothersome to you, please make an appointment to discuss treatment options, such as pessary fitting or surgery.
- A rectocele occurs when the rectal mucosa protrudes into the vaginal wall. Many patients with rectoceles have no symptoms, but some experience symptoms of heaviness in the vagina, constipation, or the need to provide support to their vagina to have a bowel movement. If these symptoms are becoming bothersome to you, please make an appointment to discuss treatment options, such as pessary fitting or surgery.

- Vaginal atrophy occurs when there is a lack of estrogen lubricating the vaginal walls, either from medications such as tamoxifen or progesterone-only birth control, menopause, breastfeeding, or hysterectomy with removal of both ovaries. Most patients have no symptoms, but some may experience painful intercourse, vaginal itching or soreness, burning on urination, urinary incontinence, or vaginal spotting. If these symptoms are becoming bothersome to you, please make an appointment to discuss treatment options, such as hormone replacement, if indicated.
- Cervical stenosis occurs when there is a lack of estrogen lubricating the cervix or when there is a surgical procedure or radiation that has caused the cervical opening to become small. Symptoms of cervical stenosis for patients who still are getting their periods include dysmenorrhea (painful periods), pelvic pain, abnormal uterine bleeding, amenorrhea (no period), or infertility. Postmenopausal patients usually have no symptoms but can experience abdominal cramping or pain from collections of blood or fluid in the uterus. This is very rare. If you are experiencing any of these symptoms, please make an appointment with your provider to discuss treatment options.

References

1. The American Cancer Society. The American Cancer Society Guidelines for the prevention and early detection of cervical cancer. Accessed at: https://www.cancer.org/cancer/types/cervical-cancer/detection-diagnosis-staging/cervical-cancer-screening-guidelines.html. Last revised April 22, 2021 on 4 Feb 2024.
2. Kirby A, Lentz GM. Pelvic organ prolapse, abdominal hernias and inguinal hernias: diagnosis and management. In: Gershenson DM, Lentz GM, Lobo RA, Valea FA, editors. Comprehensive gynecology. 8th ed. Philadelphia: Elsevier; 2022. p. 428–60.
3. Smith RP. Vaginitis: atrophic genitourinary symptoms of menopause. In: Smith RP, editor. Netter's obstetrics and gynecology. 4th ed. Philadelphia: Elsevier; 2024. p. 262–3.
4. Dolan M, Hill C, Valea FA. Benign gynecologic lesions: vulva, vagina, cervix, uterus, oviduct, ovary, ultrasound imaging of pelvic structures. In: Gershenson DM, Lobo RA, Lentz GM, Valea FA, editors. Comprehensive gynecology. 8th ed. Philadelphia: Elsevier; 2022. p. 37362–408.

Chapter 7
Sexual Assault Victim Examination

Melissa Arthur and Nadine Khouzam

Introduction

The term "sexual assault" is defined as sexual contact or any other behavior that occurs without the victim's consent. Sexual assault includes the following:

- Unwanted sexual touching
- Forcing a victim physically or psychologically to perform sexual acts, such as oral sex or penetrating the perpetrator's body

Rape is defined as forced penetration of the victim's mouth, genitals, and anus by the perpetrator where the force is either physical or psychological. Eight out of 10 sexual assaults are committed by someone known to the victim, an intimate partner sexual violence, or an acquaintance rape. When the victim does not know the perpetrator at all. It will be referred to as stranger rape.

According to the Centers for Disease Control and Prevention (CDC), over half of women and almost 1 in 3 men have experienced sexual violence involving physical contact during their lifetimes. One in 4 women and about 1 in 26 men have experienced completed or attempted rape [1]. In the United States, 81.3% of women rape victims reported their first occurrence prior to age 25 [2].

In 2018, there were 734,630 reported victims of rape, attempted rape, or sexual assault in the United States. The rate of reporting sexual assault increased from 23%

M. Arthur (✉)
St Joseph's Family Medicine Residency, Professor, Departments of Psychiatry,
Upstate Medical University Syracuse, NY, USA
e-mail: melissa.arthur@sjhsyr.org

N. Khouzam
St Joseph's Family Medicine Residency, Syracuse, NY, USA
e-mail: nadine.khouzam@sjhsyr.org

S. M. Sulik, C. B. Heath (eds.), *Primary Care Procedures in Women's Health*,
https://doi.org/10.1007/978-3-032-07061-6_7

in 2016 to 43% in 2017 [3] perhaps reflecting an increased empowerment of people who have been victimized by nonconsensual sex.

When a victim of rape presents to the Emergency Department or private office for examination, it is important to collect and preserve all forensic evidence to ensure that there are few impediments to prosecution. It is important to be complete and thorough in the exam and evidence gathering, while at the same time being sensitive to the fact that the victim has likely already endured a lengthy process prior to arriving for her physical examination.

The number of examiners and interviews should be kept to a minimum with as much history as possible being obtained from law enforcement personnel, social workers, and family members. The use of the team approach toward evaluation and treatment is effective in minimizing the trauma of the emergency department setting [4]. With that background, a more focused interview can be obtained from the victim using as many of the victim's own words as possible in recording the history. The interview process need not be duplicated, except as it pertains to specific evidence that needs to be collected for a more in-depth, directed physical exam or specimen collection. Offering to have a support person present (who is not suspected of the abuse) may be reassuring to victims of all ages [5].

It is important to have a nurse or aid assist during the exam and evidence collection as it will help to provide materials and also label evidence promptly as it is collected, minimizing disruption, and it will also expedite the process by allowing the examiner to continue wearing gloves during the entire examination without having to change them for record-keeping.

DNA collection is an important part of the examination and can assist in bringing perpetrators to justice. Specially trained nurses in the Sexual Assault Nurse Examiner (SANE) program help coordinate all the team members and minimize further trauma to the victim [5]. For more extensive resources on the examination of sexual assault victims, see below resources for health care providers.

The Rape Kit

Rape kits vary by location, but commonly include the following items:

- Detailed instructions
- Paper bags in various sizes and sheets for evidence collection
- Swabs for collecting fluids from the lips, cheeks, thighs, vagina, anus, and buttocks
- Sterile urine collection containers
- Sterile sample containers
- Blood collection devices
- Comb used to collect hair and fiber from the victim's body
- Clear glass slides

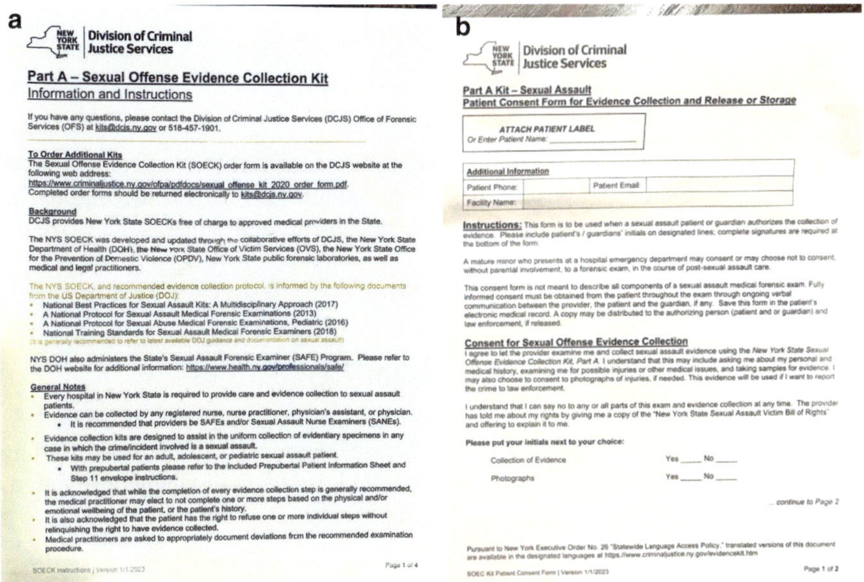

a

New York State | Division of Criminal Justice Services

Part A – Sexual Offense Evidence Collection Kit
Information and Instructions

If you have any questions, please contact the Division of Criminal Justice Services (DCJS) Office of Forensic Services (OFS) at kits@dcjs.ny.gov or 518-457-1901.

To Order Additional Kits
The Sexual Offense Evidence Collection Kit (SOECK) order form is available on the DCJS website at the following web address:
https://www.criminaljustice.ny.gov/ofpa/pdfdocs/sexual_offense_kit_2020_order_form.pdf.
Completed order forms should be returned electronically to kits@dcjs.ny.gov.

Background
DCJS provides New York State SOECKs free of charge to approved medical providers in the State.

The NYS SOECK was developed and updated through the collaborative efforts of DCJS, the New York State Department of Health (DOH), the New York State Office of Victim Services (OVS), the New York State Office for the Prevention of Domestic Violence (OPDV), New York State public forensic laboratories, as well as medical and legal practitioners.

The NYS SOECK, and recommended evidence collection protocol, is informed by the following documents from the US Department of Justice (DOJ):
- National Best Practices for Sexual Assault Kits: A Multidisciplinary Approach (2017)
- A National Protocol for Sexual Assault Medical Forensic Examinations (2013)
- A National Protocol for Sexual Abuse Medical Forensic Examinations, Pediatric (2016)
- National Training Standards for Sexual Assault Medical Forensic Examiners (2018)

(It is generally recommended to refer to latest available DOJ guidance and documentation on sexual assault)

NYS DOH also administers the State's Sexual Assault Forensic Examiner (SAFE) Program. Please refer to the DOH website for additional information: https://www.health.ny.gov/professionals/safe/

General Notes
- Every hospital in New York State is required to provide care and evidence collection to sexual assault patients.
- Evidence can be collected by any registered nurse, nurse practitioner, physician's assistant, or physician.
  - It is recommended that providers be SAFEs and/or Sexual Assault Nurse Examiners (SANEs).
- Evidence collection kits are designed to assist in the uniform collection of evidentiary specimens in any case in which the crime/incident involved is a sexual assault.
- These kits may be used for an adult, adolescent, or pediatric sexual assault patient.
  - With prepubertal patients please refer to the included Prepubertal Patient Information Sheet and Step 11 envelope instructions.
- It is acknowledged that while the completion of every evidence collection step is generally recommended, the medical practitioner may elect to not complete one or more steps based on the physical and/or emotional wellbeing of the patient, or the patient's history.
- It is also acknowledged that the patient has the right to refuse one or more individual steps without relinquishing the right to have evidence collected.
- Medical practitioners are asked to appropriately document deviations from the recommended examination procedure.

SOECK Instructions | Version 1/1/2023 Page 1 of 4

b

New York State | Division of Criminal Justice Services

Part A Kit – Sexual Assault
Patient Consent Form for Evidence Collection and Release or Storage

ATTACH PATIENT LABEL
Or Enter Patient Name: ______________

Additional Information			
Patient Phone:		Patient Email:	
Facility Name:			

Instructions: This form is to be used when a sexual assault patient or guardian authorizes the collection of evidence. Please include patient's / guardians' initials on designated lines; complete signatures are required at the bottom of the form.

A mature minor who presents at a hospital emergency department may consent or may choose not to consent, without parental involvement, to a forensic exam, in the course of post-sexual assault care.

This consent form is not meant to describe all components of a sexual assault medical forensic exam. Fully informed consent must be obtained from the patient throughout the exam through ongoing verbal communication between the provider, the patient and the guardian, if any. Save this form in the patient's electronic medical record. A copy may be distributed to the authorizing person (patient and or guardian) and law enforcement, if released.

Consent for Sexual Offense Evidence Collection
I agree to let the provider examine me and collect sexual assault evidence using the *New York State Sexual Offense Evidence Collection Kit, Part A*. I understand that this may include asking me about my personal and medical history, examining me for possible injuries or other medical issues, and taking samples for evidence. I may also choose to consent to photographs of injuries, if needed. This evidence will be used if I want to report the crime to law enforcement.

I understand that I can say no to any or all parts of this exam and evidence collection at any time. The provider has told me about my rights by giving me a copy of the "New York State Sexual Assault Victim Bill of Rights" and offering to explain it to me.

Please put your initials next to your choice:

Collection of Evidence Yes ____ No ____

Photographs Yes ____ No ____

... continue to Page 2

Pursuant to New York Executive Order No. 26 "Statewide Language Access Policy," translated versions of this document are available in the designated languages at https://www.criminaljustice.ny.gov/evidencekit.htm

SOEC Kit Patient Consent Form | Version 1/1/2023 Page 1 of 2

Fig. 7.1 (**a**, **b**) Instructions sheet and consent form (Reprinted with permission from the New York State Division of Criminal Justice Services)

- Self-sealing envelopes for preserving the victim's clothes, head hair, pubic hair, and blood samples
- Nail pick for scraping debris from beneath the nails
- White sheets to catch physical evidence stripped from the body
- Documentation and consent forms (Fig. 7.1)
- Labels

Case Study

A 22-year-old woman was at a party with her friends where alcohol was being served. She recalls drinking two beers within a time span of 3 hours but denies taking any drugs. She remembers dancing with several young men, but she now has a headache, her clothing is disheveled, and she is experiencing vaginal spotting. She suspects that she may have been a victim of unwanted sexual advances, but her memory is fuzzy about the event. She is presently on oral contraceptives; her last menstrual period was 1 week ago.

Indications (Algorithm 7.1)

Suspected Rape

The rape kit provides a very elaborate and thorough form for recording various aspects of the history and physical exam. An additional note for the hospital or office record may make a reference to these documents and should summarize the major findings.

The Examination Process (Algorithm 7.1)

We will focus on the medical and some forensic components of the exam starting with the initial contact with the sexually assaulted patient to discharge instructions and follow-up.

Equipment

- Speculum
- Lubricant
- Light source
- Rape kit: as determined by local law enforcement agencies (This includes envelopes, swabs, and slides for evidence collection, as well as forms with routine questions and diagrams.) (Fig. 7.2)
- GC/*Chlamydia* test kit with swabs, depending on local custom
- Venipuncture materials: needle, vacutainer collection tubes, alcohol prep, gloves, and gauze
- Urine collection container with cleansing wipes
- Rapid pregnancy test kit
- Pencil for labelling specimens on glass slides
- Pen for recording findings and labelling envelopes and paper bags
- Nonsterile latex-free exam gloves
- Clean sheet for the patient to stand on while collecting clothing for evidence
- Hospital gown for the patient to wear during the exam and a clean sheet for cover-up
- Water for dampening swabs to collect evidence
- Paper bags in various sizes to collect clothing
- Extra clothing for the victim, preferably "street clothes" as opposed to a hospital gown

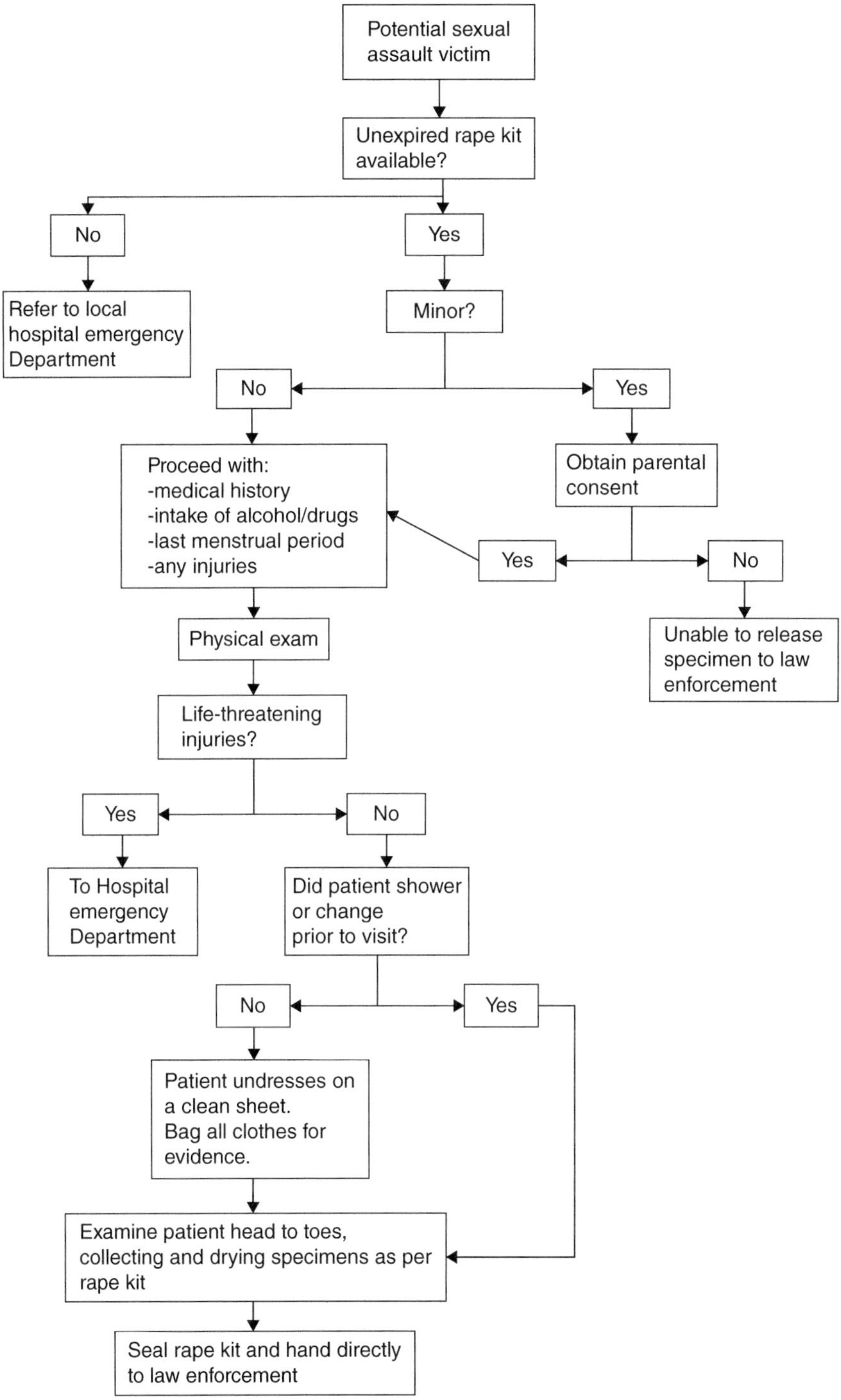

Algorithm 7.1 Decision tree for a sexual assault victim

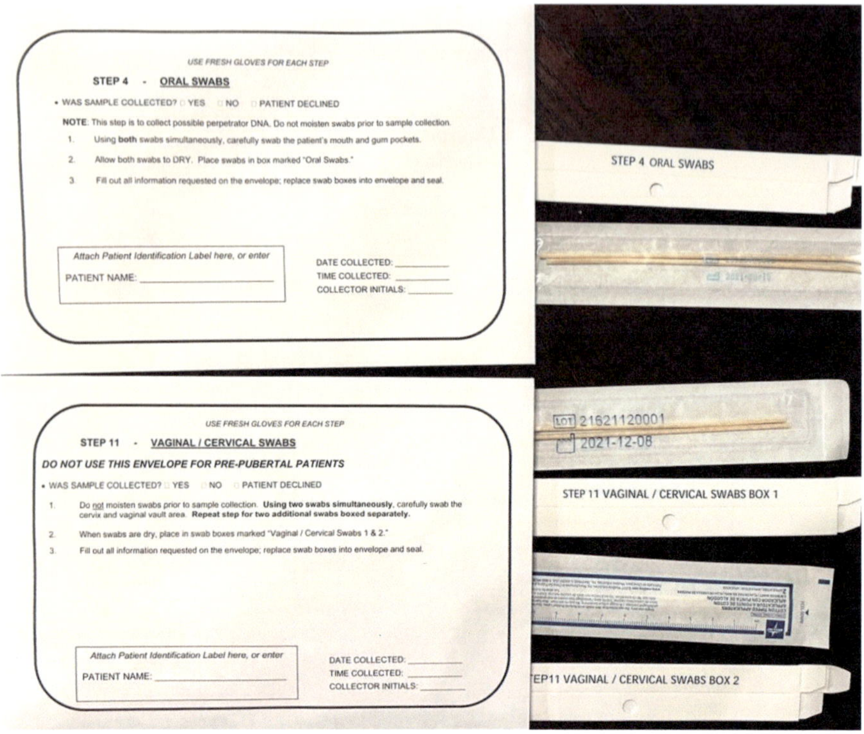

Fig. 7.2 Closer look at some of the envelopes and their contents. (Reprinted with permission from the New York State Division of Criminal Justice Services)

Optional Equipment

- UV light colposcope with video capabilities to record the evidence as collected

1. *Triage and intake*: When a patient presents to the office or ER, consider the sexual assault patient a priority regardless of whether physical injuries are evident. Address acute injury and trauma care and patient safety before collecting evidence. Discuss with the patient if they would like a family member or an advocate to be present. Observe and record the general appearance and demeanor of the patient.
2. *Documentation*: Examiners are responsible for the completion of all appropriate documentation and need to ensure the accuracy and objectivity of all the reports. Be precise, thorough, and accurate. Examiners should obtain consent from the victim or parent/legal guardian if the victim is a minor.
3. *Gather medical forensic history*: Ask the patient detailed medical and forensic questions related to the assault. The rape kit forms are very thorough in assessing the circumstances of sexual assault.

    - Any pertinent medical history, medications, allergies

- Date and time of the assault and any alcohol or drug intake if applicable
- Injuries or complaints related to sexual assault, the nature of the physical assault, and the description
- Any recent consensual sexual activity, post sexual activities

4. *Photography*: consider taking photos as necessary with patient's permission.
5. *Physical exam*: Using the rape kit (Fig. 7.3) as a guide, proceed from head to toe gathering specimens as appropriate and placing them in the appropriately labelled envelopes. Check the expiration date on the rape kit prior to proceeding.

    - Place a clean white sheet on the floor. Have the patient undress on the sheet, which will prevent any contamination of clothing and secure any fibers or

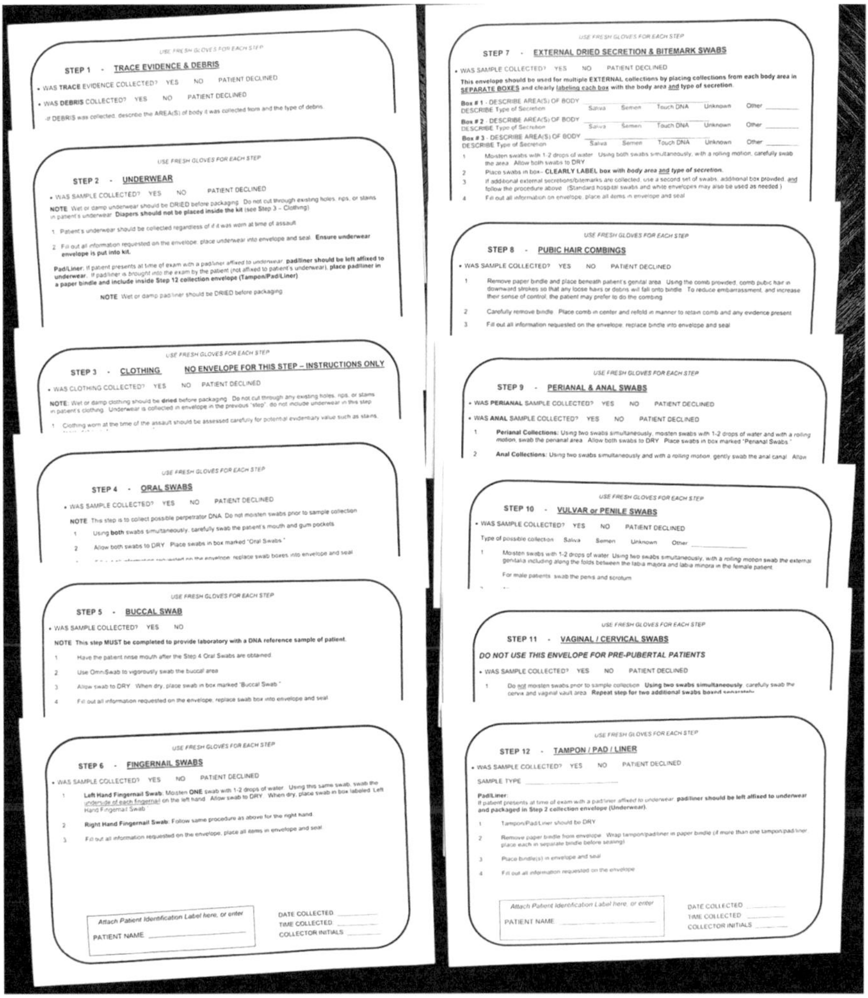

Fig. 7.3 Rape kit contents envelopes with step-by-step collection instructions (used with permission New York State Division of Criminal Justice Services).

evidence that may be on clothing, lodged in the patient's hair, or under fingernails. Package each piece of clothing individually in a paper bag, which should then be sealed. If the victim has showered and changed clothing after the sexual assault has occurred, this step may be unnecessary. Provide the patient with a hospital/office gown and a sheet.

- Perform a complete physical exam with special attention directed to the oral cavity, the skin around and near the breasts, and the perineal area and document findings on a body diagrams form. Plucked specimens of the victim's scalp hair and pubic hair can be obtained either at this step or at any follow-up visit under less stressful circumstances. Combed specimens should be obtained at the time of the exam.
- Thoroughly dry all specimens prior to packaging to avoid the destruction of samples by mold growth. Avoid the use of a hair dryer or other heat source, as this may degrade specimens.
- Obtain cervical swabs to be sent to the local laboratory for gonorrhea and chlamydia
- Collect blood and urine for toxicology screening and deliver specimens to the local lab for analysis. Specimens may also be sent for Hepatitis B, Hepatitis C, and HIV.
- Discuss the probability of pregnancy with a childbearing age female, and administer a rapid and/or quantitative β-HCG pregnancy test. Offer emergency contraception, if indicated.
- Offer patients information about the risk of STI, encourage them to accept prophylaxis, follow-up examinations and treatments as per CDC guidelines.
- Offer postexposure prophylaxis for HIV to patients at high risk of exposure per CDC guidelines.
- Seal the rape kit with the stickers provided and sign off each sticker with time and date and initials of the examiner (Fig. 7.2). The kit must be handed directly to a law enforcement officer in order to preserve the chain of evidence (Fig. 7.4). Sign each page (usually 15–20 pages, not including duplicates) and hand over the originals to the officer, keeping copies for the chart and sexual abuse management (SAM) clinic.

6. *Discharge and follow-up*: It is important to ensure that patients are fully informed about post-exam care, discharge instructions, and follow-up appointments. Provide patients with oral and written medical discharge instructions that include the summary of the exam, evidence and tests collected, provided medications if any, and their scheduled follow-up appointments and referrals. For patients with evidence of acute trauma, a short-term follow-up appointment usually in 24–48 hours is necessary to reexamine the injury and another exam in 2–4 weeks later to document resolution or healing of the injury. All patients should have a discussion about the importance of repeating the STI exam. Make sure patients' medical and mental health needs related to the assault have been addressed, and discuss the best method and time to contact them.

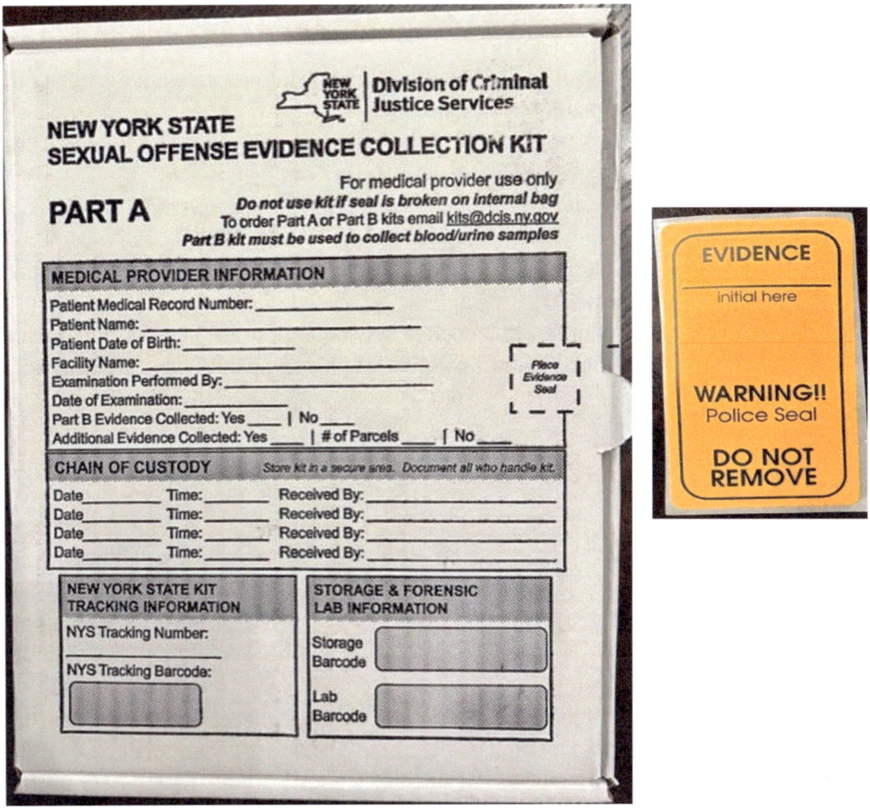

Fig. 7.4 Chain of custody sealed rape kit and evidence sealed label: State of New York. (Used with permission from the NY Division of Criminal Justice Services)

Tricks and Helpful Hints

- UV light has been used in the past to highlight areas of semen on skin and in hair; however, studies have recently shown that this yields confusing results, as many common items (such as K-Y jelly and powder) will fluoresce. It is no longer recommended.
- It is *very important* to check the date of expiration on the seal of the rape kit before proceeding. Otherwise, all evidence collected may be considered invalid and the case may not be able to be prosecuted. However, in the absence of an alternative, the kit may still be used to collect specimens to be used in patient care.
- Many of the "date-rape" drugs do not have metabolites that can be detected on routine toxicology screens. However, some drugs may be possible to detect if special instructions are given to the laboratory. Check with local law enforcement as some specimens can be sent to the state lab for testing of metabolites.

The length of time from drug ingestion to collection of the specimen also plays a role in the likelihood of detection.

- It is the patient's choice regarding whether they wish to receive emergency contraception, even if the patient is a minor.
- Special handling and special consent may be needed for HIV serology and for nonoccupational postexposure prophylaxis (nPEP) to be initiated.
- A support person or an advocate may be present during the exam.
- A normal physical exam does not exclude the possibility that a sexual assault did indeed occur. This should be discussed with the patient and with the authorities and documented in the chart.
- In some areas of the country, a colposcope may be used to aid in recording details in the vaginal examination, including bruising or bleeding consistent with trauma.

Mental Health

It is well documented that a history of abuse of any kind impacts health, both physically and psychologically. Having a history of sexual abuse, in particular, can increase the patient's risk for health conditions such as irritable bowel, chronic pelvic pain, chronic pain, asthma, migraine headaches, and fibromyalgia [6, 7]. Patients who were sexually assaulted are more likely to engage in unhealthy coping behaviors such as smoking, substance abuse with alcohol, marijuana, cocaine, or heroin.

Mental health conditions can include posttraumatic stress disorder (PTSD), anxiety, depression, sexual dysfunction, and substance use disorders. The most common sequela for survivors is PTSD, with rates that range from 30% to 65% [8]. Victims may have long-term effects and may continue to struggle psychologically based on the trauma. Both relationships and functioning can be negatively affected [9]. Compared to others who have been victimized by violent crimes, sexual assault victims are at a 70% higher risk for psychological complications [10]. Thirty percent of rape victims continue to experience PTSD symptoms 9 months after assault [10]. Depression symptoms must be monitored regularly by health care providers. Suicide ideation and death by suicide are common. Thirty-three percent of rape victims experience suicide ideation, and 13% of sexual assault survivors have made a suicide attempt [11, 12].

Communication

For patients with an acute crisis of sexual abuse and for patients who disclose a previous history of sexual abuse, the physician can play a crucial role in their process of healing. Survivors of sexual abuse often experience a lack of control, guilt, and shame. The health care professional must be cognizant of these common reactions and conduct the exam and interview accordingly. Providing emotional support, avoiding blame, and offering resources have been shown to decrease survivors' PTSD symptoms [13]. One way to avoid blame is to leave questions related to the specific circumstance to law enforcement. Never comment on the situation in which the abuse occurred—for instance, if the patient was drinking, using drugs, or permitted a stranger into their apartment. These circumstances do not give abusers permission to violate the patient. You can inquire if the patient would like to report the incident to law enforcement but allow the survivor the autonomy to decide for themselves.

Tips for communication to promote psychological safety by taking a trauma-informed approach:

1. Be compassionate, listen, use empathy, and be nonjudgmental. Use a gentle tone and convey support with your words rather than physical touch. Even a kind touch on the shoulder to comfort can be emotionally triggering for a sexual abuse survivor.
2. Thank the patient for telling you their story. It takes courage for survivors to disclose sexual abuse to you. For some, it takes many years to disclose that they were sexually abused [13]. Helpful, validating statements include: "This is not your fault." and "You did not deserve this."
3. Provide ongoing support—Statements include the following:

   "You are not alone."
   "I am here to listen and support you."
   "I care about your health, and your mental health."
   Have a close follow-up to see the patient back in 1–2 weeks.

4. Assess the patient's support network—Inquire if they have supportive people in their lives they can talk to about the abuse.
5. Assess for safety—Are they safe to return home? If a minor is being sexually abused by a family member, child protection must be contacted. If a child is being abused by an adult, then law enforcement needs to be contacted. Are they suicidal?
6. Provide resources—counseling and rape crisis

Preparation for the Exam

A sensitive approach to the exam includes preparing to have extra time with the patient. While the patient is dressed, sit down, make eye contact, and clearly explain every aspect of the procedure. This allows the patient to mentally prepare and eliminates any unforeseen physical contact that is necessary for the procedure. Ask the patient how you can be helpful. Offer the patient a cold or warm washcloth, extra gown, and water [13].

During the Exam

It is crucial to remember there is always a hierarchical difference between the patient and the provider. Procedures that include the insertion of medical instruments such as a speculum during a pelvic exam, can be a psychologically triggering event. Triggering may occur since parts of the exam may stimulate memories and feelings related to the sexual abuse. Give the patient permission to stop or take a break if needed during the exam. Ask the patient whether it would help to have her self-insert the speculum. Check in with the patient regularly throughout the encounter. These strategies will help the patient to feel empowered to care for themselves. If the exam is causing psychological triggers. The patient may become anxious and overwhelmed which can even lead to emotional flooding and dissociation. Dissociation is the process of psychologically being detached, a sense of leaving one's body from the current experience. Narrating each part of the exam and talking about nonmedical issues can help lower anxiety and help decrease the possibility of flooding and dissociation. This can help decrease flashbacks and assist the patient in staying in the present moment.

Communication and Interviewing Tips Regarding Past Sexual Abuse History

Help patients understand that inquiring about past and current abuse is connected to their overall health and mental health. This approach also lets the patient know the provider is someone they can disclose the abuse to, when and if they are ready.

Ask directly about sexual violence—for instance, "Many of my patients have experienced violence and sexual violence. Has anything like that ever happened to you?" [11]

American College of Obstetricians (ACOG) recommends the following screening questions [14]:

Has anyone ever touched you against your will or without your consent?
Have you ever been forced or pressured to engage in sexual activities when you did not want to?
Have you ever had unwanted sex while under the influence of alcohol or drugs?
Do you feel that you have control over your sexual relationships and will be listened to if you say "no" to sexual activities?
Is your visit today because of a sexual experience you did not want to have happen?

Knowing a patient has a history of sexual abuse may help you recognize barriers to nonadherence regarding certain medical procedures such as pelvic exams, colonoscopies, or endoscopies [15]. The provider can then further discuss ways to help lower the patient's anxiety and encourage the patient to follow up on these procedures in the future. If the provider is conducting the pelvic exam with a sexual assault survivor, they can ask the patient if there is anything you can do to help them make the exam more comfortable. (Follow the tips described above.)

Case Study

Cheif Complaint: A 22-yo female c/o alleged sexual assault 12 hours prior to admission. Patient consumed one beer at 1:00 am. Patient has voided and brushed her teeth but has not showered, douched, or defecated since the event. She changed her clothing prior to going to the police station. No other injuries. LMP 9/13/07 G1P0010 sexually active, one partner, on oral contraceptives. No significant past medical history. No other meds, no known allergies.

Physical Exam: Small abrasion of left labia minora with no active bleeding; exam otherwise normal. (See rape kit sheets.)

Assessment/Plan: Alleged sexual assault. STD and pregnancy prophylaxis offered. Hepatitis, HIV, GC/chlamydia pending. Patient to follow up with Sexual Abuse Management (SAM) Clinic.

Case Study Outcome

The patient was evaluated by the clinician in the emergency room for rape. She has elected to be treated for sexually transmitted infections. She decided to follow up with her primary care clinician and is planning on going to the next meeting of the support group for women who have been sexually abused.

Coding

ICD 10-CM-Diagnostic Codes (International Classification of Diseases, Tenth Revision, Clinical Modification, Centers for Disease Control and Prevention)	
Z04.41	Examination for alleged rape or sexual assault

Postprocedure Patient Handout

(*Provider to customize as necessary.*)

You have just been evaluated for sexual assault (rape). Remember that what happened is not your fault. *No one* "deserves this" or was "asking for it." Rape is a crime. You have the right to report this to the police and to be treated fairly during the justice process.

Many people experience a widely varying set of emotions, including rage, depression, anxiety, and fear. Recovering from this is a process; it may take weeks, months, or years. This is normal. In addition, it is very common for loved ones to have similar reactions. It is important not to "take the law into your own hands," as these actions will likely end in more hardship to you and to your loved ones. Allow the law to do its job. Law enforcers are specialists and are there to assist you in bringing the perpetrator to justice.

Some women prefer private counselling with a psychologist or mental health/clinical social worker. Many people find support groups quite helpful. These local support groups often have trained therapists and other women who have gone through similar circumstances. Talking with people who have also experienced sexual assault often helps people understand their own feelings and emotions. There are also national groups to help support women through the crisis of rape. (See references for patients below.)

It is also important to follow up on the medical issues surrounding sexual assault. This can be done by a local sexual abuse management team or at your primary care physician's office.

If you are on birth control and are taking it regularly, the likelihood of pregnancy is low. If you wish to be treated for prevention of pregnancy, you may be given a series of pills to take. It is important to take them as directed. If you are concerned about the possibility of infection, you may be treated for gonorrhea, chlamydia, and syphilis. If you are concerned about contracting HIV, understand the risk of this is less than 1%. However, if you elect to be treated, be sure to take the medication as directed.

Resources for Health Care Providers: Legal and Clinical Considerations

The US Department of Justice publishes "A National Protocol for Sexual Assault Medical Forensic Examinations Adult/Adolescents," which is a comprehensive guide on this examination.

Responding to Intimate Partner Violence and Sexual Violence Against Women: WHO Clinical and Policy Guidelines. 2013. https://www.ncbi.nlm.nih.gov/books/NBK174251/. Accessed.

Centers for Disease Control and Prevention: https://www.cdc.gov/violenceprevention/sexualviolence/fastfact.html. Sample Sexual Assault Screening Questions

World Health Organization. Guidelines for medico-legal care for victims of sexual violence. 2003. https://www.who.int/violence_injury_prevention/publications/violence/med_leg_guidelines/en/.

AGOC, Sexual Assault. Committee Opinion 777. April 2019. https://www.acog.org/clinical/clinical-guidance/committee-opinion/articles/2019/04/sexual-assault [14]

Resources for Patients

RAINN (Rape, Abuse & Incest National Network): https://www.rainn.org/about-rainn

RAINN Hotline: 800-656-HOPE (4673)

National Sexual Violence Resource Center: https://www.nsvrc.org offers directory of support.

National Sexual Assault Hotline (1-800-656-4673)

Referrals to local rape crisis centers.

References

1. Centers for Disease Control and Prevention (CDC). Sexual violence. www.cdc.gov/violenceprevention/sexualviolence/fastfact.html. Updated 2022. Accessed Feb 2024.
2. Sexual Assault [website]. United States Department of Justice, Office on Violence Against Women. https://www.justice.gov/ovw/sexual-assault#sa. Updated 2019. Accessed 26 Jan 2024.
3. Cantu M, Coppola M, Lindner AJ. Evaluation and management of the sexually assaulted woman. In: Coppola M, Della Giurstina D, editors. Emergency medicine clinics of North America: obstetric and gynecological emergencies, vol. 21. Philadelphia: WB Saunders; 2003. p. 3.
4. Morgan R, Truman J. Crime victimization. US Department of Justice, Bureau of Justice Statistics; 2019. https://www.bjs.gov/content/pub/pdf/cv17.pdf. Accessed Mar 2024.
5. Crawford-Jakubiak J, Alderman E, Leventhal J. Care of the adolescent after an acute sexual assault. Pediatrics. 2017;139(3):e20164243. https://doi.org/10.1542/peds.2016-4243.
6. A national protocol for sexual assault medical forensic examinations adults/adolescents. 2nd ed. [website]. U.S. Department of Justice Office on Violence Against Women; 2013. https://www.ncjrs.gov/pdffiles1/ovw/241903.pdf. Accessed Jan 2024.
7. Basile KC, Smith SG, Kresnow M, et al. The National Intimate Partner and Sexual Violence Survey (NISVS): 2016–2017 state report. National Center for Injury Prevention and Control, Centers for Disease Control and Prevention: Atlanta; 2022.
8. Walsh K, Danielson CK, McCauley JL, Saunders BE, Kilpatrick DG, Resnick HS. National prevalence of posttraumatic stress disorder among sexually revictimized adolescent, college, and adult household-residing women. Arch Gen Psychiatry. 2012;69(9):935–42.
9. Thurston RC, Chang Y, Matthews KA, von Kanel R, Koenen K. Association of sexual harassment and sexual assault with midlife women's mental and physical health. JAMA Intern Med. 2019;179(1):48–53.
10. Langton L, Truman J. Department of Justice, Office of Justice Programs, Bureau of Justice Statistics, Socio-emotional Impact of Violent Crime. 2014. https://bjs.ojp.gov.library.publications.Socio-emotional, Impact of Violent Crime.
11. Davidson JT, Foa EB, editors. Posttraumatic stress disorder: DSM-IV and beyond. Washington, DC: American Psychiatric Press. p. 23–36.

12. US Department of Veterans Affairs: https://www.ptsd.va.gov/professional/treat/type/sexual_trauma. Accessed 15 Feb 2024.
13. Sherman MD, Hooker S, Doering A, Walther L. Communication tips for caring for survivors of sexual assault. Fam Pract Manag. 2019;26(4):19–23. https://www.aafp.org/pubs/fpm/issues/2019/0700/p19.html.
14. AGOC, Sexual Assault. Committee Opinion 777. 2019. Accessed 6 Feb 2024. https://www.acog.org/clinical/clinical-guidance/committee-opinion/articles/2019/04/sexual-assault.
15. Farahi N, McEachem M. Sexual assault of women. Am Fam Physician. 2021;103(3):168–76. Accessed 12 Feb 2024. https://www.aafp.org/pubs/afp/issues/2021/0201/p168.html.

Chapter 8
Pap Smear and HPV Testing

DeAnn Cummings

Introduction

The Pap smear for cervical cancer screening Pap smear was first introduced in the 1940s. Since then, the incidence of cervical cancer in the USA has decreased from 14/100,000 to 7.1/100,000 in 2022 [1]. In 2023, there were an estimated 13,960 new cervical cancer diagnoses with 4310 deaths. Racial disparities continue with rates higher among Black, Hispanic/Latino, and Asian patients. In developed countries such as the USA, the decline in incidence and deaths is thought to be from effective screening and higher incidence of human papillomavirus (HPV) vaccination rates [2]. Persistence of HPV is a major factor in the development of cervical cancer. Ninety-five percent of tumors and 75–95% of high-grade cervical intraepithelial lesions (CIN) are derived from HPV, most commonly squamous cell carcinoma, adenocarcinoma, and adenosquamous types [2].

This observation has led to new options for prevention, screening, and management of cervical cancer and its precursors. Vaccines against HPV types 6, 11, 16, 18, 31, 33, 45, 52, and 58 have been introduced to reduce HPV infection. Vaccination against HPV is an essential tool in the primary prevention of cervical cancer. Available since 2006 for women and 2009 for both men and women in the USA, the 9-valent Gardasil 9 is the only HPV vaccine currently available in the USA.

HPV DNA testing is utilized in the management of the abnormal Pap smear and cervical dysplasia as well as for primary screening. HPV testing has a sensitivity of 94.6% and a specificity of 94.1% for the detection of high-grade cervical disease. In comparison, the Pap smear has a sensitivity of 55.4% and a specificity of 96.8%. The combination of Pap smear and HPV testing has been approved by the FDA for screening women over age 24 every 5 years. Combination screening improves the

D. Cummings (✉)
Department of Family Medicine, St. Joseph's Hospital Health Center, Syracuse, NY, USA
e-mail: Deann.Cummings@sjhsyr.org

S. M. Sulik, C. B. Heath (eds.), *Primary Care Procedures in Women's Health*,
https://doi.org/10.1007/978-3-032-07061-6_8

sensitivity but decreases the specificity, potentially resulting in an increased need for colposcopy [3]. There are now two FDA-approved primary high-risk HPV screening tests that are approved for use without co-testing in women > aged 24. There are five FDA-approved high-risk HPV screening tests approved for use with co-testing.

Liquid-based cytology (LBC) (ThinPrep®, SurePath™) as an alternative to the conventional Pap smear was introduced in 1996 to improve the sensitivity of the Pap smear (40–80%). The liquid-based samples allow for a monolayer smear with decreased obscuring artifact and decreased inflammatory and hemorrhagic cells leading to decreased screening time in the lab. Instead of applying the cervical specimen to a slide, the specimen collected in the same fashion is instead inserted into a vial of fluid which is later spun in the lab to remove excess material. With the SurePath™ method, the brush is detached and sent in the specimen container along with the sample. ThinPrep® specimens are collected with the cytobrush or broom and do not require detaching the brush.

Several studies have compared the conventional pap to LBC for efficiency and diagnosis of precancerous lesions. In developing countries, LBC has virtually replaced the conventional pap; however, the conventional pap still provides cost-effective screening in underdeveloped countries [4–6]. One meta-analysis found that LBC is as good or even better than a conventional Pap smear for the detection of high-grade cervical disease [7]. Another benefit is the ability to obtain reflex HPV DNA testing from the same Pap test. Comparison between the two methods of liquid-based cytology shows that SurePath™ may have a higher specimen adequacy rate (therefore decreasing the number of unsatisfactory Pap smear results) [8]. Other studies have shown that the SurePath™ system may handle adverse limiting factors such as blood better than the ThinPrep® system [9].

Primary HPV testing can be used on low- or average-risk patients, as the test is highly sensitive for CIN 3 or above. It also decreases the incidence of false positives that occur from cytology and thus decreases the number of cervical screening procedures within a patient's lifetime [10]. The two currently approved by the FDA are the Roche CobasHPV test and BD OnclarityHPV™ Assay testing. High-risk patients are those aged 30–65 with a cervix who are on immunosuppressants, have HIV/AIDS, have postcoital bleeding, or have been diagnosed previously with HPV positivity and are under surveillance per ASCCP guidelines. In May 2024, the US Food and Drug Administration approved the use of primary HPV testing collected by the patients themselves. This was approved to be performed with a swab or a brush by the patient within a medical facility such as a primary care office, urgent care, pharmacy, or mobile clinic or by a patient aged 30 or above at home. The intention is to decrease barriers to screening for cervical cancer [11].

New guidelines for the interpretation of the Pap smear results have been published and provide different options for following minor cytological abnormalities based on age and risk of cervical cancer. The 2024 recommendations for management after colposcopy can be found in Chapter 24.

Case Study

A healthy 32-year-old G2P2 presents for her yearly physical exam. The patient has had a negative Pap smear every 3 years since starting screening at age 21. She has not been exposed to diethylstilbestrol and is not immunocompromised (low risk). She is otherwise healthy and has had the same partner for the past 5 years.

Diagnosis

Normal exam

Differential Diagnosis (Algorithm 8.1)

- Cervical dysplasia
- Human papillomavirus

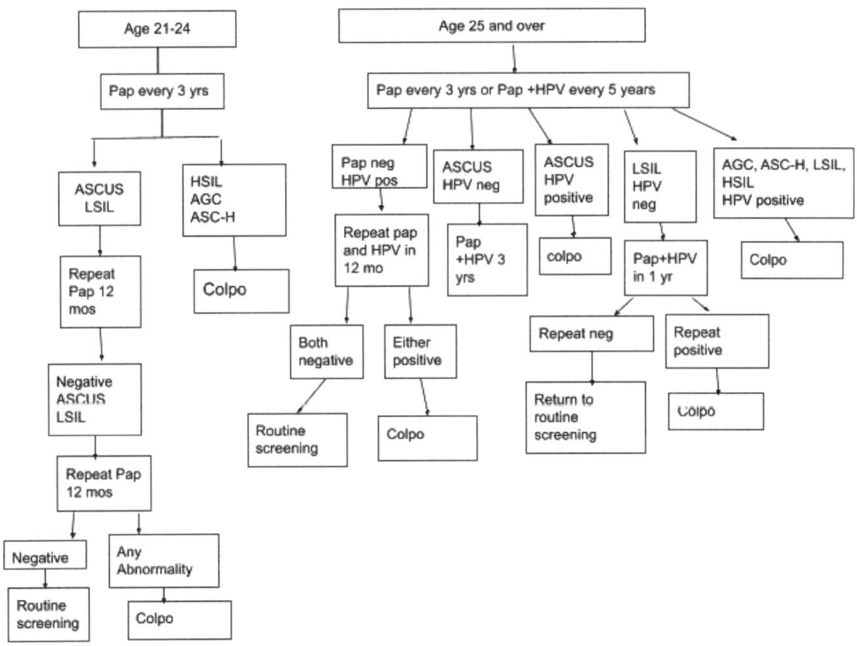

Legend: ASCUS - Atypical Squamous Cells of Undetermined Significance
LSIL - Low grade intraepithelial lesion
HSIL - High grade intraepithelial lesion
AGC - Atypical glandular cells
ASC-H - Atypical Squamous Cells - cannot rule out a High grade lesion
HPV - Human papilloma virus

Algorithm 8.1 Algorithm for interpretation of Pap smear

Indications [3, 10–15]

Clinicians should describe the differences listed with their patients using shared decision making regarding the following recommendations

- *Adolescents*: Recommendations from the American College of Obstetricians and Gynecologists (ACOG), American Society of Colposcopists and Cervical Pathologists (ASCCP), US Preventive Services Task Force (USPSTF), all state that *screening should begin at age 21.* The American Cancer Society (ACS) recommends that screening start at age 25.
- *Patients Aged 21–24*: All guidelines except ACS (ACOG, ASCCP, and USPSTF) recommend regular screening for cervical cancer with a *Pap smear alone (no HPV testing) every 3 years for women aged 21–24.*
- *Patients Aged 25–29*: The ACS recommends screening with primary HPV testing every 5 years in this age range. All other guidelines recommend a Pap smear every 3 years, with the option to consider primary HPV testing every 5 years.
- *Patients Ages 30–64:* Three options
  - Pap smear every 3 years
  - Pap smear and high-risk HPV testing every 5 years
  - High-risk HPV testing alone every 5 years
- *Patients Ages 65 and older:*
  - All guidelines agree that *screening is not indicated* for women 65 and older who have had regular cervical cancer screening and have no history of cervical cancer or high-grade dysplasia.
  - Regular adequate cervical cancer screening is defined as two consecutive HPV tests or co-tests within the past 10 years.
- *Patients with a history of hysterectomy:*
  - All guidelines agree that *screening is not indicated* for women who have undergone hysterectomy with removal of the cervix for reasons other than cervical cancer.

Contraindications

- Age less than 21
- Reluctant patient (relative contraindication)—it is important to assess the reasons that a patient may have in obtaining a gynecologic examination in a non-judgmental fashion. If indicated by age group, consider offering self-swab Primary HPV and STI screening (if indicated)
- Patients who have never been sexually active or who have experienced sexual violence may need additional time and emotional support. Some patients may

need to undergo anesthesia to perform a pap smear and/or HPV testing. Consider self-administered high-risk HPV testing as an alternative.

Equipment (Fig. 8.1)

- Exam table equipped to place the patient in the lithotomy position
- Vaginal speculum (metal or plastic)
- Light source
- Nonsterile latex-free gloves
- Large cotton swabs
- Pap broom (cytobroom) *or* extended tip spatula plus endocervical brush
- Liquid transport medium
- HPV collection kit (if using Pap smear slide with fixative)

Procedure

1. Place the patient in the dorsal lithotomy position.
2. Insert the speculum to visualize the entire transformation zone.
3. If sexually transmitted infection (STI) testing is indicated, then perform it prior to performing the Pap smear. If using liquid-based cytology, HPV testing and the STI testing for gonorrhea and chlamydia can be ordered with the cytology sample and does not require a separate sample.
4. Look for warts, lesions, erosions, or leukoplakia on the cervix.

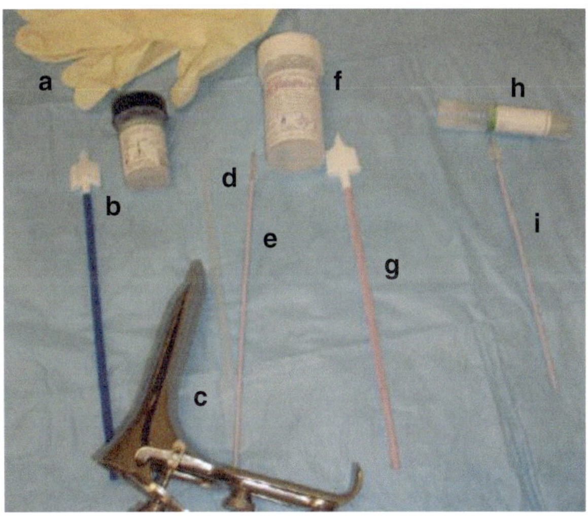

Fig. 8.1 Equipment setup with Pap smear tools: (**a**) gloves; (**b**) SurePath™ (TriPath, Burlington, NC) Pap jar with detachable broom; (**c**) Graves speculum; (**d**) spatula; (**e**) endocervical brush; (**f**) ThinPrep® (Hologic, Bedford, MA) Pap jar with cervical broom; (**g**) cervical broom; (**h**) HPV specimen container; (**i**) HPV collection brush

5. Obtain a Pap smear either with a broom device or spatula plus endocervical brush:
   - Must obtain a sample from both the endocervix and ectocervix.
   - If using cytobroom, rotate 360°, making sure that the long bristles in the center extend into the cervical os and rotate at least three times.
   - If using the spatula, take an ectocervical sample first by rotating the spatula (long end into the os) and rotating the shorter end 360° around the ectocervix. Then, insert the endocervical brush and rotate 360°. Use a plastic spatula for liquid-based cytology.
6. Avoid using a swab on the cervix before Pap unless there is a large amount of blood or discharge.
7. For a slide-based Pap smear, smear specimen onto a prelabelled slide by sliding down the slide, turning the cytobroom over, and sliding down the slide again, and then apply fixative immediately. Both ectocervical and endocervical samples can go on the same slide (Fig. 8.2).
8. For liquid-based cytology, place the collection device in the liquid transport medium and vigorously twirl the device in the liquid (Fig. 8.3).
9. HPV testing can be done with the liquid transport medium, or a separate testing brush can be used. For the latter, insert the brush two-thirds of the way into the cervical os so that part of the brush is on the ectocervix and a part is in the endocervix, and rotate 360°. Place the brush into the transportation device and break off the stem.
10. Upon removal of the speculum, observe the vaginal walls and vulva for any lesions.

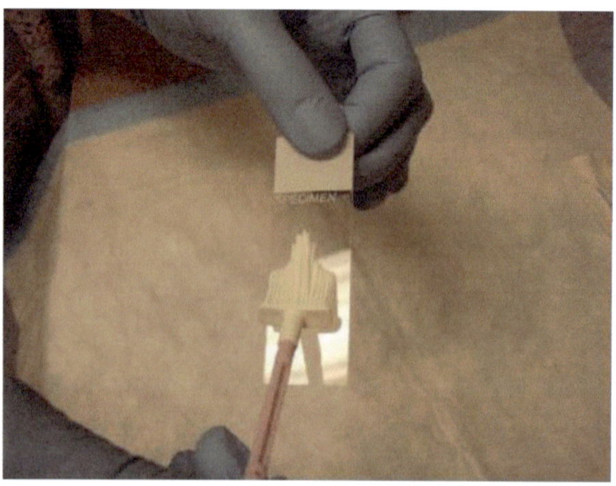

Fig. 8.2 Conventional Pap smear collection onto a glass slide

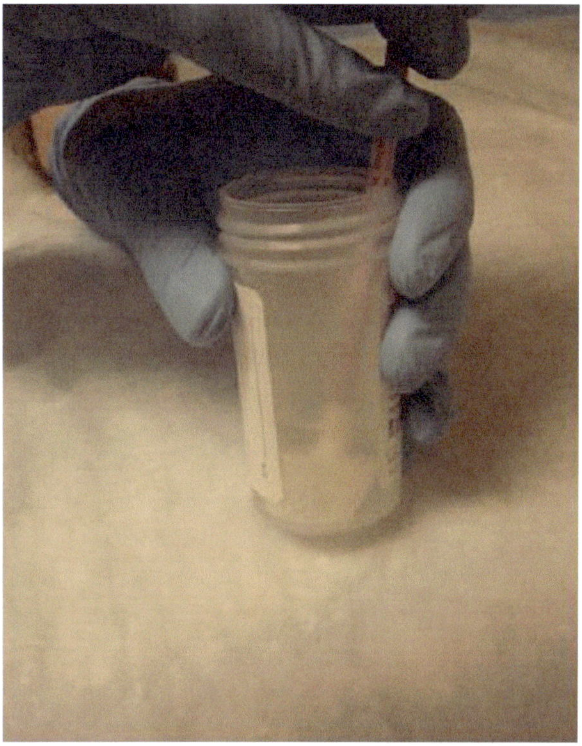

Fig. 8.3 Swish the broom in the liquid cytology jar

Complications and Risks

- False-positive result with unnecessary additional tests.
- Bleeding with use of the broom or cytobrush can occur, usually self-limited.

Tricks and Helpful Hints

- Difficult to visualize the cervix:
  - Move the patient down on the table so that her pelvis is just at the edge.
  - Have the patient press down on her lower abdomen to raise the cervix into view.
  - Place a folded towel under the patient's hips.
  - Try a larger or longer speculum.
  - If using a plastic speculum, try a metal speculum.
  - If the vaginal wall blocks the view, try placing a condom with a small hole in the end over the blades of the speculum, or use vaginal wall spreaders

- Stenotic cervical os:
  - Have the patient use estrogen cream intravaginally for 2–3 weeks prior to a Pap smear.
  - Use an endocervical brush.
- No endocervical cells on previous Paps: Use endocervical brush.
- Excessive cervical discharge or bleeding: Use a large cotton swab to clear away exudate or blood,

Interpretation of Results for Low-Risk Women (No History of Cervical Dysplasia) [10, 13, 14] (Algorithm 8.1)

- Unsatisfactory cytology: Pap must be repeated in 2–4 months.
- Absence of transformation zone (endocervical cells):
  - Age 21–29—Repeat pap in 3 years.
  - Age >29—Reflex HPV testing preferred, but repeat Pap smear in 3 years is also acceptable.
- Negative Pap smear but HPV positive: Repeat Pap and HPV in 12 months; if either repeat test is positive, refer for colposcopy. If high-risk HPV positive (types 16 or 18), refer for colposcopy
- ASC-US (atypical squamous cells of undetermined significance). 5–17% will be diagnosed with CIN 2 or greater.
  - Age >24 years—Reflex HPV typing.
    (a) If high-risk HPV positive, refer for colposcopy.
    (b) If high-risk HPV negative, return to routine screening.
  - Age 21–24 years—Repeat Pap at 12 months
    (a) If Pap Atypical squamous cells -cannot rule out high grade squamous intraepthtelial lesion (ASC-H), Atypical Glandular cells of uncertain significance (AGUS), or High grade squamoue intraepithelial lesion (HSIL), refer for colposcopy.
    (b) If Pap is normal, low grade intraepithelial lesion (LSIL), or Atypical squamous cells of uncertain significance (ASCUS), repeat Pap again at 12 months. If pap again shows any abnormality, refer for colposcopy.
  - HPV testing should not be done in women <25 years.
  - Pregnant patients—Defer to 6–8 weeks postpartum.
- ASC-H 24–94% will be diagnosed with CIN 2 or greater.
  - Refer for colposcopy in all ages and all pregnant women.

- Atypical Glandular cells - not otherwise specified (AGC-NOS). 9–38% will be diagnosed with CIN 2, adenocarcinoma insitu (AIS), or greater. 3–17% will have invasive cancer.
  - Refer for colposcopy with endocervical sampling and endometrial biopsy if over age 35.
  - If atypical endometrial cells on Pap, perform an endometrial biopsy prior to colposcopy.
- AGC favor neoplasia or AIS. 27–96% will be diagnosed with CIN 2 or greater.
  - Refer all patients for colposcopy with endocervical sampling.
  - Endometrial biopsy if indicated. (See previous discussion in this section.)
  - If testing negative for neoplasia, refer for diagnostic excisional procedure.
  - Following up with repeat Pap smears is unacceptable.
- Low grade intraepithelial lesion (LSIL) 12–16% will be diagnosed with CIN 2 or greater.
  - Age >24 years.
    (a) Test for high-risk HPV.
    (b) If HPV negative, repeat Pap and HPV tests in 12 months. If both are negative, return to routine screening. If either test is abnormal, refer for colposcopy.
    (c) If HPV positive, refer for colposcopy.
  - Age 21–24 years
    (a) Repeat Pap in 12 months (no HPV testing)
    (b) If Pap negative, ASC-US, or LSIL, repeat Pap again at 12 months. If repeat Pap is abnormal, refer for colposcopy. If repeat Pap is normal, return to routine screening.
    (c) If Pap HSIL, ASC-H, or AGUS, refer for colposcopy.
- HSIL (high-grade intraepithelial lesion). High grade intraepithelial lesion (HSIL) 70–75% will be diagnosed with CIN 2 (moderate dysplasia) or greater.
  - Refer all patients for colposcopy regardless of age or pregnancy.
    (a) In patients <25, if colposcopy is negative for CIN 2 or 3, close observation is recommended instead of a diagnostic excisional procedure.
    (b) In patients <25 with limited CIN 2, close observation may be an option.
    (c) In patients greater, if colposcopy is negative, consider a diagnostic excisional procedure.
    (d) In patients 25 or older, if colposcopy shows CIN 2 or 3 (severe dysplasia), an excisional procedure is preferred.
- Endometrial cells
  - If premenopausal, no further action is required.
  - If postmenopausal, perform an endometrial biopsy.

Procedure Note

(Provider to fill in blanks/circle applicable choice when given multiple choices and customize as needed.)

The patient was placed in the dorsal lithotomy position, and a speculum was inserted. The cervix was well visualized. Pap smear was obtained using ________ (insert collection device) and __________________________ (insert either conventional Pap processing or liquid based cytology). No cervical, vaginal, or vulvar lesions were seen.

Coding

Pap and Physical

CPT® Codes (Current Procedural Terminology, AMA, Chicago, IL)
99395 (age 18–39), 99396 (age 40–64), 99397 (age 65 or greater)
Medicare Pap and Pelvic Codes
G0101 and Q0091
ICD 10-CM-Diagnostic Codes (International Classification of Diseases, 10th Revision, Clinical Modification, Centers for Disease Control and Prevention)
Z12.4 for any Pap done

Post-procedure Patient Instructions

Instruct the patient that the results will be sent to her with instructions on when she should have the next testing. Reassure her that spotting can be normal after a Pap smear.

Case Study Outcome

The patient is at low risk for cervical cancer and has a history of consistent Pap smears. She may decrease her Pap frequency to every 3 years or get HPV testing and Pap smear every 5 years or get HPV testing alone every 5 years.

Patient Handout

(*Provider to customize as needed.*)

- What is a Pap smear and HPV testing?
  - It is a test in which cells are taken from the cervix and examined under a microscope to look for signs of cancer or precancer. HPV checks for the presence of human papillomavirus (HPV) types that can cause cervical changes
- How is it done?
  - An instrument called a speculum is inserted into the vagina to see the cervix. A brush is then rotated over the cervix to collect a sample.
- How often do I need to have a cervical cancer screening?
  - If you are less than 30, you should have a Pap smear every 3 years.
  - If you are 30 or over and have had regular Pap smears, you may be able to get a Pap smear every 3 years or Pap with HPV testing every 5 years, or a high-risk HPV test every 5 years, depending on your risk factors for cancer.
- When should I start getting cervical cancer screening?
  - Women should begin getting Pap smears at age 21.
- When can I stop getting cervical cancer screening?
  - If you have had regular screening with a Pap smear and/or high-risk HPV testing and are not at high risk for cervical cancer, you can stop Pap smears at age 65.
- What are the risk factors for cervical cancer?
  - Almost all cervical cancers are caused by the HPV virus, which is sexually transmitted.
  - Risk factors include multiple sexual partners, early age of the first sexual intercourse, personal history of HPV infection, partner with HPV infection, previous abnormal Pap smear, illnesses that suppress the immune system, and smoking.
- If I have had a hysterectomy, do I still need to get cervical cancer screening?
  - You do not need to get cervical cancer screening unless you have a history of cervical cancer or still have your cervix.
- What is HPV?
  - HPV stands for human papillomavirus. It is the virus that causes genital warts. Certain types can also cause precancer and cancer of the cervix. HPV is transferred from person to person through sex.

- What can I do to keep from getting HPV?
  - Practice safe sex using condoms
  - There is now a vaccine for HPV approved for people between the ages of 9 and 26 that protects against the most common types of the virus that cause cancer. The vaccine is recommended for all 9- to 26-year-olds, whether they have had HPV infections or not, and works best for those prior to exposure to the virus. The vaccine is approved for those up to age 45 depending on their risk factors for HPV.
- Should I be tested for HPV?
  - Your doctor may recommend HPV testing as part of a screening program.
  - A test for HPV is also often done to monitor abnormal Pap smears.
- Is there a treatment for HPV?
  - There is no medicine that will get rid of the virus. Most of the time, your body's immune system will fight off the virus over time. If there are severe changes in the cells on your Pap smear, the abnormal cells can be surgically removed or frozen.
- What can I expect after cervical cancer testing?
  - Some women have a small amount of spotting; consider wearing a sanitary pad for the next 24 h.
  - Expect either a phone call or a letter from your provider describing the results of your Pap smear and/or HPV testing and when you should return to the office for your next Pap or HPV testing.

References

1. SEER preliminary cancer incidence rate estimates for diagnosis years 2000 to 2022. Bethesda: National Cancer Institute. https://seer.cancer.gov/statistics/preliminary-estimates/, based on the February 2024 SEER data submission. Posted to the SEER web site and SEER Explorer, November 2024.
2. Abu-Rustum NR, Yashar CM, Arend R, Barber E, Bradley K, Brooks R, Campos SM, Chino J, Chon HS, Crispens MA, Damast S, Fisher CM, Frederick P, Gaffney DK, Gaillard S, Giuntoli R, Glaser S, Holmes J, Howitt BE, Lea J, Mantia-Smaldone G, Mariani A, Mutch D, Nagel C, Nekhlyudov L, Podoll M, Rodabaugh K, Salani R, Schorge J, Siedel J, Sisodia R, Soliman P, Ueda S, Urban R, Wyse E, McMillian NR, Aggarwal S, Espinosa S. NCCN guidelines® insights: cervical cancer, version 1.2024. J Natl Compr Cancer Netw. 2023;21(12):1224–33. https://doi.org/10.6004/jnccn.2023.0062. PMID: 38081139.
3. Naucler P, Ryd W, Tomberg S, et al. Human papillomavirus and pap tests to screen for cervical cancer. N Engl J Med. 2007;357(16):1589–97.
4. Honarvar Z, Zarisfi Z, Salari Sedigh S, Masoumi Shahrbabak M. Comparison of conventional and liquid-based Pap smear methods in the diagnosis of precancerous cervical lesions. J Obstet Gynaecol. 2022;42(6):2320–4. https://doi.org/10.1080/01443615.2022.2049721. Epub 2022 May 17. PMID: 35579303.

5. Dasgupta S. The efficiency of cervical pap and comparison of conventional Pap smear and liquid-based cytology: a review. Cureus. 2023;15(11):e48343. https://doi.org/10.7759/cureus.48343. PMID: 38060751; PMCID: PMC10698710.
6. Patel N, Bavikar R, Buch A, Kulkarni M, Dharwadkar A, Viswanathan V. A comparison of conventional Pap smear and liquid-based cytology for cervical cancer screening. Gynecol Minim Invasive Ther. 2023;12(2):77–82. https://doi.org/10.4103/gmit.gmit_118_22. Erratum in: Gynecol Minim Invasive Ther. 2024 Feb 23;13(1):68. PMID: 37416097; PMCID: PMC10321340.
7. Bernstein SJ, Sanchez-Ramos L, Ndubisi B. Liquid-based cervical cytologic smear study and conventional Papsnicolaou smears: a metaanalysis of prospective studies comparing cytologic diagnosis and sample adequacy. Am J Obstet Gynecol. 2001;185:308–17.
8. Nance KV. Evolution of pap testing at a community hospital – a ten-year experience. Diagn Cytopathol. 2007;35:148–53.
9. Sweeny BJ, Haq Z, Happel JF, Weinstein B, Schneider D. Comparison of the effectiveness of two liquid based papanicoleau systems in the handling of adverse limiting factors, such as excessive blood. Cancer. 2006;108(1):27–31.
10. Harper DM, Bettcher CM, Young AP. It is time to switch to primary HPV screening for cervical cancer. Am Fam Physician. 2024;109(1):8–9. Online.
11. NCI News. FDA approves HPV tests that allow for self-collection in a health care setting. HPV tests with self-collection in a health setting approved – NCI. Accessed 5 Feb 2025.
12. Melnikow J, et al. Screening for cervical cancer with high risk human papilloma virus testing, updated evidence report and systematic review. USPSTF. JAMA. 2018;320(7):687–705.
13. American College of Obstetricians and Gynecologists Practice Advisory. Updated guidelines for the management of cervical cancer screening abnormalities. ACOG; 2020.
14. Perkins RB, et al. 2019 ASCCP-Risk-based management guidelines for abnormal cervical cancer screening tests and cancer precursors. J Low Genit Tract Dis. 2020;24:102–31.
15. American Cancer Society. Cervical cancer screening for individuals at average risk 2020 guideline update from the ACS. CA Cancer J Clin. 2020;70:321–46.

Additional Resources

www.ahrq.gov.
www.asccp.org.
www.cancer.gov.
www.cancer.org.

Chapter 9
Vaginal Discharge

Kenya M. Lyons and Barbara Jo McGarry

Introduction

The complaint of vaginal discharge is the most common diagnosis involving gynecological complaints in the primary care office. [1] Symptoms include discharge with or without odor, which may be accompanied by dysuria, vulvar and/or vaginal itching or burning. Most Patients will have at least one vaginal infection during their lifetime. A careful history that includes inquiry of new or multiple sexual partners, type of birth control, sexually transmitted infection (STI) prevention measures, current health status, medications used, vaginal hygiene practices, and vaginal preparations used will help with the diagnosis. Symptoms alone cannot make the diagnosis of vaginitis. The practitioner must evaluate the vaginal mucosa with a speculum exam and obtain a sample of the vaginal discharge. The discharge should be evaluated by doing a pH test, a whiff test, and saline and potassium hydroxide (KOH) wet mount slides viewed under the microscope. There are several commercial kits available that help to identify the most common causes of vaginal discharge. Commercial tests for the evaluation of *Trichomonas vaginalis* have higher sensitivity and specificity than the wet mount. The most common identified pathological causes of

K. M. Lyons (✉)
Planned Parenthood California Central Coast, Santa Monica, US
e-mail: kenya.lyons@ppcentralcoast.org

B. J. McGarry
Department of Family Medicine and Community Health,
Rutgers Robert Wood Johnson Medical School, New Brunswick, NJ, USA
e-mail: mcgarrbj@rwjms.rutgers.edu

S. M. Sulik, C. B. Heath (eds.), *Primary Care Procedures in Women's Health*,
https://doi.org/10.1007/978-3-032-07061-6_9

vaginal discharge are vulvovaginal candidiasis (VVC; 20–25% of cases), bacterial vaginosis (BV; 40–50% of cases), and trichomoniasis (15–20% of cases) [1–3]. While VVC and BV are not sexually transmitted, *Trichomonas vaginalis* is a sexually transmitted protozoan organism. Allergic reactions, atrophic vaginitis, vaginal irritants, and inflammatory conditions are noninfectious causes which can occur but are much less common. For further information regarding causes of other STIs, see Chapter 10.

Vulvovaginal Candidiasis

- The vaginal discharge is classically thick, white, and of a cottage cheese consistency
- The vaginal mucosa is generally erythematous
- Patients complain of itching and/or burning
- Generally, there is no odor
- Vaginal pH < 4.5
- KOH wet mount shows buds and hyphae
- Risk factors: diabetes, antibiotic use, corticosteroid use, immune compromise
- Organisms: *Candida albicans* (62–88%), other Candida species (12–38%) [4, 5].

Microscopic examination of the discharge associated with VVC (Fig. 9.1a, b) will show hyphae and buds when the discharge is combined with 10% KOH solution.

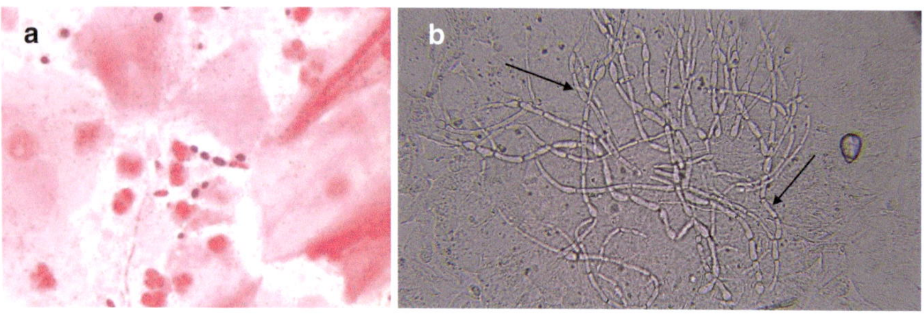

Fig. 9.1 (**a**) Budding yeast (dark oval and linear) and hyphae (lines) on a Gram-stained specimen. (**b**) Numerous hyphae on KOH wet mount black arrows. (All courtesy of Dr. Nancy Phillips, MD)

Bacterial Vaginosis

- The hallmark complaint is discharge with a fishy odor [6].
- The discharge is generally thin and white-gray.
- The vaginal mucosa is either normal or may be mildly inflamed.
- Vaginal pH > 4.5.
- Clue cells noted on saline wet mount (Fig. 9.2).
- Generally, patients do not complain of vaginal itching or burning.
- Risk factors: smoking, douching, low socioeconomic status, new or multiple sex partners, unprotected intercourse, patients who have sex with same sex partners [1].
- Organisms: polymicrobial anaerobes: *Gardnerella vaginalis*, Prevotella, Mobiluncus, Ureaplasma, Mycoplasma [7, 8, 9].

Diagnosis of BV is done using Amsel's Criteria. Three of the following four criteria are required to make a diagnosis:

- A thin, non-clumping, homogeneous gray-white discharge.
- A vaginal pH > 4.5.
- More than 20% of cells are clue cells (Fig. 9.2a, b) that are present on a saline wet mount (most reliable single indicator of BV).
- A positive whiff test (presence of fishy amine odor with addition of KOH to the discharge) [8].

When at least three out of four factors are met, the sensitivity and specificity of the Amsel's Criteria are 37–70% and 94–99%, respectively [8].

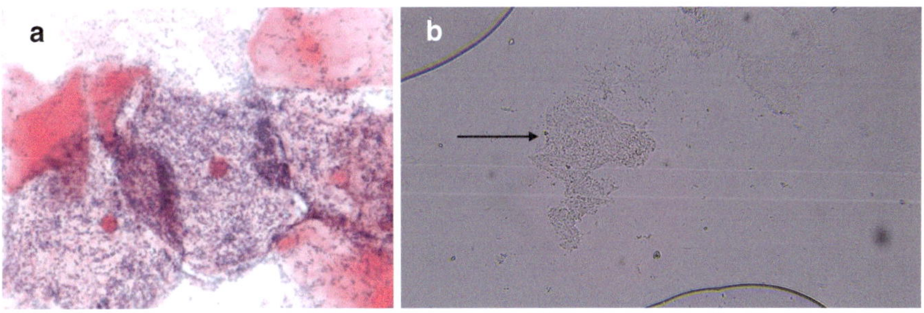

Fig. 9.2 (**a**) Clue cells on vaginal smear on a Gram-stained specimen. Note the classic stippled appearance of the epithelial cells due to the presence of numerous coccobacilli [9]. These cells appear clear on a non-stained specimen. (**b**) Clue cell on normal saline wet mount. Note the classic stippled appearance of the epithelial cells due to the presence of numerous coccobacilli [9]. (All courtesy of Dr. Nancy Phillips, MD)

Trichomoniasis [18]

- Discharge is classically frothy, green or yellow.
- Foul odor—may be fishy smelling.
- Itching and burning may be present.
- Strawberry cervix (areas of hemorrhagic punctuation) seen in 10% patients (Fig. 9.3) [10].
- Vaginal pH > 5.4.
- Saline wet mount shows pear-shaped motile organisms.
- Risk factors: low socioeconomic status, multiple sex partners, unprotected intercourse, smoking, drug use [1].
- Organism: *Trichomonas vaginalis*.
- Nucleic acid amplification tests (NAAT) are highly sensitive (88–100%) and specific (98–100%) for *T. vaginalis* and recommended [11]. NAAT detects 3–5 times more *T. vaginalis* than wet mount microscopy [7].
- Wet mount microscopy may be performed in the office for immediate results and is inexpensive; however, sensitivity (44–68%) is low compared to culture [7].

In trichomoniasis (Fig. 9.4a, b), a saline wet mount will show the motile pear-shaped organisms.

Fig. 9.3 Strawberry cervix

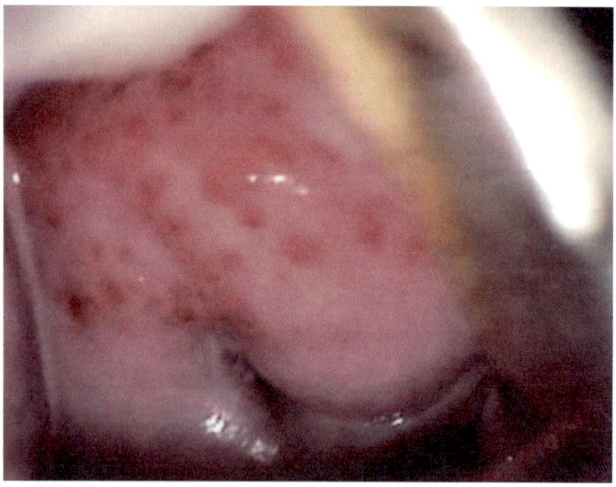

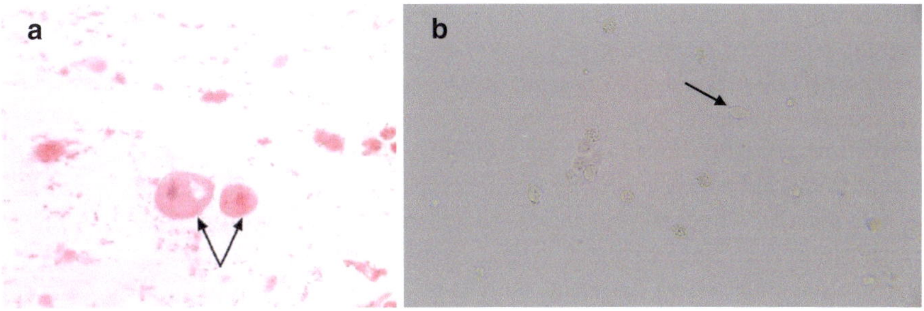

Fig. 9.4 (**a**) Trichomonads on vaginal smear on a Gram-stained specimen. (**b**) Trichomonad on normal saline wet mount. (All courtesy of Dr. Nancy Phillips, MD)

Fig. 9.5 Gram stain of normal vaginal discharge

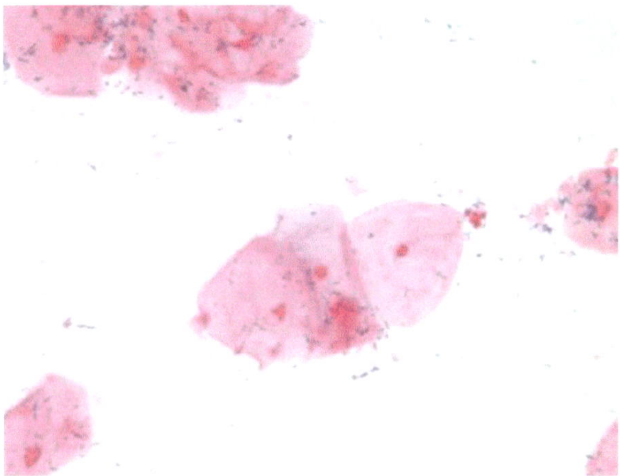

Healthy patients have varying amounts of healthy, normal vaginal discharge during their menstrual cycles. A Gram stain will demonstrate smooth squamous epithelial cells and lactobacillus (Fig. 9.5).

Commercially Available Tests

There are several commercial kits available to assist in the diagnosis of vaginitis.

The Affirm™ VPIII Microbial Identification Test (Becton, Dickinson, & Co., Sparks, MD) [15] is a DNA probe test intended for use in the detection and identification of *Candida* species, *Gardnerella vaginalis*, and *Trichomonas vaginalis* in vaginal fluid specimens from patients with symptoms of vaginitis/vaginosis. The results are available in 45 min, and the sensitivity and specificity are 63% and 99.9%, respectively [7]. A speculum exam without water or lubricant should be performed to obtain a sample of vaginal fluid from the posterior vagina and the lateral walls of the vagina. The sample is then processed in the office if the equipment is purchased or alternatively sent to the lab for testing.

The APTIMA Bacterial Vaginosis RNA assay (Hologic Gen-Probe, San Diego, CA) detects bacterial vaginosis with a sensitivity and specificity of 95.0% and 89.6%, respectively. Similarly, the APTIMA Candida/*T. vaginalis* assay detects Candida species with a sensitivity and specificity of 91.7% and 94.9%, respectively; *T. vaginalis* is detected with a sensitivity and specificity of 96.5% and 95.1%, respectively [12]. The urine and vaginal swabs have up to 100% concordance.

For identification of bacterial vaginosis, the OSOM BV Blue test (Sekisui Diagnostics, Framingham, MA) detects vaginal sialidase activity and has sensitivities of 92–100% and specificities of 92–98% compared with Gram stain [13].

Case Studies

Case A

A 32-year-old G3P3 comes in complaining of a 2-week history of foul-smelling vaginal discharge. She describes the discharge as whitish and profuse. She feels the need to wear a panty liner at times. She denies having any vaginal sores or bumps. She does not find her vagina to be particularly itchy or sore. She emphatically insists that her only sexual partner is her husband of 12 years. She is otherwise well, has no chronic medical problems, and does not take any medications. Her LMP was 2 weeks ago and was normal. She denies any other associated symptoms.

Case B

A 29-year-old patient is complaining of multiple episodes of vaginal discharge and itching. She has used multiple over-the-counter preparations to try and help her symptoms. She has found these products moderately helpful in the past, but this time she feels that the usual creams are not helping. She describes the discharge as thick and white. She finds her vaginal area to be very itchy. She has had two sexual partners in the past year, but insists that she always uses condoms for protection. She denies any other associated symptoms.

Case C

This is an 18-year-old patient who comes in for an emergency visit to your office for an itchy vaginal discharge that began 4 days ago. She is very concerned about "this smelly, constant discharge." She also complains of itching and burning in her vaginal area. She is healthy and is on no medications. She has had several sexual partners in the past year. She denies any other associated symptoms.

Diagnosis (Algorithm 9.1)

Vaginal discharge

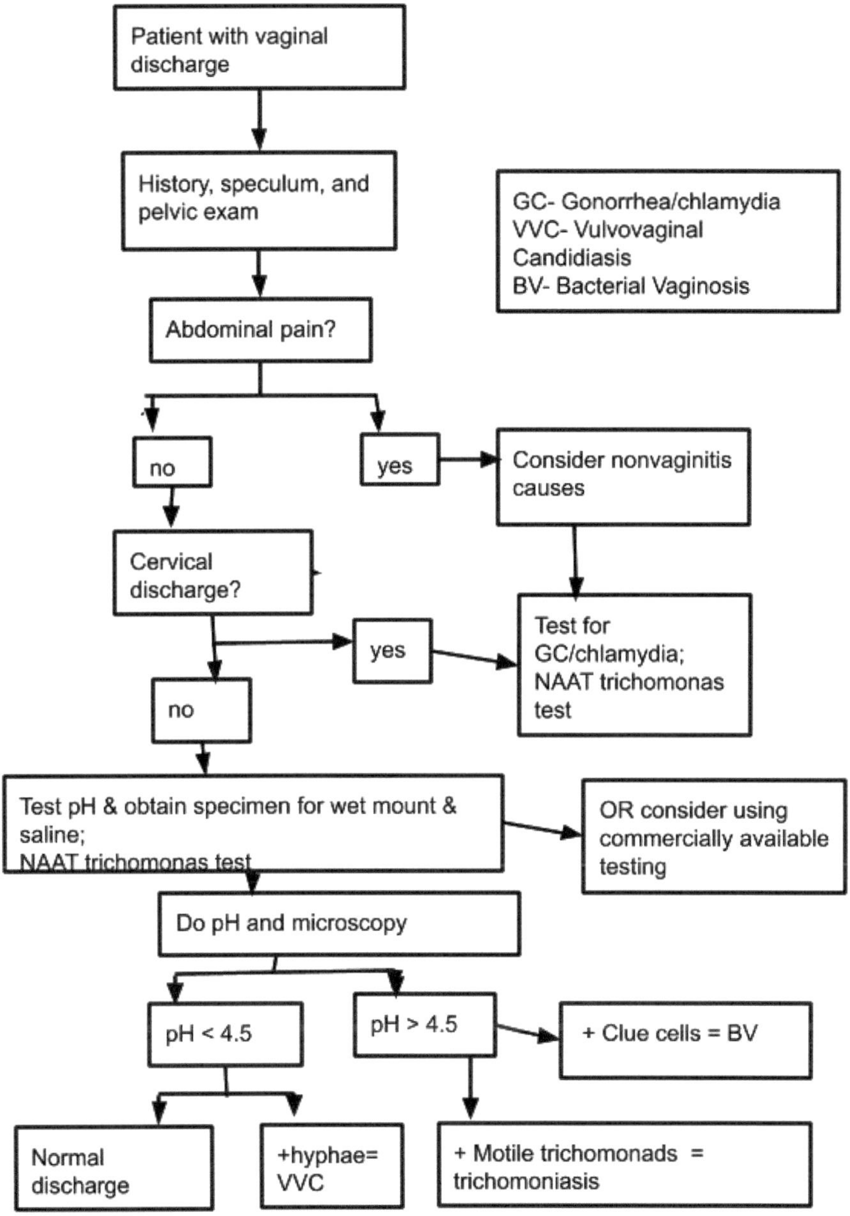

Algorithm 9.1 Decision tree for diagnosis of vaginitis [16]

Differential Diagnosis (Algorithm 9.1) [16]

- Vulvovaginal candidiasis
- Bacterial vaginosis
- Trichomoniasis
- Gonorrheal cervicitis
- Chlamydial cervicitis
- Noninfectious causes of vaginitis:
  - Atrophic vaginitis
  - Irritant/chemical vaginitis
  - Normal physiologic discharge

Indications (Algorithm 9.1)

- Vaginal discharge
- Vaginal irritation
- Vaginal odor

Contraindications

None.

Always use sensitive exam techniques, especially in persons who have never had penetrative intercourse, postmenopausal patients, and patients with a history of sexual assault or trauma. Consider avoiding the speculum exam if it is not tolerated, and do a vaginal swab.

Equipment (Fig. 9.6)

- Vaginal speculum
- Nonsterile gloves
- Cotton swab applicators
- Test Tube with saline
- Microscope with 10× and 40× magnification
- 10% KOH solution
- Microscope glass slides and coverslips
- Nitrazine paper—narrow range PH paper
- Gonorrhea and chlamydia antigen culture tubes

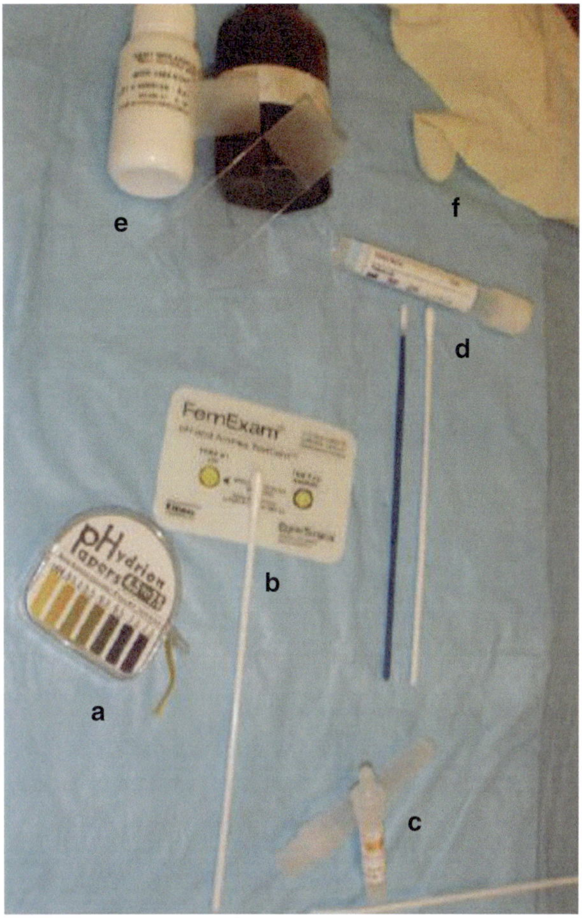

Fig. 9.6 Nonsterile equipment set-up for vaginal discharge: (**a**) ph paper (pHydrion™ Papers, Micro Essential Labs, Brooklyn, NY); (**b**) FemExam® (Cooper Surgical, Trumbull, CT) specimen card with swab; (**c**) Affirm® (Becton, Dickinson, & Co, Franklin Lakes, NJ) specimen collection container, KOH, swab; (**d**) Gonorrhea/chlamydia collection container with swabs; (**e**) saline and KOH for microscopic evaluations with glass slides; (**f**) gloves

- Commercial kits (optional): - FemExam Cards [17]
  - BD Affirm™ VPIII Microbial Identification Test
  - APTIMA
  - OSOM BV, OSOM Trichomonas Test

Procedure (Algorithm 9.1)

1. Place the patient in the dorsal lithotomy position after noting any abdominal or pelvic tenderness on abdominal examination.
2. Carefully note any irritation of the labia. Note any discharge, smell, open sores, or masses.
3. Insert the speculum into the vagina.

4. Note quality, color, and character of discharge. Also note erythema or open sores in the vagina or on the cervix. Note whether the discharge is primarily coming from the cervical os or whether it is diffusely in the vagina.
5. Use a cotton swab to take a sample of discharge from the lateral vaginal walls. Consider whether it is useful to do a chlamydia and gonorrhea culture. If the discharge is primarily coming from the os, and if the patient has had unprotected intercourse, consider doing a culture.
6. Place the cotton swab into a test tube that contains a few drops of saline solution. Cap the test tube.
7. Use a cotton swab to take another sample of discharge from lateral vaginal walls, and then, use nitrazine paper to determine the pH of the discharge sample. Normal vaginal pH is 3.8–4.5. Bacterial vaginosis (BV), trichomoniasis, and atrophic vaginitis often increase the vaginal pH above 4.5. Obtain cultures for gonorrhea and chlamydia, if indicated. Remove the speculum and perform a bimanual pelvic exam. If there are symptoms of pain or if the patient is at risk for sexually transmitted infections, send the cultures for gonorrhea and chlamydia.
8. Take the test tube to your office laboratory while your patient is changing.
9. Perform the whiff test. Add several drops of potassium hydroxide (KOH) to a sample of the vaginal discharge. Using gloved hands, hold the slide within 4–6 inches of your nose and inhale through your nose. A strong fishy odor from the mixture suggests bacterial vaginosis or Trichomonas vaginalis.
10. Make the KOH slide by placing a sample of the vaginal discharge on the slide and mix with a few drops of the 10% KOH solution. The KOH destroys bacteria and cells from the vagina, leaving yeast hyphae and spores (if present) that indicate a yeast infection. Place a cover slip on the slide, then view under the microscope.
11. Make the wet mount slide by placing a sample of the vaginal discharge on a slide and mix with saline solution. Place a cover slip on the slide. The prepared slide is then examined under a microscope for bacteria, yeast cells, trichomonads, white blood cells that indicate an infection, or clue cells that indicate bacterial vaginosis (BV). These are best seen by 40× magnification.

Complications and Risks

- Pain and tenderness during exam
- Extreme anxiety (assess for history of trauma sexual abuse, sexual assault, etc. prior to performing sensitive exams). It may be helpful to ask the patient how they have tolerated pelvic exams in the past and if there are particular techniques that would make them feel more comfortable (i.e. self-insertion of the speculum, a support person present).

Tricks and Helpful Hints

- Patients with some forms of vaginal discharge, especially candida vaginitis, may actually have very little lubrication. Consider using extra time when inserting the speculum.
- Many patients have more than one sexually transmitted infection (STI) at the same time. Consider doing cultures on those who are at risk for STIs.
- Patients with trichomoniasis should be instructed to avoid intercourse with sex partner until after both partners have been fully treated.
- Patients should be counseled to avoid alcohol when taking metronidazole.
- Notify patients that clindamycin vaginal cream is oil-based and can weaken latex condoms or diaphragms during use of the cream and for 5 days after use.
- VVC is usually not sexually transmitted; therefore, male partners do not need treatment.
- All vaginal creams/suppositories used for VVC can weaken latex condoms and diaphragms.
- pH may be elevated (more alkaline) due to menstrual blood and semen [14]
- Assays sent to laboratories for evaluation may not be covered by all insurance companies and can be very expensive. Consider reviewing the patient's insurance coverage prior to sending.

Interpretation of Results

See Algorithm 9.1 for the decision tree for the diagnosis of vaginitis.

Treatment

The following treatments are recommended by the CDC 2021 STI Treatment Guidelines:

Candida Vaginalis
Oral regimen: fluconazole (Diflucan) 150 milligrams (mg) orally ×1 dose

Over-the-counter (OTC) intravaginal regimens:

- Clotrimazole:

  (a) 1% cream—5 grams (g) intravaginally daily ×7–14 days OR
  (b) 2% cream—5 g intravaginally daily ×3 days

- Miconazole:

  (a) 2% cream—5 g intravaginally daily ×7 days OR
  (b) 4% cream—5 g intravaginally daily ×3 days OR

(c) 100 mg vaginal suppository daily ×7 days OR
(d) 200 mg vaginal suppository daily ×3 days OR
(e) 1200 mg vaginal suppository ×1 day

- Tioconazole 6.5% ointment—5 g intravaginally once

Prescription intravaginal regimens:

- Butoconazole 2% cream—5 g intravaginally once
- Terconazole 0.4% cream:

  (a) 5 g intravaginally daily ×7 days OR
  (b) 0.8% cream 5 g intravaginally daily ×3 days OR
  (c) 80 mg vaginal suppository daily ×3 days

Recurrent VVC

- Definition: three or more episodes in less than 1 year
- Prevalence: <5% of patients
- May be primary or secondary (related to another condition such as diabetes mellitus)
- Initial treatment:
  - Topical therapy for 7–14 days (see above)
  - Oral fluconazole every 72 hours ×3 doses (may use 100, 150, or 200 mg dose)
- Maintenance: Oral fluconazole 100, 150, or 200 mg weekly ×6 months

Non-Albicans Candida Species

- Optimal treatment regimen is unknown. Longer duration of therapy recommended. [14]
- Topical or oral treatment with a non-fluconazole azole drug for 7–14 days.
- May respond to boric acid 600 mg intravaginally daily for 3 weeks.
- Referral to specialists is recommended if symptoms recur.

Bacterial Vaginosis

- Metronidazole 500 mg orally twice a day for 7 days; Efficacy 86% at 5–7 days; 78% at 4 weeks.
- Metronidazole 0.75% gel 5 g vaginally once daily for 5 days; Efficacy 81% at 5–7 days; 71% at 4 weeks.
- Clindamycin 2% cream 5 g vaginally nightly for 7 days; Efficacy 85% at 5–7 days; 82% at 4 weeks.
- Alternative regimens:

  (a) Clindamycin 300 mg orally twice a day for 7 days
  (b) Clindamycin 100 mg ovules inserted into the vagina nightly ×3 days
  (c) Secnidazole 2 g orally once
  (d) Tinidazole 2 g orally once daily for 2 days
  (e) Tinidazole 1 g orally once daily for 5 days

The 2021 CDC guidelines recommend that patients use condoms consistently or avoid sexual activity while undergoing treatment for bacterial vaginosis. The guidelines also suggest that douching increases the risk of relapse.

Recurrent BV

- Initial recurrence: repeat any of the above regimens. A recent randomized controlled trial in the New England Journal of Medicine found that the addition of combined oral and topical treatment for male partners of woman with recurrent BV had a lower recurrence rate than standard care [19].
- Multiple recurrences:
  - 0.75% metronidazole gel or 750 mg metronidazole vaginal suppository twice weekly for greater than 3 months
  - Oral nitroimidazole (metronidazole or tinidazole) 500 mg BID × 7 days, followed by 21 days of intravaginal boric acid (600 mg daily) in addition to 0.75% metronidazole gel twice a week for 4–6 months
- 2 g Metronidazole with 150 mg fluconazole monthly

Trichomoniasis

- Preferred regimen: 500 mg PO metronidazole BID for 7 days
- Alternative regimens: Tinidazole 2 g PO once
- Recurrent infection:
  - If due to re-exposure to untreated partner: Repeat 500 mg PO metronidazole BID for 7 days.
  - If not due to re-exposure to untreated partner: metronidazole or tinidazole 2 g daily for 7 days.
  - For persistent recurrence in the absence of exposure, consider requesting a test kit for drug resistance from the CDC.

https://www.cdc.gov/laboratory/specimen-submission/detail.html?CDCTestCode=CDC-10239

- There is evidence the following treatment methods are NOTeffective and therefore should be avoided: intravaginal betadine (povidone-iodine), clotrimazole, acetic acid, furazolidone, gentian violet, nonoxynol-9, and potassium permanganate

Procedure Note

(Provider to fill in blanks/circle applicable choice when given multiple choices and customize as needed.)

On speculum examination of the vagina and cervix, samples of vaginal discharge were obtained with cotton-tipped applicators. The whiff test was performed. The sample was examined with a KOH slide and with a saline wet mount preparation.

Microscopy revealed clue cells, trichomonads, or yeast and hyphae. Nitrazine paper revealed the pH to be ___.

Coding

CPT® Codes (Current Procedural Terminology, AMA, Chicago, IL)
87210 Smear, primary source with interpretation; wet mount for infectious agents using KOH or Saline
Medicare Codes
Q0111 (HCPCS code) Wet mounts, including preparations of vaginal, cervical, or skin specimens for saline slide
Q0112 For the slide with KOH

ICD 10-CM-Diagnostic Codes
N76.0 Vaginitis NOS
B37.3 Candida vaginitis
N76.0 Bacterial vaginosis
A59.01 Trichomonas vaginitis
N95.2 Atrophic vaginitis
N89.8 Vaginal discharge
R94.81 Vulvar pain
R10.2 Vaginal pain

Case Study Outcome

Case A

The nitrazine paper showed a pH of 5.0. The KOH slide did not show any buds or hyphae. The whiff test released a strong fishy odor. The saline wet mount showed many clue cells. The diagnosis of bacterial vaginosis was made, and the patient was treated with metronidazole 500 mg PO twice daily for 7 days. She was advised to abstain from alcohol during the time of treatment to avoid nausea, vomiting, and abdominal pain.

Case B

The nitrazine paper showed a pH of 3.5. The KOH slide showed many buds and hyphae. The whiff test did not produce any strong odors. The saline wet mount showed some white blood cells, but no clue cells. The diagnosis of Candida vaginitis was made, and the patient was treated with Diflucan 150 mg orally one time.

Case C

The nitrazine paper showed a pH of 5.4. The KOH slide did not show any buds or hyphae. The whiff test did not produce any strong odors. The saline wet mount showed many motile pear-shaped organisms. The diagnosis was trichomoniasis, and the patient was treated with 500 mg PO metronidazole BID for 7 days. She was advised that trichomoniasis is a sexually transmitted infection, and so her sexual partner should be treated at the same time. She was advised to abstain from sexual contact with her partner until they both are fully treated. She was also advised to abstain from alcohol during the time of treatment to avoid nausea, vomiting, and abdominal pain.

Postprocedure Patient Handout

(*Provider to customize as needed.*)

Candida

You have an infection of *Candida albicans*, commonly known as yeast. Yeast is *not* a sexually transmitted infection (STI); you did *not* catch it from anyone, and your partner does not need to be treated. It is caused by a change in the pH of the vagina, which is usually acidic and keeps yeast from growing. A variety of antibiotics, diabetes, pregnancy, and your menstrual period may change the pH and make it more likely for yeast to grow. In addition, there are some preventive measures that may help in avoiding another infection. Wearing cotton underwear, wiping front to back after urination, and avoiding douching may help. The medications are safe to use while pregnant and nursing.

Occasionally, people develop chronic yeast infections. If you have not improved after the course of medication given to you, please return to your clinician.

Bacterial Vaginosis

You have bacterial vaginosis, also known as Gardnerella vaginitis. It is the most common vaginal infection. It is caused by an overgrowth of the anaerobic bacteria that are commonly present in the vagina. BV is *not* an STI; you did *not* catch it from anyone, and your partner does not need to be treated. The infection can cause a thin vaginal discharge and sometimes a distinct fishy odor. It can be treated with oral pills or vaginal creams or gels. While it is safe to take the medication in pregnancy, there is less information about using the medication while nursing. If you are nursing, please discuss with your clinician.

If you are taking metronidazole by mouth, be sure not to drink alcohol while on the medication and for 24 h after you take the last dose of medication. If you are using the clindamycin vaginal cream or ovules, be aware that the cream may cause condoms to break. Use another form of birth control while on the cream and for 3 days afterward.

Some people may experience a yeast infection at the same time or after the treatment of bacterial vaginosis. If so, you may need treatment with an antifungal medication after the treatment of the BV. If you have any questions, please call your clinician.

Trichomonas vaginalis

You have an infection of *T. vaginalis* ("trich" or "tric"). Trich is a protozoan organism that is sexually transmitted. Trich causes a thin, watery, yellow-greenish discharge that can have a fishy odor. It can cause itching of the vagina and vulva ("lips") and burning during urination. It can also be present with very few symptoms for a very long time.

You and your partner should be treated for Trich at the same time to avoid passing the infection back to each other. It is important to avoid drinking alcohol while you are on the medication and for 24 h afterward. Trich infections can be avoided by having your partner use condoms. Treatment is safe in pregnancy. Please let your clinician know if you are nursing.

Trich can be present with other vaginal infections and other STIs. Please make an appointment with your clinician to discuss screening for other STIs if you have not done so during your visit today or if other symptoms occur after treatment. Please make a follow-up visit in 3 months for retesting.

References

1. Paladine HL, Desai UA. Vaginitis: diagnosis and treatment. Am Fam Physician. 2018;97(5):321–9.
2. Danby CS, et al. Nucleic acid amplification testing compared with cultures, gram stain, and microscopy in the diagnosis of vaginitis. J Low Genit Tract Dis. 2021;25(1):76.
3. Broache M, et al. Performance of a vaginal panel assay compared with the clinical diagnosis of vaginitis. Obstet Gynecol. 2021;138(6):853.
4. Paulitsch A, et al. A 5-year (2000-2004) epidemiological survey of Candida and non-Candida yeast species causing vulvovaginal candidiasis in Graz, Austria. Mycoses. 2006;49:471–5.
5. Bignoumba M, et al. High diversity of yeast species and strains responsible for vulvovaginal candidiasis in South-East Gabon. J Med Mycol. 2023;33(2):101354.
6. Anderson MR, Klink K, Cohrssen A. Evaluation of vaginal complaints. JAMA. 2004;291(11):1368–79.

7. CDC. Diseases characterized by vulvovaginal itching, burning, irritation, odor or discharge. In: 2021 Sexually transmitted infections treatment guidelines. Updated 22 July 2021. https://www.cdc.gov/std/treatment-guidelines/vaginal-discharge.htm. Accessed 2 Feb 2024.
8. Amsel R, Totten PA, Spiegel CA, Chen KC, Eschenbach D, Holmes KK. Nonspecific vaginitis: diagnostic criteria and microbial and epidemiologic associations. Am J Med. 1983;74:14.
9. Majeroni BA. Bacterial vaginosis: an update. Am Fam Physician. 1998;57(6):1285. -9, 1291
10. Preethi V, et al. Trichomoniasis: an update. Trop Parasitol. 2011;1(2):73–5.
11. Hobbs MM, Sena AC. Modern diagnosis of Trichomonas vaginalis infection. Sex Transm Infect. 2013;89(6):434–8.
12. Schwebke JR, et al. Clinical validation of the Aptima bacterial vaginosis and Aptima Candida/Trichomonas vaginitis assays: results from a perspective multicenter clinical study. J Clin Microbiol. 2020;58(2):e01643-19.
13. Kampan NC, Suffian SS, Ithnin NS, Muhammad M, Zakaria SZ, Jamil MA. Evaluation of BV(®) Blue Test Kit for the diagnosis of bacterial vaginosis. Sex Reprod Healthc. 2011;2(1):1–5.
14. Sobel JD, Chaim W, Chaim W, Nagappan V, Leaman D. Treatment of vaginitis caused by candida glabrata: use of topical boric acid and flucytosine. Am J Obstet Gynecol. 2003;189(5):1297–300.
15. Brown HL, Fuller DD, Jasper LT, Davis TE, Wright JD. Evaluation of the affirm VPIII test in the detection and identification of Trichomonas vaginalis, Gardnerella vaginalis, and Candida species in vaginitis/vaginosis. Infect Dis Obstet Gynecol. 2004;12(1):17–21.
16. Nyirjesy P, Sobel JD. Advances in diagnosing vaginitis: development of a new algorithm. Curr Infect Dis Rep. 2005;6:458–62.
17. West B, Morison L, Schim van der Loeff M, Gooding E, Awasana AA, Demba E, Mayaud P. Evaluation of a new rapid diagnostic kit (FemExam) for bacterial vaginosis in patients with vaginal discharge syndrome in The Gambia. Sex Transm Dis. 2003;30(6):483–9.
18. Wölner-Hanssen P, Krieger J. Clinical manifestations of vaginal trichomoniasis. JAMA. 1989;261:571–6.
19. Vodstrcil LA, Plummer EL, Fairley CK, Hocking JS, Law MG, Petoumenos K, Bateson D, Murray GL, Donovan B, Chow EPF, Chen MY, Kaldor J, Bradshaw CS; StepUp Team. Male-Partner Treatment to Prevent Recurrence of Bacterial Vaginosis. N Engl J Med. 2025;392(10):947–57. https://doi.org/10.1056/NEJMoa2405404. PMID: 40043236.

Chapter 10
Sexually Transmitted Infections

Sara-Ann Fox and DeAnn Cummings

Introduction

Clinicians play a critical role in encouraging vaccination, preventing STIs, and counseling patients about contraception as they see their patients for both well-child/adult exams as well as for acute illnesses. Primary care providers need to understand prevention, screening, symptoms, and treatment of sexually transmitted infections (STIs), particularly in at-risk populations. In the 2022 STI Surveillance report, the US Centers for Disease Control and Prevention (CDC) reported an increase in the number of STIs from 2.45 million cases in 2018 to 2.50 million cases in 2022. Particularly concerning is the increase in primary and congenital syphilis [1]. Two-thirds of cases are found in adolescents and young adults, while 2.5% of cases are found in older adults. Seven percent of the total cases of primary and secondary syphilis are found in the older population with gay, bisexual, and other men who have sex with men (MSM) accounting for approximately 50% of the cases [2]. Untreated STIs not only lead to the continued spread of disease but can also have personal serious life-long health consequences. In 2020, the WHO estimated 374 million new infections with one of four STIs: chlamydia (129 million), gonorrhea (82 million), syphilis (7.1 million), and trichomoniasis (156 million) [3].

This chapter is not meant to be all-inclusive but will review common STIs, screening recommendations, and current treatment guidelines. The chapter is divided into infections causing urethritis and cervicitis followed by infections causing genital lesions, HIV and ectoparasitic infections. Genital warts are covered in Chapter 22. Hepatitis testing should be considered when screening for STIs but is also not covered in this chapter.

S. Fox (✉) · D. Cummings
St. Joseph's Family Medicine Residency, Syracuse, NY, USA
e-mail: Sara-Ann.Fox@sjhsyr.org; Deann.Cummings@sjhsyr.org

S. M. Sulik, C. B. Heath (eds.), *Primary Care Procedures in Women's Health*,
https://doi.org/10.1007/978-3-032-07061-6_10

Risk Factors

Individual risk stratification for sexual behaviors is important to update regularly, as increased screening and preventative counseling can be provided to those at high risk. People at high risk include those that are sexually active with more than one person, have a new partner, or do not practice consistent condom usage. Populations that are at high risk for sexually transmitted infections include those with a past history of sexual abuse, low-income individuals living in urban areas, those with a former or current incarceration, former or current injection drug usage, military recruits, and individuals with psychiatric diseases or disabilities [4].

Prevention

Preventing patients from contracting a sexually transmitted infection starts with education and counseling, with the goal of making them feel empowered to make safe sex decisions. The US Preventive Services Task Force (USPSTF) recommends that providers engage in behavioral counseling for all sexually active adolescents and high-risk adults. There has been no evidence found that behavioral counseling increases sexual activity among teens nor does it result in forgoing later medical care or make the patient feel stigmatized or embarrassed. Counseling should include basic information about STIs, including route of transmission, symptoms, and reasons to get tested. It should also include instructions regarding proper condom usage and how to start a conversation with a partner about safe sex and routine testing [4]. Review vaccination records to ascertain whether the patient has been vaccinated for Human Papillomavirus (HPV) and offer the vaccine if unvaccinated or partially vaccinated. For more information regarding HPV vaccination, see Chapter 8.

Safe sex counseling strategies should be tailored to the age group and included in well adult exams as well as with acute visits for vaginal complaints or STI exposure concerns.

CDC recommends screening for chlamydia, gonorrhea, and syphilis every 3–6 months in persons at high risk for infection including MSM, transgender patients, and persons with HIV. Annual chlamydia and gonorrhea screening in patients under 25 is recommended at each site of contact except for oropharyngeal chlamydia which is considered rare. Syphilis screening should be done in all patients at increased risk (recent incarceration, transactional or sex work) and at least annually for MSM. HIV screening should be offered once to all individuals aged 13–64 and to older individuals at risk. MSM should be screened annually if their partner's HIV status is unknown or if they have had more than one partner since last screened [5].

Collection Methods

The standard of care previously was for patients to present to their clinician with complaints, and an exam and testing by the clinician were performed. With the advent of newer testing methods using urine collection and self-swabbing, patients can self-test with similar accuracy of results.

A number of studies have compared vaginal swabs to urine collection for chlamydia and gonorrhea and have shown that vaginal swabs are superior. Yet, self-swabbing is underutilized. Patient-collected vaginal samples have been found to be as sensitive as clinician-collected samples [6]. The instructions for self-swabbing and clinician swabbing are similar [7].

Chlamydia and gonorrhea should be tested together commonly using nucleic acid amplification testing (NAAT) and are both reportable infections in every state. NAAT can be performed on vaginal, pharyngeal, and rectal sites or by urine testing [8].

Indications

- Routine well teen/adult exam
- Abdominal/pelvic pain
- Vaginal discharge
- Dyspareunia
- Abnormal bleeding
- Sexual assault

Contraindications

- Patient refusal of exam or testing; consider offering self-swabbing

Equipment (Fig. 10.1)

For clinician exam:

- Appropriately sized gown
- Sheet
- Light source
- Non-sterile non-latex gloves
- Water-based lubricant
- Large vaginal swabs
- Speculum
- If performing wet mount: glass slide, cotton swab, small test tube, saline, pH paper, glass slide
- Appropriate culture collection devices

For patient self-swab:

- Appropriate collection devices
- Written and/or verbal directions for the collection of swab

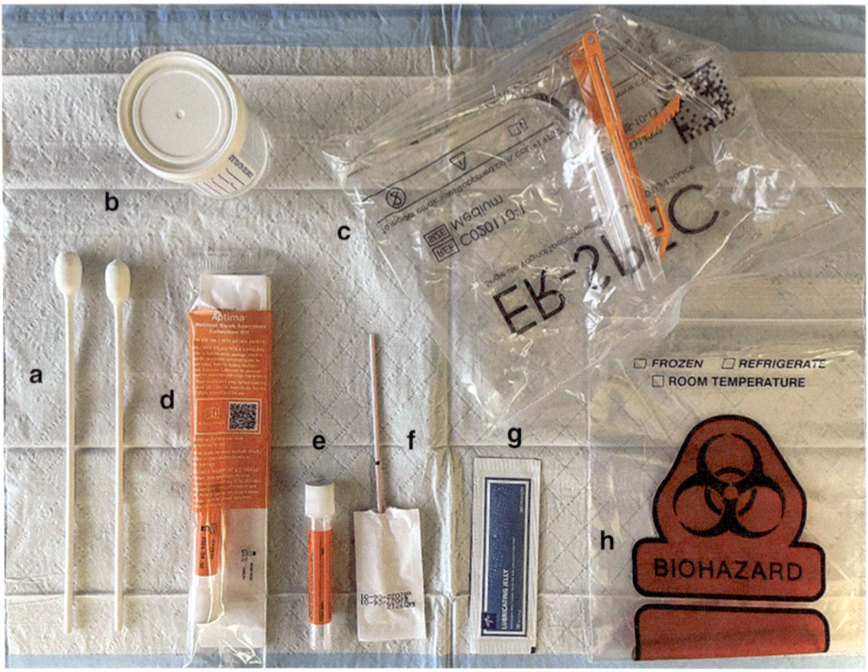

Fig. 10.1 Non-sterile equipment setup for STI collection: (**a**) large cotton swabs, (**b**) specimen collection container (if performing Pap smear), (**c**) disposable speculum, (**d**) Aptima® Multitest Swab Specimen Collection Kit, (**e**) Aptima® Collection transport tube, (**f**) Aptima® Collection Swab, (**g**) lubricant, (**h**) specimen transport bag

Procedure

Patient instructions for self vaginal swabbing:

1. Wash hands with soap and water.
2. Open the testing kit and read any instructions available.
3. Peel back the seal on the test tube and place it on a flat surface.
4. Remove the swab and hold at mid-shaft.
5. Insert the swab approximately 2 inches into the vagina.
6. Swirl the swab for 10–30 s with the intention of it touching each side of the vaginal wall.
7. Remove the swab from the vagina without letting it touch the skin.
8. Place the swab into the test tube with the sample side down.
9. Break off the swab at the marked perforated line.
10. Screw the top back on the test tube tightly leaving the swab inside.
11. Label the test tube with your name and the date.

Provider collected vaginal or endocervical sample:

1. Place the patient on the exam table in the dorsal lithotomy position.
2. Inspect for any erythema, discharge, or lesions on the exterior.
3. Insert the speculum into the vagina.
4. Inspect for any erythema, discharge, or lesions in the vagina.
5. For a vaginal swab, insert the swab into the vagina, and with a swiping motion move the swab along the lateral vaginal walls for 10–30 s.
6. For an endocervical swab, first with a cleansing swab remove any excessive mucus, then insert the swab into the endocervical canal and rotate in a circular motion for 10–30 s.
7. Remove the swab, and place into the test tube, with careful attention that it is sealed properly.
8. Send to lab.

Provider collected pharyngeal swab:

1. Obtain an endocervical, if a pharyngeal is not available.
2. Instruct the patient to open her mouth as wide as possible.
3. Inspect for any growths, erythema, discharge, or lesions.
4. Insert the swab into the oropharyngeal cavity and brush it along the posterior pharynx and tonsillar area for 5 s on each side.
5. Remove the swab and place into the test tube, with careful attention that it is sealed properly.
6. Send to lab for N Gonorrhea testing.

Instructions to provide to the patient for pharyngeal self-swabbing:

1. Wash hands with soap and water.
2. Open the testing kit and read any instructions available.
3. Peel back the seal on the test tube and place it on a flat surface.
4. Remove the swab and hold at mid-shaft.
5. Say “aah” to open up the throat so that the swabbing is in the back of the throat.
6. Move the swab up and down in the back of the throat, left and right five times.
7. Remove the swab from the throat without letting it touch.
8. Place the swab into the test tube with the sample side down.
9. Break off the swab at the marked perforated line.
10. Screw the top back on the test tube tightly leaving the swab inside.
11. Label the test tube with your name and the date.

Provider collected rectal swab:

1. Obtain an endocervical if a rectal is not available.
2. Consider the most appropriate patient positioning; if obtaining vaginal swabs patient may be in dorsal lithotomy position already, but if not, the patient may be offered to place forearms on the exam table in a bent over position.
3. Inspect for any growths, erythema, discharge, or lesions.
4. Insert the swab into the rectum approximately 2–4 inches.

5. Rotate the swab in a wide circular motion, with the goal of obtaining a sample from all sides of the rectal mucosa.
6. Remove the swab and place into the test tube, with careful attention that it is sealed properly.
7. Send to lab.

Instructions to provide to the patient for rectal self-swabbing:

1. Wash hands with soap and water.
2. Open the testing kit and read any instructions available.
3. Peel back the seal on the test tube and place it on a flat surface.
4. Remove the swab and hold at mid-shaft.
5. Insert the swab approximately 2 inches into the rectum.
6. Swirl the swab for 10–30 s with the intention of it touching each side of the rectal wall.
7. Remove the swab from the rectum without letting it touch the skin.
8. Place the swab into the test tube with the sample side down.
9. Break off the swab at the marked perforated line.
10. Screw the top back on the test tube tightly leaving the swab inside.
11. Label the test tube with your name and the date.

Swabbing a potential vesicular HSV lesion:

1. Obtain a viral test kit or viral culture medium and a swab.
2. Using a sterile instrument, such as an 18-gauge needle, puncture the lesion allowing the fluid to escape.
3. With the swab, apply pressure to the lesion allowing it to absorb the fluid.
4. With the same swab, brush the perimeters of the lesion.
5. Insert the swab into the test tube containing viral medium.
6. Label specimen.
7. Refrigerate until transport.

Swabbing a potential crusted HSV lesion:

1. Obtain a viral test kit or viral culture medium and a swab.
2. Moisten a sterile piece of gauze with water.
3. Gently wipe away crusting with the moist piece of gauze.
4. With the swab, apply pressure to the base of the lesion allowing it to absorb any fluid or viral cells present.
5. Insert the swab into the test tube containing viral medium.
6. Label specimen.
7. Refrigerate until transport.

Swabbing a potential Mpox lesion:

1. Contact the local health department to verify the exact method of testing and collection.
2. Full personal protective equipment must be worn during collection.

3. Vigorously swab two skin lesions with a synthetic swab (not cotton), collecting two specimens from both skin lesions.
4. Send to lab for PCR analysis.

Complications and Risks

- Patients with a history of sexual trauma may be unable to be examined or perform a self-swab; offer urine testing if necessary.

Tricks and Helpful Hints

- Post written instructions for urine collection in the bathroom and self-swabbing in exam rooms.
- If doing urine testing for GC/chlamydia first morning void is the best sample but may be performed if a patient hasn't urinated for 1–2 h prior to collection.

Procedure Note

(*Provider to fill in blanks/circle applicable choice when given multiple choices and customize as necessary.*)

Patient placed in a dorsal lithotomy position. External genitalia examined without lesions or abnormalities. Speculum inserted without difficulty; cervix visualized; cultures obtained. Bimanual examination performed with uterus noted to be in ____________ (anteverted, retroverted) position. Approximately ___________ cm in size. Vaginal discharge present/absent in the vaginal vault. Mucopurulent discharge noted from cervical os yes/no. Adnexae without masses or tenderness. Rectal examination (performed, not performed) with no noted lesions.

Coding

CPT Codes (Current Procedural Terminology, AMA, Chicago, IL)

- If testing is done during a preventive visit, use CPT codes 99381-99387 (new patient) or 99391-99397 (established patient), depending on the age of the patient.
- If done for STD exposure of symptoms, use appropriate CPT code for an office visit.

ICD-10-CM Codes

- If testing is done during a preventive visit, use ICD-10 codes Z01.411 (OB-Gyn exam with abnormal findings) or Z01.419 (OB-Gyn exam without abnormal findings).
- If screening for STIs only, use code Z11.3.
- If testing after a possible exposure to STIs, use code Z20.2.

Urethritis and Cervicitis

(*See Table 10.1 for symptoms, diagnosis, treatment, and aftercare.*)

Urethritis usually presents with dysuria, urethral itching or burning, and/or visible penile discharge. Patients with cervicitis are often asymptomatic but can present with vaginal discharge. The clinical exam can show hyperemia, mucopurulent

Table 10.1 Caption

	Urethritis/cervicitis: *Chlamydia trachomatis* [9]	Urethritis/cervicitis: *Neisseria gonorrhea* [4, 5, 10]	Urethritis/cervicitis: *Mycoplasma genitalium* [10]
Symptoms	Vaginal discharge, abdominal pain, pyuria, dysuria, and urinary frequency, although most are asymptomatic	Vaginal discharge, menorrhagia, pelvic pain, pyuria, dysuria, and urinary frequency, although 95% of women are asymptomatic	Vaginal discharge, pelvic pain, dysuria, and urinary frequency
Physical exam	Mucopurulent endocervical discharge and cervical friability; cervical motion or adnexal tenderness raises suspicion for PID. Serovars L1, L2, and L3 can cause painful ulcers known as lymphogranuloma venereum	Swollen Bartholin's glands, greenish-yellow endocervical discharge, and cervical friability; cervical motion or adnexal tenderness raises suspicion for PID	Mucopurulent or purulent endocervical discharge and cervical friability; cervical motion or adnexal tenderness raises suspicion for PID
Extragenital infections	Conjunctivitis, uveitis, pharyngitis, proctitis, and reactive arthritis; all can be swabbed and tested with NAAT	Conjunctivitis, pharyngitis, proctitis, and disseminated (purulent arthritis, dermatitis, tenosynovitis, and polyarthritis are most common, although can present as endocarditis or meningitis); all can be swabbed and tested with NAAT	None

(continued)

Table 10.1 (continued)

	Urethritis/cervicitis: *Chlamydia trachomatis* [9]	Urethritis/cervicitis: *Neisseria gonorrhea* [4, 5, 10]	Urethritis/cervicitis: *Mycoplasma genitalium* [10]
Diagnosis	Nucleic acid amplification testing (NAAT) from a first stream urine sample or clinician or patient collected vaginal/ endocervical sample	Nucleic acid amplification testing (NAAT) from a first stream urine sample or clinician- or patient-collected vaginal/ endocervical sample	Nucleic acid amplification testing (NAAT) from a first stream urine sample or clinician- or patient-collected vaginal/ endocervical sample
Treatment	Doxycycline 100 mg, twice a day for 7 days; due to macrolide resistance, azithromycin 1 g once should only be used in certain patients such as those with poor compliance	High-dose IM ceftriaxone; 500 mg for patients less than 150 kg and 1 g for patients great than or equal to 150 kg	Doxycycline 100 mg twice daily for 7 days followed by moxifloxacin 400 mg daily for 7 days
After care	Patients should abstain from sexual intercourse for 7 days following the single-dose antibiotic or following completion of the 7 day course only if asymptomatic and if partner has been treated	Patients should abstain from sexual intercourse for 7 days following the single-dose injection only if asymptomatic and if partner has been treated	
Follow up	CDC recommends retesting 3 months following treatment, not as a test of cure, but to screen for reinfection. Test of cure is not generally recommended unless the patient is pregnant, continues to be symptomatic, and is at high risk for non-compliance or a second-line antibiotic was used	Re-testing is recommended 3 months after completion of treatment. Test of cure is recommended for any oropharyngeal infections 14 days following treatment or if there are persistent symptoms. If the test of cure is positive, a culture should be sent for susceptibilities	Retesting not recommended
Other			No screening recommendations. Testing is recommended for patients with ongoing urethritis, cervicitis, or PID symptoms following empiric treatment for other STIs

cervical discharge, and friability. The most common causes of urethritis and cervicitis are *Chlamydia trachomatis*, *Neisseria gonorrhoeae*, and *Trichomonas vaginalis* (see vaginitis chapter 9); less common are Herpes Simplex Virus and *Mycoplasma genitalium*. If treating presumptively for urethritis and symptoms persist, testing for *Mycoplasma genitalium* is recommended.

The US Preventive Services Task Force (USPSTF) recommends screening all sexually active women under age 24 and all women over age 25 with risk factors for chlamydia and gonorrhea [10].

Untreated infections can lead to pelvic inflammatory disorder (PID), reactive arthritis triad (cervicitis/urethritis, conjunctivitis/uveitis, and arthritis), Fitz-Hugh-Curtis syndrome (perihepatitis), chronic pelvic pain, fallopian tube scarring leading to infertility and ectopic pregnancy, and vertical neonatal transmission [9].

Expedited partner therapy is recommended and legal in most states in the United States, with state-specific guidelines found on the CDC website. Clinical manifestations and diagnosis of *Chlamydia trachomatis* infections [11].

Chlamydia trachomatis

Chlamydia remains the most reported STI in the United States. Infections are more common in females than males with the highest rates among the 15–24 female population [12]. Signs and symptoms of chlamydia may include vaginal discharge, abdominal pain, pyuria, dysuria, and urinary frequency. Most patients are asymptomatic [9]. NAAT testing is recommended, and patients should avoid urination for at least 1 h prior to testing urine and avoid douching prior to vaginal swabbing. Chlamydia is not typically associated with pharyngeal infection and is rarely considered the cause of pharyngitis.

Neisseria gonorrhoeae

A dramatic rise in infection rates of gonorrhea was seen from 2009 to 2021, with rates decreasing by 9.2% in 2022. Decreased rates were most pronounced in women [4]. Many patients with gonorrhea are asymptomatic; when symptoms do occur, they include vaginal discharge, pelvic pain, and pharyngitis. Infection resistance to the only current antibiotic recommended for treatment (Ceftriaxone) of gonorrhea is a concern worldwide. Any clinician who suspects that a patient has developed resistance to ceftriaxone should contact the CDC in the United States and national health agencies in their countries (Fig. 10.2).

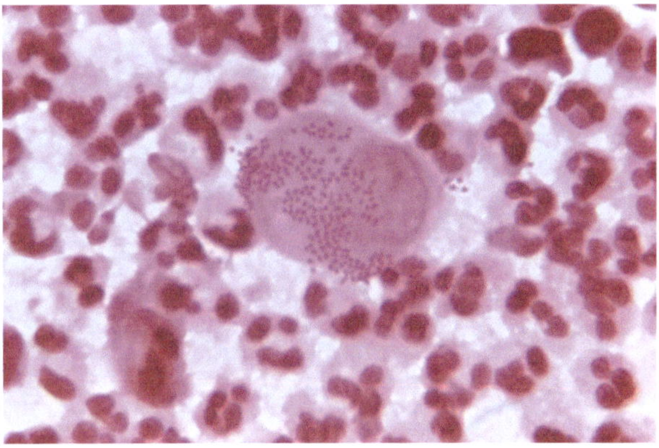

Fig. 10.2 *Neisseria gonorrhea* gram-negative diplococci. (Provided by: CDC/Dr. Caldwell)

Mycoplasma genitalium

Assessment for *Mycoplasma genitalium* (*M. genitalium*) is done if a patient continues to have symptoms of cervicitis or urethritis and has been tested negative for gonorrhea and chlamydia. Prevalence of *M. genitalium* in the US population aged 15–49 was 1.7% [13]. It is not associated with pharyngeal infection. There are some studies showing a correlation of male infertility with *M. genitalium* infections [14]. *M. genitalium* has also been associated with preterm birth, but there are no current recommendations for routine screening or treatment of asymptomatic infections during pregnancy [15].

Genital Lesions

(*See Table 10.2 for symptoms, diagnosis, treatment, and after care.*)

Genital lesions or ulcers can present in a variety of ways and locations including the vagina, perianal, and anorectal locations. Lesions can be infectious or non-infectious. The most common causes of ulcers in the United States are genital herpes and syphilis. Both can present as oral or perianal ulcers. Less common ulcer-presenting causes are Granuloma inguinale (*Klebsiella granulomatis*), chancroid (*Haemophilus ducreyi*), and mpox (Orthopox virus).

Non-infectious causes of genital ulcers include Behçet syndrome, Crohn's disease, neoplasms, psoriasis, fixed drug eruptions, and sexual trauma. A sexual history including recent travel is essential when diagnosing genital ulcers as the predominant infectious cause differs among geographical locations. A complete evaluation should include serologic testing for syphilis and HSV-specific typing from the lesion. Based on history, presumptive treatment should be initiated. NAAT is preferred to culture especially in healing genital lesions and recurrent disease as it is more sensitive [18].

Table 10.2 Caption

Genital lesions: Syphilis Primary [16]	Genital lesions: herpes simplex virus 1 & 2 [17]	Genital lesions: granuloma inguinale (*Klebsiella granulomatis*) [18]	Genital lesions: chancroid (*Haemophilus ducreyi*) [19]	Genital lesions: monkey pox [20, 21]	HIV [22, 23]
SYMPTOMS: Painless ulcer (chancre) 10–90 days after exposure	Painful lesions with the primary outbreak likely to include fever, myalgias, lymphadenopathy, and fatigue. Subsequent outbreaks may include fewer lesions and less pain.	Pruritic papules with slow progression to painless ulcers on the genitals or perineum, which may bleed easily	Painful ulcers with swollen and/or draining lymph nodes	Rash similar to chicken pox, begins with maculopapules which evolve into vesicles, pseudopustules that crust over and cause atrophic scars	HIV is often asymptomatic. Symptoms may develop 2–4 weeks after exposure and include non-specific symptoms such as fatigue, headache, fever, myalgias/arthralgias, rash, sore throat, diarrhea, and weight loss
PHYSICAL EXAM: Primary: an ulcerated papule with a clean base and smooth but rigid borders.	Two to four grouped vesicles measuring 1–3 mm on an erythematous base, followed by eruption to an ulcer with scalloped margins	One or more papules that transition to 5–10 mm red ulcers with rolled margins of granulation tissue and extensive vascularity as well as subcutaneous granulomas and typically without lymphadenopathy	One to three 10–20 mm painful non-indurated ulcers with a friable base and serpiginous borders with overlying purulent or necrotic exudate, as well as unilateral painful lymphadenopathy that can proceed to a buboes in half of patients	Lesions start as 2-5 mm maculopapules which then evolve. Papular, pustular, or vesicular rash. May be isolated lesions (predominate on the face) or diffuse rash	Minimal findings on exam. Patients with acute HIV may have a maculopapular rash, pharyngeal erythema, lymphadenopathy or mucocutaneous ulcers in the mouth, esophagus, genitalia, or anus. Occasionally there may be evidence of oral candidiasis

Genital lesions: Syphilis Primary [16]	Genital lesions: herpes simplex virus 1 & 2 [17]	Genital lesions: granuloma inguinale (*Klebsiella granulomatis*) [18]	Genital lesions: chancroid (*Haemophilus ducreyi*) [19]	Genital lesions: monkey pox [20, 21]	HIV [22, 23]
EXTRAGENITAL INFECTIONS: Secondary: symmetric maculopapular rash on the palms and soles and in some cases the trunk or verrucous lesions called condyloma lata. Teritary: can occur 1–20 years following the initial infection presents with granulomatous gummas, neurological dysfunction, meningitis signs and decreased cardiac reserve.	Meningitis, encephalitis, sacral radiculitis leading to urinary retention and proctitis	Inoculation of any other body part, as well as hematogenous spread to organs			
DIAGNOSIS: Serological testing with a non-treponemal test (RPR, VRDL or TRUST) followed by a confirmatory treponemal test (FTA-ABS, MHA-TP, TPPA, TP-EIA, CIA).	Physical exam with viral testing of active lesions with a viral culture or PCR. PCR-based testing has the highest sensitivity and specificity	Probable diagnosis requires that a patient has one or more genital ulcers that are painful and clinically consistent with chancroid, negative Syphilis testing, which includes dark field examination or NAAT testing of the lesion or serological testing 7–14 days following the onset of symptoms and negative HSV NAAT or culture of the lesion		Mpox viral DNA testing of two skin lesions.	Preferred initial test is the HIV-1/HIV-2 immunoassay which tests for HIV IgG/IgM antibodies and HIV-1 p24 antigen. Intermediate test results should get reflex nucleic acid testing (HIV RNA)

(continued)

Table 10.2 (continued)

Genital lesions: Syphilis Primary [16]	Genital lesions: herpes simplex virus 1 & 2 [17]	Genital lesions: granuloma inguinale (*Klebsiella granulomatis*) [18]	Genital lesions: chancroid (*Haemophilus ducreyi*) [19]	Genital lesions: monkey pox [20, 21]	HIV [22, 23]
TREATMENT: Primary and secondary syphilis treatment: Penicillin G benzathine 2.4 million units intramuscular injection once. Alternative therapy for primary and secondary infections are doxycycline 100 mg orally twice daily for 2 weeks or ceftriaxone 1 g daily IV or IM for 10–14 days. Tertiary syphilis: Penicillin G benzathine 2.4 million units intramuscular injection weekly for 3 weeks if a dose is missed by more than 2 weeks, the treatment course is restarted. Alternative therapy for tertiary infections are doxycycline 100 mg orally twice daily for 4 weeks or ceftriaxone 2 g daily IV or IM for 10–14 days.	Primary outbreak treatment: Acyclovir 400 mg three times a day, Famciclovir 250 mg three times a day and Valacyclovir 1000 mg twice a day for 7–10 days. For disseminated disease IV acyclovir is recommended. Recurrent episodic treatment: Antivirals to be started with onset of prodromal symptoms. Acyclovir 800 mg three times a day for 2 days or 800 mg twice daily for 5 days. Famciclovir 1000 mg twice daily for 1 day or 125 mg twice daily for 5 days or 500 mg once then 250 mg twice daily for 2 days. Valacyclovir 500 mg twice daily for 3 days or 1000 mg once daily for 5 days	Azithromycin 1 g once weekly or 500 mg daily until complete resolution of lesions	Azithromycin 1 g once or Ceftriaxone 250 mg IM injection once. Fluctuant inguinal lymph nodes should undergo needle aspiration	Most patients will require only supportive care and pain control. Patients who are immuno-compromised, pregnant or have a severe mpox infection may benefit from anti-viral treatment with tecovirimat. Contact infectious disease or your local health department	Patients who test positive for HIV should be referred to infectious disease for treatment

Genital lesions: Syphilis Primary [16]	Genital lesions: herpes simplex virus 1 & 2 [17]	Genital lesions: granuloma inguinale (*Klebsiella granulomatis*) [18]	Genital lesions: chancroid (*Haemophilus ducreyi*) [19]	Genital lesions: monkey pox [20, 21]	HIV [22, 23]
AFTER CARE: In the 24 h following initial treatment patients may experience flu-like symptoms called a Jarisch-Herxheimer reaction, which is a result of the killing of spirochetes. These symptoms can be treated with NSAIDs.	Possibility of latent disease with reoccurrences should be discussed with patients. Frequency of reoccurrence has multiple variables including viral strain and hosts immune system. Viral shedding can occur during asymptomatic periods	Treatment may be prolonged based on the rate of healing. Relapse may occur 6–18 months following treatment. Patients should abstain from sexual intercourse until all ulcers are healed	Relief of pain typically occurs 3–5 days after treatment, with healing of ulcers occurring at about a week after treatment. If this does not occur, an alternative diagnosis should be considered. Patients should abstain from sexual intercourse until all ulcers are healed		
FOLLOW UP: Follow-up should take place at 6 and 12 months with a clinical exam and non-treponemal testing (4 fourfold decrease in titers is considered negative).					

(continued)

Table 10.2 (continued)

Genital lesions: Syphilis Primary [16]	Genital lesions: herpes simplex virus 1 & 2 [17]	Genital lesions: granuloma inguinale (*Klebsiella granulomatis*) [18]	Genital lesions: chancroid (*Haemophilus ducreyi*) [19]	Genital lesions: monkey pox [20, 21]	HIV [22, 23]
OTHER: Any sexual partner in the 90 days prior to diagnosis should be empirically treated.	Testing of asymptomatic patients is not recommended. Chronic suppressive treatment: Recommended for patients with frequent outbreaks, 6 or more a year or those that have severe symptoms with outbreaks. Acyclovir 400 mg twice daily. Famciclovir 250 mg twice daily. Valacyclovir 500 mg daily or 1000 mg daily for patients that have more than 10 outbreaks a year.	Any sexual partner that had contact with the patient during symptoms or 60 days prior to symptoms should be encouraged to seek evaluation. Autoinoculation is possible; therefore, hygiene precautions are essential to stop the spread. Untreated lesions increase the risk of squamous and basal cell carcinoma	Any sexual partner that was encountered during symptoms or 10 days prior should receive treatment despite being symptomatic or not		Correct condom use should be encouraged and people should not share IV drug equipment

Syphilis

In 2022, 207,255 cases of syphilis, all stages, including congenital syphilis were reported in the United States representing a 21% increase over 2021. The rates have been steadily increasing since 2000. Rates of primary and secondary syphilis have increased in both men and women in all regions of the United States. Syphilis is a systemic disease caused by the organism *Treponema pallidum.*

Primary infection typically occurs 10–90 days after infection and presents as a single painless ulcer called a chancre. Secondary infection typically occurs at 4–8 weeks following the chancre and presents as flu-like symptoms with fever, headache, fatigue, and lymphadenopathy accompanied by a non-pruritic rash or wart-like growths. Tertiary infection, which can occur 1–20 years following the initial infection, presents with granulomatous gummas, neurological dysfunction, meningitis signs, and decreased cardiac reserve. Latent syphilis is a concern if a patient had exposure and no symptoms but tested positive (Figs. 10.3, 10.4, and 10.5).

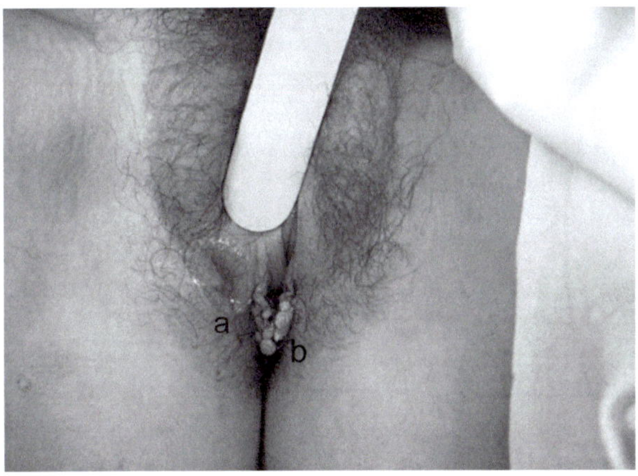

Fig. 10.3 (a) Primary syphilis ulcer, (b) genital warts. (Photo provided by CDC/Susan Lindsley)

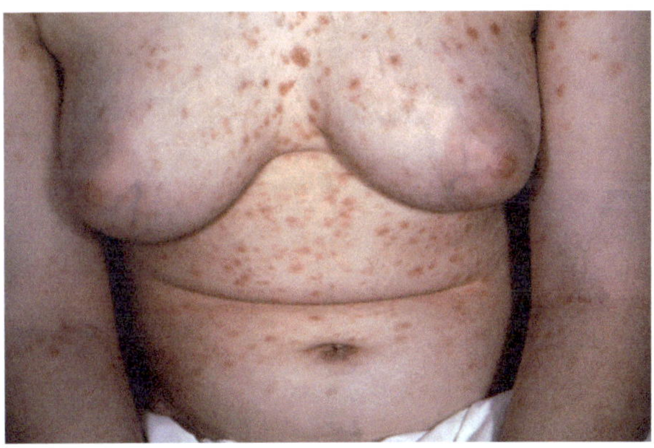

Fig. 10.4 Secondary syphilis. (Photo provided by CDC)

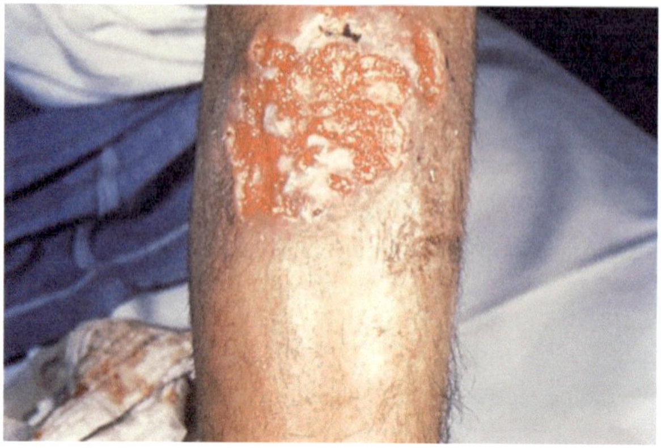

Fig. 10.5 Large cutaneous lesion of the forearm due to tertiary syphilis. (Photo provided by CDC)

On physical exam, the primary infection presents as a chancre, which is an ulcerated papule with a clean base and smooth but rigid borders. Secondary infection findings include a symmetric maculopapular rash on the palms and soles, and in some cases, the trunk or verrucous lesions called condyloma lata. Tertiary infection findings include granulomatous gummas which can be described as rubbery growths that often ulcerate in a destructive pattern. Neurosyphilis presents with posterior column degeneration; therefore, pain sensation is decreased, peripheral reflexes are diminished, and ataxia is present. Argyll Robertson pupil may be present. The pupil will constrict to accommodation but is not reactive to light. Tertiary syphilis also affects the heart and can lead to findings of aortic regurgitation due to aneurysms, as well as aortitis. Penicillin G benzathine is the treatment of choice. In those with documented penicillin allergy, desensitization is recommended particularly for tertiary symptoms and during pregnancy or for patients who have failed therapy. Treatment response should be monitored and a fourfold change in titer to confirm treatment response preferably using the same test and the same laboratory.

Persons who have had sexual contact with the patient diagnosed with primary or secondary syphilis should be treated presumptively even if the serologic testing is negative [16].

Herpes Simplex Virus (HSV-1 and HSV-2)

Genital herpes, HSV-1 and HSV-2, is the most common ulcerative disease worldwide. In 2018, there were an estimated 18.6 million cases prevalent cases and approximately 500,000 incident cases in patients 18–49 in the United States [24]. While most cases of genital herpes are HSV-2, there is an emerging number of first episode HSV-1 cases especially in the higher income population. Women account for a higher percentage of cases compared to men, and seroprevalence increases with age and number of sexual partners. Both HSV-1 and HSV-2 are transmitted through intimate skin and mucosal contact. HSV-2 infection is generally transmitted

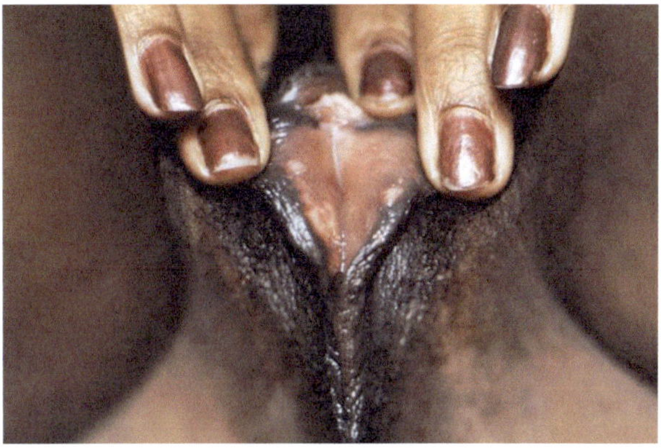

Fig. 10.6 Herpes Genitalia on the female perineum. (Photo provided by CDC/Susan Lindsley)

through genital-to-genital contact while HSV-1 can be transmitted through either oral or genital contact with either the oral or genital compartment of the partner. Clinical manifestations usually occur within 1 week of exposure with the primary exposure causing more pronounced symptoms. Recurrences are generally mild to moderate in severity. Transmission of HSV to a neonate occurs most commonly peripartum. The greatest risk to the neonate is when the primary infection occurs during pregnancy. Suppressive therapy should be started at 36 weeks of gestation to prevent recurrence of infection and need for cesarean section. HSV-2 serologic screening is not recommended [24] (Fig. 10.6).

*Granuloma Inguinale (***Klebsiella granulomatis***)*

Granuloma inguinale is a bacterial infection caused by *Klebsiella granulomatis*. It is very rare in the United States with approximately 100 cases reported yearly. It is more commonly seen in the tropical and subtropical climates (India, South America, Africa).

The lesions start as a painless papule or subcutaneous nodules and develop into a beefy red, friable ulcer. Diagnosis is difficult in non-endemic areas and is made by identifying Donovan bodies in a tissue sample. PCR and serologic tests are not accurate [25]. A tissue biopsy of the ulcer should be obtained. There is a risk of a false-negative biopsy early in the disease; therefore, tissue crush preparation with staining can be used. A small piece of tissue should be obtained from the base or edge of the ulcer with a punch biopsy or curettage, followed by taking the specimen between two glass microscope slides and applying pressure. It should then be separated and air-dried. The following stains could be used to elicit Donovan bodies: toluidine blue, Wright-Giemsa, Leishman, or Warthin-Starry stain. Donovan bodies are encapsulated thin rods found in macrophages [18].

*Chancroid (***Haemophilus ducreyi***)*

Chancroid is an extremely rare STI both in the United States and globally. The causative organism is *Haemophilus ducreyi*. Chancroid primarily affects younger individuals 21–30 years of age, more commonly in career sex workers and young men. Incubation is often 4–10 days after microabrasion or trauma during sex. An erythematous papule develops that quickly becomes a painful ulcer with soft, irregular borders [26]. Kissing ulcers can be seen.

Diagnosis is difficult; the CDC recommends two categories: confirmed with culture or probable based on history. Culture requires a culture medium with hemin and serum rich in CO2 at high humidity to grow. It is not readily available and has a sensitivity of 80%. There is no PCR test available. Probable chancroid diagnosis requires a patient with one or more painful genital ulcers with negative syphilis testing of the lesion, or serological testing 7–14 days after onset of symptoms and negative HSV NAAT or culture of the ulcer [19].

Monkey Pox (Mpox)

Mpox is caused by Orthopoxvirus, a group of dsDNA viruses. It can be transmitted by rodents to humans or via human-to-human transmission through direct contact with infected sores or through contact with infected materials. It can also be transmitted through the placenta. The incubation period is usually 5–13 days from contact with the disease. There is often a prodrome of fever, headache, myalgia, and lymphadenopathy followed by a rash which evolves from papules and vesicles to pustules and scabs. The rash can occur anywhere on the body, but it is most common on the face and extremities, especially the palms and soles.

Transmission of Mpox can occur from animals to humans via direct contact with diseased parts of animals or bodily fluids. Person-to-person transmission occurs when in contact with someone infected with the virus via respiratory secretions, skin lesions, prolonged face-to-face contact along with bedding and clothing. There is limited data on infection during pregnancy, but one study did show vertical transmission [20].

People at very high risk for exposure to mpox (e.g., MSM, occupational exposure) may benefit from pre-exposure vaccination with the smallpox/mpox vaccine (Jynneos). The vaccine is a two-dose vaccine given 4 weeks apart. People who have been exposed to mpox should get the mpox vaccine as post-exposure prophylaxis within 4–14 days of contact [21].

Human Immunodeficiency Virus (HIV)

(*See Table 10.2 for symptoms, diagnosis, treatment, and after care.*)

- HIV is an RNA retrovirus that can be transmitted by sexual intercourse, exposure to infected blood, or via perinatal transmission. Men who have sex with men (MSM), use of illicit IV drugs, lack of condom use with >1 sexual partner, anal sex, and history of other STIs are the greatest risk factors.
- HIV is often asymptomatic. It is estimated that one in eight people with HIV do not know they have the virus. Symptoms may develop 2–4 weeks after exposure and include non-specific symptoms such as fatigue, headache, fever, myalgias/arthralgias, rash, sore throat, diarrhea, and weight loss. Consider HIV if the above symptoms are prolonged or the patient also has mucocutaneous ulcers.

The CDC recommends that all people ages 13–64 be tested at least once in their lifetime. People with ongoing risk factors should be tested more frequently [22].

- Prevention—Correct condom use should be encouraged, and people should not share IV needles or syringes. There are also two medication options for the prevention of HIV transmission. Labs to check prior to starting the meds include HIV, Hep B, Hep C, syphilis, gonorrhea, chlamydia, pregnancy test, serum creatinine, and liver enzymes.
  - Pre-exposure prophylaxis (PrEP)—This is indicated for people who are HIV negative but are at high risk for acquiring HIV (see risk factors above). HIV should be tested every 3 months on PrEP. There are three FDA-approved options:
    - Tenofovir 300 mg daily combined with emtricitabine 200 mg daily.
    - (Truvada or generic combination)—can be used for GFR > 60.
    - Tenofovir alafenamide 25 mg daily combined with emtricitabine 200 mg daily (Descovy)—can be used for GFR > 30.
    - Cabotegravir 600 mg IM every 8 weeks (Apretude).

- Post-exposure prophylaxis (PEP)—This is indicated for people at very high risk, within 72 h of possible exposure. PEP will often be started prior to the return of the HIV result. If HIV is positive, the patient will need referral to an infectious disease specialist. Labs to check are the same as for PrEP.
  - Three-drug regimen—tenofovir DF 300 mg daily plus emtricitabine 200 mg daily (Truvada or generic version) PLUS either raltegravir 400 mg bid or dolutegravir 50 mg daily [23].

Ectoparasitic Infections

Pediculosis pubis (pubic lice) and scabies are both sexually transmitted in adults. Often presenting with profound pubic itching, diagnosis can be made by visual exam of brown nits or adult mobile crab-shaped lice or burrows or mites seen in scabies [27]. Dermoscopy can be helpful to identify burrows of scabies. Scabies among adults is usually sexually acquired while in children it is not. The initial sensitization of scabies can take weeks to present, but with reinfection, pruritus can develop in less than 24 h [28].

Genital Warts

See Chap. 22.

Pregnancy STI Screening (See Table 10.3)

Screening for STIs is an integral part of prenatal care. Recommendations for screening and for treatment are listed in the tables below.

With the rise of syphilis infections, early syphilis testing of all pregnant women with repeat testing at 36 weeks of gestation is recommended.

CDC recommends screening all pregnant women under the age of 25 and women older than 25 at increased risk. Retesting in the third trimester in the same group of women as well as a test of cure for chlamydia is also recommended [29].

Table 10.3 [29, 30]

SS	Chlamydia	Gonorrhea	Syphilis	HSV	HIV	Hepatitis B	Hepatitis C
Screening	All pregnant women less than the age of 25 or anyone at high risk in the first trimester If positive, perform a test of cure no sooner than 4 weeks and retest in 3 months Rescreen in the third trimester for anyone at increased risk	All pregnant women less than the age of 25 or anyone at high risk in first trimester Retest in 3 months if positive	All pregnant women are to be tested in the first trimester Rescreening is recommended in the third trimester and at delivery	Serological testing is not recommended for asymptomatic patients	All pregnant women are to be tested in the first trimester Rescreening is recommended in the third trimester and at delivery for high-risk patients	All pregnant women are to be tested in the first trimester for HBsAg	All pregnant women are to be tested in the first trimester for Hepatitis C antibody
Treatment	Azithromycin 1 g orally once Amoxicillin 500 mg three times a day for 7 days	Ceftriaxone 500 mg for patients less than 150 kg and 1 g for patients greater than or equal to 150 kg	1°/2° infection and post-exposure: Penicillin G benzathine 2.4 million units intramuscular injection once 3°: Penicillin G benzathine 2.4 million units intramuscular injection once weekly for 3 weeks	Acyclovir 400 mg three times a day Valacyclovir 500 mg twice a day	Immediate ID consult, as antiviral is recommended to start during the pregnancy	Passive and active immunization of newborns in the first 12 h of life HBV to be tested at 26–28 weeks if >200,000 international units/mL, antiviral should be considered	Antiviral recommended to start postpartum

References

1. Centers for Disease Control and Prevention. Sexually transmitted infections surveillance. 2022. Last Update: Jan 2024. https://www.cdc.gov/std/statistics/2022/.
2. Van Epps P, Musoke L, McNeil CJ. Sexually transmitted infections in older adults: increasing tide and how to stem it. Infect Dis Clin N Am. 2023;37(1):47–63. https://doi.org/10.1016/j.idc.2022.11.003. PMID: 36805014.
3. World Health Organization. Sexually transmitted infections fact sheets. https://www.who.int/news-room/fact-sheets/detail/sexually-transmitted-infections-(stis). Accessed Apr 2024.
4. American Academy of Family Physicians. Prevention and management of sexually transmitted infections. Oct 2023. https://www.aafp.org/about/policies/all/prevention-sti.html. Accessed Jan 2024.
5. Center for Disease Control and Prevention. STI and HIV infection risk assessment – STI treatment guidelines. 2021 [Online]. Available at: (STI and HIV Infection Risk Assessment – STI Treatment Guidelines (https://www.cdc.gov/std/treatment-guidelines/clinical-risk.htm). Accessed Jan 2024.
6. Aaron KJ, Griner S, Footman A, Boutwell A, Van Der Pol B. Vaginal swab vs urine for detection of *Chlamydia trachomatis*, *Neisseria gonorrhoeae*, and *Trichomonas vaginalis*: a meta-analysis. Ann Fam Med. 2023;21(2):172–9. https://doi.org/10.1370/afm.2942. PMID: 36973065; PMCID: PMC10042575.
7. Lunny C, Taylor D, Hoang L, et al. Self-collected versus clinician-collected sampling for chlamydia and gonorrhea screening: a systematic review and meta-analysis. PLoS One. 2015;10(7):e0132776.
8. Lee K, Ngo Metzger Q, Wolff T, et al. Sexually transmitted infections: recommendations from the US Preventive Services Task Force. Am Fam Physician. 2016;94(11):907–15.
9. Centers for Disease Control and Prevention. Detailed STD fact sheet. https://www.cdc.gov/std/chlamydia/stdfact-chlamydia-detailed.htm. Accessed Jan 2024.
10. United States Preventive Services Task Force. Chlamydia and gonorrhea: screening. Sept 2021. https://www.uspreventiveservicestaskforce.org/uspstf/recommendation/chlamydia-and-gonorrhea-screening. Accessed Jan 2024.
11. Hsu K, Marrazzo J, Bloom A. Clinical manifestations and diagnosis of Chlamydia trachomatis infections. UpToDate; 2022. Accessed 4 Nov 2024.
12. Tapp J, Hudson T. Sexually transmitted infections prevalence in the United States and the relationship to social determinants of health. Nurs Clin North Am. 2020;55(3):283–93. https://doi.org/10.1016/j.cnur.2020.05.001. Epub 2020 Jul 15. PMID: 32762850.
13. NHANES National Health and Nutrition Examination Survey, Torrone EA, Kruszon-Moran D, Philips C, Morris MR, Bowden KE, Papp J, Bachmann LH, Weinstock H, Kersh EN. Prevalence of urogenital Mycoplasma genitalium infection, United States, 2017 to 2018. Sex Transm Dis. 2021;48(11):e160–2. https://doi.org/10.1097/OLQ.0000000000001394.
14. Cheng C, Chen X, Song Y, Wang S, Pan Y, Niu S, Wang R, Liu L, Liu X. Genital mycoplasma infection: a systematic review and meta-analysis. Reprod Health. 2023;20(1):136. https://doi.org/10.1186/s12978-023-01684-y. PMID: 37700294; PMCID: PMC10496402.
15. Frenzer C, Egli-Gany D, Vallely LM, Vallely AJ, Low N. Adverse pregnancy and perinatal outcomes associated with *Mycoplasma genitalium*: systematic review and meta-analysis. Sex Transm Infect. 2022;98(3):222–7. https://doi.org/10.1136/sextrans-2021-055352. Epub 2022 Mar 29. PMID: 35351816; PMCID: PMC9016252.
16. Clement M, Okeke N, Hick C. Treatment of syphilis: a systematic review. JAMA. 2014;312:1905.
17. Albrecht M. Epidemiology, clinical manifestations, and diagnosis of genital herpes simplex virus infection. Up-to-Date; 2022. https://www.uptodate.com/contents/epidemiology-clinical-manifestations-and-diagnosis-of-genital-herpes-simplex-virus-infection. Accessed Jan 2024.
18. Schmid G. Approach to the patient with genital ulcer disease. Med Clin North Am. 1880;74(6):1559–72. https://doi.org/10.1016/s0025-7125(16)30495-3.

19. Hicks C. Chancroid. Up-to-Date; 2023. https://www.uptodate.com/contents/chancroid. Accessed Dec 2023.
20. Huang Y, Mu L, Wang W. Monkeypox: epidemiology, pathogenesis, treatment and prevention. Signal Transduct Target Ther. 2022;7(1):373. https://doi.org/10.1038/s41392-022-01215-4. PMID: 36319633; PMCID: PMC9626568.
21. Deputy NP, Deckert J, Chard AN, Sandberg N, Moulia DL, Barkley E, Dalton AF, Sweet C, Cohn AC, Little DR, Cohen AL, Sandmann D, Payne DC, Gerhart JL, Feldstein LR. Vaccine effectiveness of JYNNEOS against Mpox disease in the United States. N Engl J Med. 2023;388(26):2434–43. https://doi.org/10.1056/NEJMoa2215201. Epub 2023 May 18. PMID: 37199451; PMCID: PMC10962869.
22. Centers for Disease Control and Prevention. Estimated HIV incidence and prevalence in the United States, 2015–2019. HIV Surveill Suppl Rep. 2021;26(1):1–81. http://www.cdc.gov/hiv/library/reports/hiv-surveillance.html. Accessed Jan 2024.
23. Centers for Disease Control and Prevention: US Public Health Service. Preexposure prophylaxis for the prevention of HIV infection in the United States—2021 update: a clinical practice guideline. 2021. https://www.cdc.gov/hiv/pdf/risk/prep/cdc-hiv-prep-guidelines-2021.pdf. Accessed Jan 2024.
24. Van Wagoner N, Qushair F, Johnston C. Genital herpes infection: progress and problems. Infect Dis Clin N Am. 2023;37(2):351–67. https://doi.org/10.1016/j.idc.2023.02.011. PMID: 37105647.
25. Santiago-Wickey JN, Crosby B. Granuloma inguinale. 2023. In: StatPearls [Internet]. Treasure Island: StatPearls Publishing; 2024. PMID: 30020678.
26. Irizarry L, Velasquez J, Wray AA. Chancroid. 2023. In: StatPearls [Internet]. Treasure Island: StatPearls Publishing; 2024. PMID: 30020703.
27. Zhao YK, Luo DQ. Pubic Lice. N Engl J Med. 2024;390(3):e6. https://doi.org/10.1056/NEJMicm2303713. Epub 2024 Jan 13. PMID: 38226842.
28. Bernigaud C, Fischer K, Chosidow O. The management of scabies in the 21st century: past, advances and potentials. Acta Derm Venereol. 2020;100(9):adv00112. https://doi.org/10.2340/00015555-3468. PMID: 32207535; PMCID: PMC9128908.
29. Reese P. STIs during pregnancy. Am Fam Physician. 2024;109(1):10–2.
30. American College of Obstetrics and Gynecology. Routine tests during pregnancy. 2023. https://www.acog.org/womens-health/faqs/routine-tests-during-pregnancy. Accessed Jan 2024.

Chapter 11
Barrier Contraception

Anthony L. Ciricillo

Introduction

The use of barrier methods as the primary mode of contraception has declined over several decades due to the increasing number and relative effectiveness of other available contraceptive methods. Barrier methods still have a place in providing contraception for certain carefully selected patients. Unlike other forms of contraception, some barrier methods may also provide some degree of protection against sexually transmitted infections. The use of barrier methods is generally female-controlled, although it may require partner cooperation. Many barriers are widely available without a prescription. They are not hormonally based, making them safe for many patients in whom the use of a hormonal contraceptive would be contraindicated or undesired. Barrier methods available today include male (external) and female (internal) condoms, the contraceptive sponge, diaphragms, and cervical caps.

Case Study

Kara is a 26-year-old nulliparous patient in a monogamous long-standing relationship. She presents to your office today for her Pap smear and physical exam and asks you about changing her birth control method. She and her partner have been using condoms but would like a method that allows a little more spontaneity. She intends on having children in the next 1–2 years. In the past, she gained a great deal of weight on Depo-Provera and does not want to use this method again. She is a smoker and wants to avoid oral contraceptives because she has heard about the

A. L. Ciricillo (✉)
Liberty Resources, Syracuse, NY, USA
e-mail: anthony.ciricillo@sjhsyr.org

S. M. Sulik, C. B. Heath (eds.), *Primary Care Procedures in Women's Health*,
https://doi.org/10.1007/978-3-032-07061-6_11

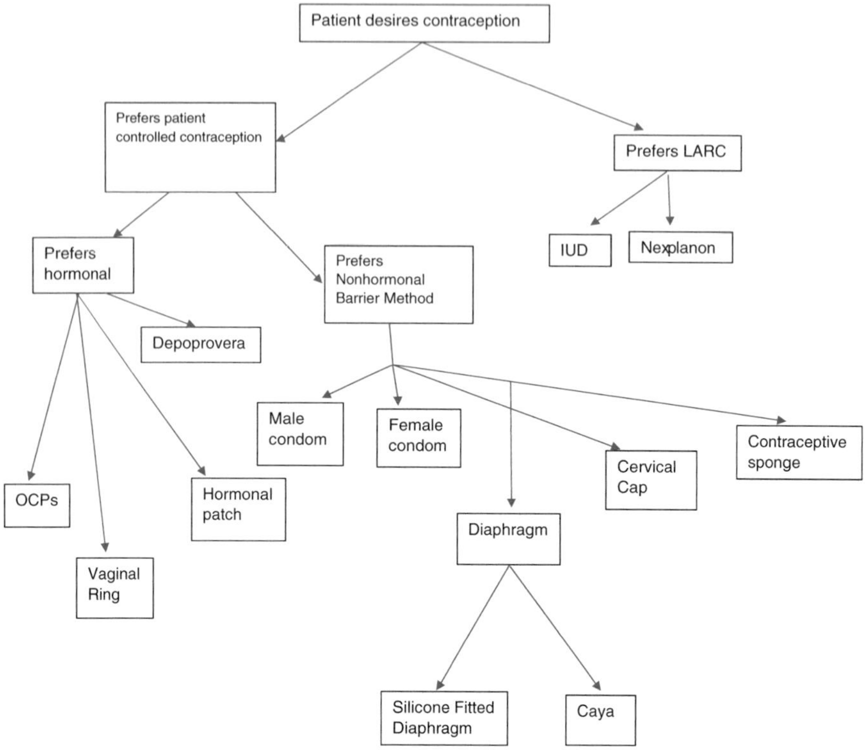

Algorithm 11.1 Decision tree for non-hormonal contraception. Long Acting Reversible Contraceptives (LARC). Intrauterine Device (IUD) Oral Contraceptive Pills (OCP)

risks. Her aunt told her about her diaphragm, and she asked if this method is still available (Algorithm 11.1).

The Male Condom

The male (external) condom has been used to prevent pregnancy since the beginning of recorded history. Early versions were made of silk and animal tissues. Currently, external condoms are available in latex (most common), polyurethane, polyisoprene, silicone, and lambskin. Widely available without a prescription and with few contraindications, condoms provide the most consistent protection against transmission of sexually transmitted infections of all barrier methods. Condoms should not be used if the packaging is damaged, open, or expired. Expiration dates are stamped on the edges of the foiled wrappers and typically last for 1-5 years.

If used properly, condoms can be quite effective with perfect use failure rates of 2%. However, they require commitment, forethought, consistent, and well-timed use, resulting in a typical use failure rate of 12% [1]. There is no evidence that condoms lubricated with nonoxynol-9 (N-9) spermicide are more effective, and potential adverse effects of N-9 include increased risk of urinary tract infections (particularly in young females) and increased rate of HIV transmission. Therefore, these condoms are no longer recommended given the potential adverse effects and lack of benefit compared to condoms without additional spermicidal lubricant [2].

Latex condoms are available in multiple sizes, textures, and colors and tend to be inexpensive. Condoms come with some variation in length and girth, and although most condoms fit most sizes, some men may need to try different sizes and brands to optimize fit. They must be used with water-based lubricants only, as the latex condom will become permeable within seconds of contact with oil-based lubricants or other oil-based products including some moisturizers. Sexually transmitted infection (STI) prevention is most effective for diseases that are transmitted in bodily fluids (HIV, chlamydia, gonorrhea, trichomoniasis) as they have not been proven to be as effective for those infections spread by skin contact (herpes and HPV) [3]. If not stored properly in a dark, cool, dry place, or if stored for more than 5 years, the latex can deteriorate and its effectiveness decreases. Patients using latex condoms may complain of decreased sensitivity, a side effect which may be utilized therapeutically to address premature ejaculation in males.

Non-latex condoms offer alternatives for those who have latex allergies or other issues that prevent their consistent use. Polyurethane condoms transmit more body heat and can be used with oil-based lubricants. While possibly less effective than latex, due to higher breakage rates [4], all but lambskin condoms offer some protection against STI transmission. Lambskin condoms have small pores on the surface that can allow the passage of viral particles such as HIV, HSV, and hepatitis B [4].

Condoms need to be applied to the erect penis, prior to penetration, allowing space for semen by pinching ½ inch at the tip while it is rolled on (Fig. 11.1). Avoiding the presence of air bubbles under the condom and wearing them throughout intercourse prevents leakage and increases effectiveness. Proper removal occurs after ejaculation but while the penis is still erect, using care to hold the rim of the condom to prevent spillage.

Indications for Use of Male Condom

- Patient desires non-hormonal contraception that provides protection against sexually transmitted infections.
- Both partners are willing to use the device properly with every act of coitus and store the device as directed prior to use.

Contraindications to Use of Male Condom

- Allergy to components in the condom (latex for latex condoms or lanolin for lambskin)

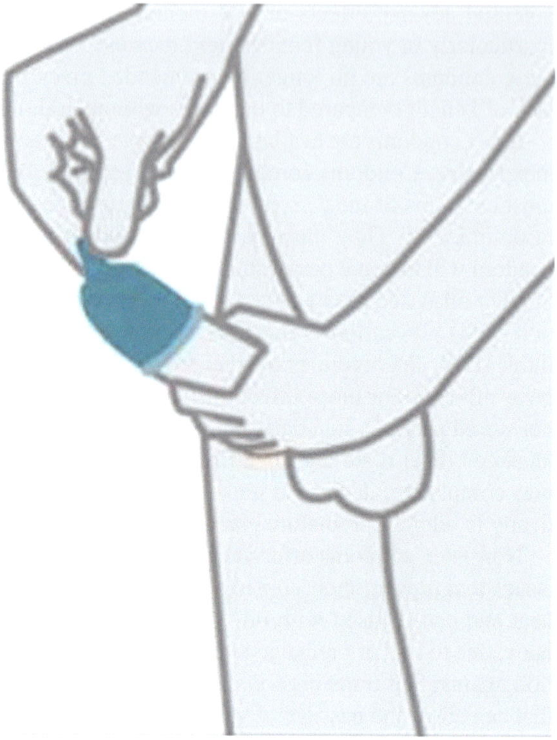

Fig. 11.1 Male condom; pinch air out of condom after application

- Improper size, application process, or removal of the condom
- Inability to store the device in a cool, dry, dark place or condom packaging is expired, open, or damaged.

Complications and Risks

- Irritation due to latex, lubricant, or spermicide.
- Slippage, breakage, or leakage of the condom.
- Increased risk of urinary tract infections (UTIs) due to alteration of normal vaginal flora with spermicide-coated condoms [5].
- Men may have decreased sensation or loss of erection.
- Errors in use may result in leakage, slippage, or breakage.
- Pre-purchasing prior to sexual intercourse and having condoms available for immediate use may be difficult for some

Procedure and Initiation of Method

1. Condoms are widely available in stores, online, and through clinics and do not require a prescription.
2. Patients choosing this method should be properly educated on selecting the correct size and type of condom; proper storage, utilization, and disposal of the condom; and safe lubricants to use with the selected type of condom. Models are available to demonstrate proper application.
3. Educate patients about the availability of emergency contraception (EC) in the event of condom failure and consider providing a prescription for EC if required for your patients using condoms as the primary method. STI testing should also be considered in this setting.
4. Prior to sexual intercourse, the condom must be carefully opened to avoid damage and placed on the tip of the erect penis. Next, it is important to pinch air out from the tip of the condom before gently unrolling the condom to the base of the penis ensuring adequate coverage of the glans and shaft. Lubrication should also be encouraged to reduce irritation and prevent breakage of the condom.
5. After ejaculation, the penis can be safely withdrawn while holding the condom at the base by the rim. It should be inspected for any defects that may have occurred during use before discarding it into the trash [6].

Tips and Helpful Hints

- Ensure that the patient is aware that they still have a risk for contracting sexually transmitted diseases and recommend routine screening.
- Encourage the patient to make condom application part of foreplay and involve both partners in the process of application if issues of erectile function and lack of spontaneity are barriers to use.
- Provide patients with a list of safely used lubricants if latex condoms are chosen as a primary contraceptive method.

Female Condom (Fig. 11.2)

The female condom has undergone several changes to address concerns regarding the initial version. Originally composed of polyurethane and available as Reality®, the new version is named FC2 and is the only FDA-approved female (or internal) condom available in the US. Composed of nitrile polymer (synthetic latex), it is a seamless soft sheath, closed at the proximal end. Flexible rings at both ends act to anchor the proximal end into the vagina and to keep the outer end in place on the perineum.

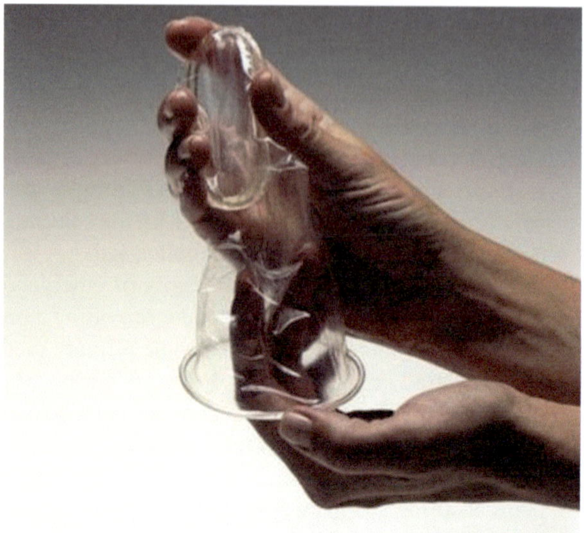

Fig. 11.2 Female condom (Courtesy of Mayer Laboratories, Inc.)

FC2 is coated with a silicone-based lubricant but can be used with both water- and oil-based lubricants. FC2 should not be used with a male condom, as friction between the devices increases the risk of displacement. Nitrile is less likely to degrade than latex and withstands storage well.

The FC2 acts as a physical barrier to skin contact and semen that can be inserted up to 8 hours prior to intercourse. It is the only barrier method that provides protection against pregnancy, is a probable barrier to HIV and sexually transmitted infections, and is completely female-controlled. However, there is no current data to directly support that the FC2 is as effective as latex external condoms at preventing transmission of STIs [7]. Any recommendations for use to prevent STI transmission are based on prior data regarding the effectiveness of polyurethane male condoms.

Unlike male condoms, the penis does not need to be erect to initiate use.

The male partner may find it less constricting, and the female partner may find the outer ring can increase enjoyment by stimulating the clitoris during intercourse.

Contraceptive effectiveness is estimated as comparable to the latex male condom, with a 5% annual pregnancy rate with perfect use and up to 21% rate with typical use [8]. Failure can occur due to device breakage; displacement, where the device slips completely into or out of the vagina during intercourse; or misdirection, if the penis is accidentally inserted next to rather than within the sheath [9]. The same events are thought to result in potentially less protection against STIs due to increased exposure to semen.

Indications for Use of Female Condom

- The patient desires a barrier method of contraception providing a degree of protection against STIs and allowing autonomous control.
- Allergy to latex or inability to use or tolerate external/male condoms.
- Willingness and ability to insert and use a new FC2 for each act of intercourse. Check for tears prior to insertion.

Contraindications to Use of Female Condom

- Allergy to nitrile
- Inability to insert the device properly due to pelvic anatomy or physical limitations

Complications and Risks

- Difficulty in inserting the FC2 properly.
- Slippage, breakage, displacement of the device, or misdirection of the penis during intercourse due to poor insertion of FC2.
- Rings may cause discomfort for either partner during intercourse.
- Noise can occur during intercourse (however, this has been improved by the change to the nitrile composition of the FC2).

Procedure and Initiation of Method

1. Female condoms can be purchased without a prescription; however, they can be prescribed for patients with many insurances to decrease the cost of the device to that of a prescription co-payment. In general, FC2s are more expensive when purchased over the counter than male condoms.
2. Insertion must occur prior to penetration and is accomplished by folding the internal ring and inserting it into the posterior fornix. FC2 does not need to be fitted to patients prior to use. Positions for insertion can include lying down or with one leg raised on a chair or toilet.
3. A new FC2 must be used for each act of coitus.
4. After intercourse, the outer ring must be twisted to close the sheath to contain semen prior to standing or removing. Remove by placing gentle traction on the twisted FC2.
5. FC2 must be thrown out, not flushed down the toilet.

6. Educate patients about the availability of emergency contraception and consider providing a prescription for EC in patients who choose condoms as the primary contraceptive method.

Tricks and Helpful Hints

- Many insurances will cover FC2 as a monthly prescription benefit.
- Male partners may find it more comfortable and less constricting than male condoms, and an erect penis is not required for application.
- A female partner may find the external ring increases enjoyment by stimulating the clitoris.
- If a mishap occurs, ensure that the patient is screened for STIs and consider the use of EC.

The Contraceptive Sponge and Other Spermicidal Agents

The contraceptive sponge is a soft, round, porous polyurethane device that is saturated with nonoxynol-9 spermicide and is inserted into the vagina prior to intercourse (Fig. 11.3).

Currently, the Today® sponge, produced by Mayer Laboratories, Inc., is the only vaginal contraceptive sponge available on the US market. Today® sponge's dimpled side fits around the cervix and works by blocking the sperm path, absorbing sperm into the sponge, and through its spermicidal activity. There is a loop on the other side of the device to facilitate removal. The Today® sponge is effective immediately on insertion, and protection lasts for a full 24 h.

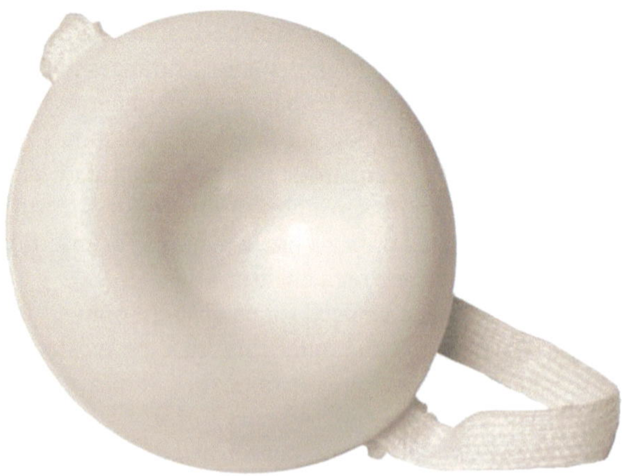

Fig. 11.3 Contraceptive sponge

In addition to the contraceptive sponge, spermicides are available in many delivery methods, including gels, creams, films, and foams. In general, the use of spermicide alone is considered less effective for pregnancy prevention than when combined with a barrier. When used alone, the failure rate in nulliparous patients with perfect use of the sponge is 9% but up to 20% in parous women. For nulliparous women, the typical use failure rate is 12% but 24% in parous women [9]. However, it should be noted that studies are very inconsistent and reported contraceptive failure rates for spermicides vary widely. Nonoxynol-9 is a surfactant that destroys the sperm cell membrane [10]. It is not a microbicidal substance. There is a risk of genital tissue irritation with the use of nonoxynol-9, which may facilitate transmission of HIV. This risk increases with the duration of exposure and the frequency of repeated use. For this reason, its use is not recommended in sex workers or others at high risk of HIV transmission [11].

Indications for Use of the Contraceptive Sponge

- Desire for non-hormonal contraception that is female-controlled, in a patient with an inability to use other available methods, or who prefers not to.
- Patient who does not require STI protection.
- Need for 24 h of uninterrupted protection without reapplication.
- Use in nulliparous patients has proven more effective.

Contraindications to Use of the Contraceptive Sponge

- High risk of exposure to HIV, HIV positivity, or current use of antiretroviral therapy
- Interrupted vaginal epithelium
- Allergy to spermicide ingredients
- History of toxic shock syndrome (TSS) in the past
- Need for protection against STIs
- Inability to properly insert the sponge
- Recurrent UTIs
- Vaginal bleeding—including menses or delivery in the last 6 weeks.

Complications and Risks

- There is a risk of developing TSS, and it is imperative that the device not be left in the vagina for more than 30 h.
- Increased risk of HIV transmission with the use of nonoxynol-9.

- Relatively high risk of pregnancy with spermicide alone.
- Risk of urinary tract infections with nonoxynol-9 use.

Procedure and Initiation of Method

1. The Today® sponge is available over the counter without a prescription. The sponge does not require fitting; it is available only in one size.
2. Before inserting the sponge, wash your hands with soap and water, then wet the sponge thoroughly with clean water to activate the spermicide.
3. Squeeze the sponge to activate foaming.
4. Insert the sponge deep inside the vagina with the dimple toward the cervix and the loop facing into the vagina (Fig. 11.4). It is effective immediately on insertion but must be in place before intercourse occurs.
5. The device should be left in place for at least 6 h after the last episode of intercourse, up to a maximum of 30 h. It provides 24 h of protection without reinsertion for repeated acts of coitus. Remove by pulling down on the loop.

Helpful Hints

- Ensure the sponge user is aware of symptoms/signs of TSS.
- Careful selection of patients for this method is crucial, taking into consideration the risk of STI transmission and acceptability of unplanned pregnancy—due to high failure rates when used alone.

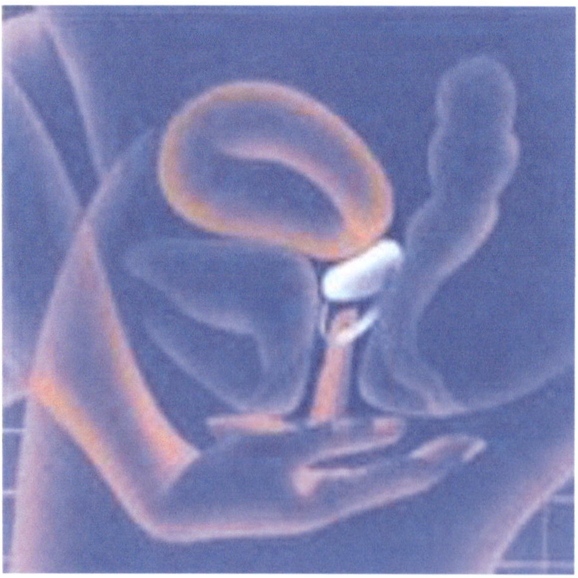

Fig. 11.4 Sponge placement

Contraceptive Diaphragm

The diaphragm is a silicone flexible dome that fits over the cervix and into the vaginal fornices during intercourse, providing a physical barrier to sperm. Inserted up to 2 hours (h) prior to intercourse, it must be left in place for at least 6 h and up to 24 h after. The options currently available for patients choosing a diaphragm include the provider-fitted traditional version (Milex®) (Fig. 11.5) or the newer single-size contraceptive barrier device called Caya® (Fig. 11.6), a product that requires a prescription but not a traditional size fitting. Janssen Pharmaceuticals ceased production of the popular Ortho All-Flex diaphragm in 2013, leaving the Milex® Wide Seal as the only available fitted diaphragm.

The traditional diaphragm type must be properly fitted to each patient by their provider and refitted as necessary due to weight change or reproductive events. Effectiveness of the diaphragm is very user-dependent, and estimated effectiveness rates range widely from 70% to 96%, assuming "perfect use" and spermicide use with the diaphragm [8].

The Milex® Wide-Seal diaphragm is available in arcing spring and coil spring versions. Both types are silicone-based and have a thin skirt of silicone around the base of the rim to improve the seal and help hold spermicide. They are supplied by Cooper Surgical® and select other medical suppliers and come in a variety of sizes ranging from 60 to 95 mm. Both types can be ordered through the provider who orders them directly from the supplier. Neither type of diaphragm can be obtained at the pharmacy.

The Milex® arcing spring-type diaphragm folds into a half-moon shape for insertion along a single plane and does not require an introducer. The arcing spring diaphragm's firm rim makes it the best choice for women with decreased pelvic support. Due to single-plane folding, if the axis rotates while inserted, some women may find it difficult to remove.

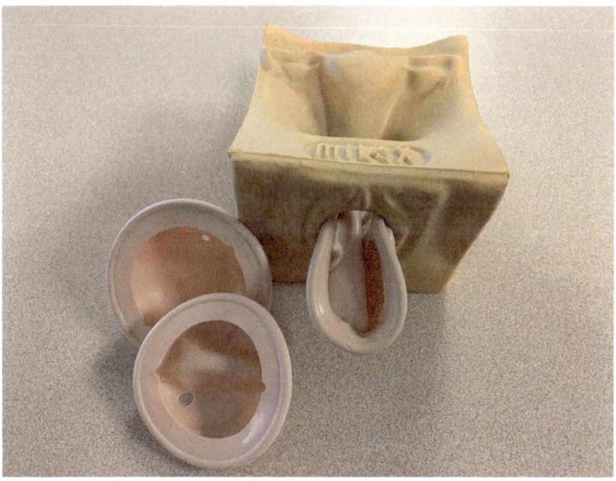

Fig. 11.5 Milex® Wide-Seal silicone diaphragm

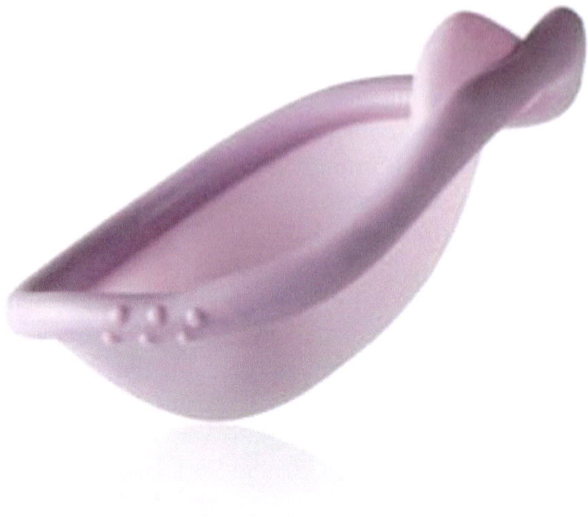

Fig. 11.6 Caya® diaphragm. (Photo—image courtesy of KESSEL MEDintim)

The coil spring version of the Milex® Wide-Seal diaphragm, the Omniflex, has a rim which is more flexible than the arcing spring, allowing for folding anywhere along the rim. It can be used with or without an introducer for insertion. It is better suited to women without pelvic muscle relaxation.

In September 2014, the Caya® was FDA approved for use in the USA. The Caya® is a silicone-based contoured-shaped diaphragm with a nylon rim. It has grip dimples to ease insertion and a dome for easy removal. It is designed to fit most patients who would normally wear between a 65- and 80-mm diaphragm. Single-use disposable test fit devices are available from the distributor, HPSRx Enterprises Inc., to allow the patient to test use prior to ordering. The device is available supplied through the provider's office by purchasing from supplier, specialty pharmacies, and several commercial pharmacies with a prescription. If a patient has already been fitted with a diaphragm in the 65–80 mm size range, there is no fitting required. Those with no prior diaphragm use may benefit from a test fit visit to ensure they are able to use the device comfortably. Caya® has a 6-month typical use failure rate of 9.6–12.5%, which is similar to the Milex® diaphragm [12].

The diaphragm is filled with spermicidal jelly or cream to increase effectiveness. One small study has shown that women who use the diaphragm without spermicide are slightly more likely to become pregnant, but due to the low power of the study, this finding was not significant [13]. If repeated acts of intercourse take place during 24 h of use, the diaphragm is left in place (Fig. 11.7) and additional spermicide is added. Acid-buffering gel has been explored as a spermicidal alternative with standard diaphragms and was found to have about the same effectiveness [14].

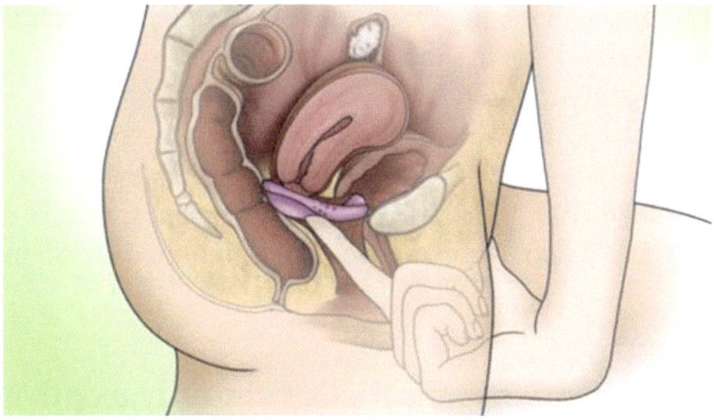

Fig. 11.7 Caya® diaphragm in vaginal vault. (Image courtesy of KESSEL MEDintim)

Effectiveness is thought to be due to a physical barrier function of the gel and to the decreased sperm motility in lower pH environments [14].

Some studies show modest protection provided against transmission of STIs, mainly due to physical protection of the cervix which is thought to be more susceptible to infections. Other studies do not show benefit and cite that there are multiple confounding factors such as the fact that diaphragm users may be at lower risk in general [15]. Frequent use of nonoxynol-9 spermicides may be associated with increased risk of HIV transmission due to the formation of small cervical and vaginal erosions or irritation from the spermicide [14].

Adolescents may not be good candidates for diaphragms because of the level of maturity required for their use and the decreased level of protection from sexually transmitted diseases and unplanned pregnancy.

Indications for Diaphragm Placement

- Patient desires a nonhormonal, immediately reversible, female-controlled method of birth control.
- Comfortable with insertion and removal of the device and is willing to reliably use the device with every act of coitus.
- Safe for use while breastfeeding.
- Safe for patients with a latex allergy history.

Contraindications to Contraceptive Diaphragm

- Significant pelvic organ prolapses, including cystocele, rectocele, or uterine prolapse (however, arching spring diaphragms may be helpful for patients with mild pelvic relaxation)
- Frequent urinary tract infections
- Allergy to spermicide or silicone

- Vaginal or cervical lacerations or significant friability
- History of toxic shock syndrome
- Inability to insert or use properly
- History of HIV or high risk of HIV transmission
- Inability to clean, store, or transport the device to the location of use
- Inability to be refit Milex® after pregnancy, weight gain >10 lbs. or abortion
- Caya® is not recommended if size required is >85 mm or <60 mm

Complications and Risks for Contraceptive Diaphragm Use

- Unintended pregnancy (not as effective as other types of contraception)
- Frequent urinary tract infection
- Toxic shock syndrome (risk is 2.4 cases per 100,000 women, particularly when left in place more than 24 h) [8]
- Improper fitting resulting in failure of the method
- Cervical or vaginal lacerations, ulcerations, or abrasions
- Dislodgement during intercourse
- Vaginal discharge or odor can develop if left in place too long
- Female or male partner awareness of the device or pain with the device
- Penile abrasions
- Requires resizing postpartum, post abortion, or with any change in weight of 10 pounds

Equipment List for Diaphragm Fitting

- Diaphragm fitting kit or fitting ring kit (sterilized) if using Milex® products
- Test fit device if using Caya®
- Nonsterile gloves
- Vaginal speculum
- Spermicidal jelly
- Vaginal lubricating gel for fitting

Procedure Steps for Diaphragm Fitting

1. The patient should be known to have normal cervical cytology prior to proceeding.
2. The patient should be at least 6 weeks postpartum or 2 weeks post abortion.
3. Have the patient empty their bladder and place them in the dorsal lithotomy position.

4. Insert vaginal speculum and examine cervix and vaginal vault for any lacerations, abrasions, polyps, or signs of infection which would contraindicate placement.
5. Insert the index and middle fingers into the vaginal vault so that the middle finger is placed at the posterior fornix.
6. Place the thumb of the same hand against the symphysis pubis (Fig. 11.8).
7. Keeping the thumb against the index finger, remove the entire measuring hand, and measure the distance from the tip of the thumb to the tip of the middle finger. This distance represents the estimated necessary diaphragm size (Fig. 11.9).
8. Choose the estimated-size diaphragm from the fitting kit and insert it into the vaginal vault by folding it in half, spring, and directing it posteriorly while separating the vulva with the other hand. Most patients fit a 70 mm size.
9. Palpate edges of diaphragm to ensure that it fits snugly behind the pubic symphysis, covers cervix entirely, and reaches the posterior fornix (Fig. 11.10). If necessary, choose a larger or smaller size to meet these criteria and try again.
10. Instruct the patient to feel for the proper placement of the diaphragm in the vagina and to remove it by hooking the index finger behind the anterior rim and pulling straight down.
11. Provide or order the diaphragm from Cooper Surgical for patients if using Milex®. If using Caya®, the patient measures 65–80 mm on exam or on previous use of a diaphragm, and test fitting is successful, write a prescription for the device.
12. Clean the Milex® fitting set between fittings by autoclaving and discard the Caya test fit device.

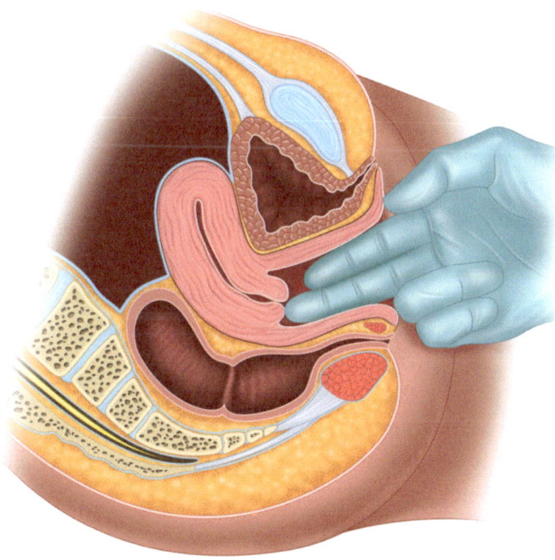

Fig. 11.8 Estimating diaphragm size by measuring distance from the posterior fornix to pubic symphysis

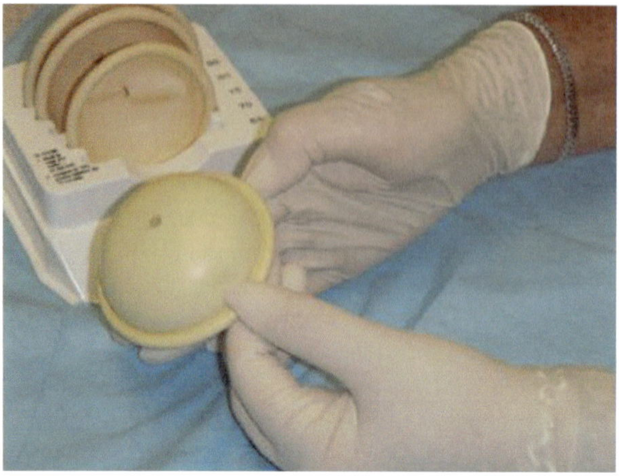

Fig. 11.9 Estimating diaphragm size for fitting

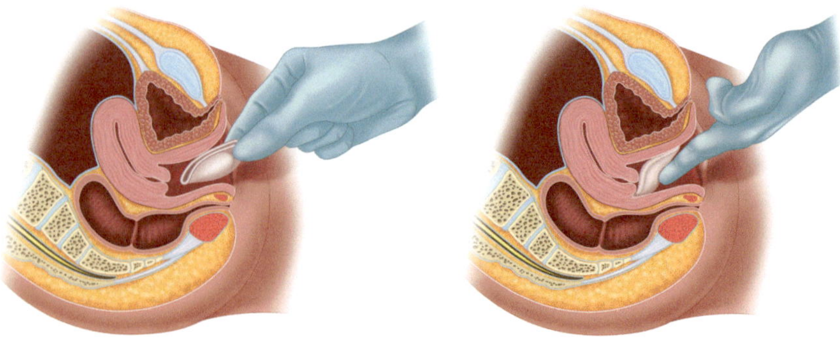

Fig. 11.10 Proper position of the diaphragm in the vaginal vault

Tricks and Helpful Hints, Diaphragm

- Have the patient perform a Valsalva maneuver and walk around the exam room after fitting to make sure there is no discomfort, and the diaphragm does not dislodge.
- Ensure that the patient is comfortable with insertion and removal of the device on their own while they are in your office, and demonstrate proper application of one tablespoon of spermicide into the dome and around the rim of the device.
- The patient should be able to feel their cervix through the membrane of the diaphragm if properly placed.
- The patient should be instructed to urinate before insertion and again after intercourse to avoid a urinary tract infection.
- If UTIs occur, consider changing diaphragm type, size, or switching to a cervical cap [16].

- Provide a prescription for or inform the patient of the availability of emergency contraception, given the higher failure rate of barrier devices.
- Milex and Caya diaphragms should be replaced every 2 years.

Cervical Cap

First approved by the FDA in 1988, the cervical cap is smaller than a diaphragm and more thimble-shaped with a deeper well (Fig. 11.11). Many types of caps are in production worldwide, but only the silicone FemCap™ is FDA approved for use in the US. The second-generation FemCap™ device had several upgrades to the first and was released in 2003. The device is available today through the office of a provider who stocks them or with a prescription through the FemCap™ website or designated specialty pharmacies.

Cervical caps are sized by a provider based on exam and patient history. They are available in three sizes, namely, small (22 mm), medium (26 mm), and large (30 mm). Requiring less spermicide than a diaphragm, the cap is placed more tightly around the cervix. The FemCap™ dome covers the cervix, and the brim fits into the vaginal fornices to collect semen [17]. There is a strap to facilitate removal. Like the diaphragm, it must be left in place for at least 6 hours after intercourse. Additional spermicidal gel should be inserted for subsequent episodes of intercourse. The FemCap™ is approved for continuous use up to 48 h in the US. The FemCap is 92.4% effective with typical use and 96-98% effective with perfect use. Failure rates with typical use 7.6/100 women years [18].

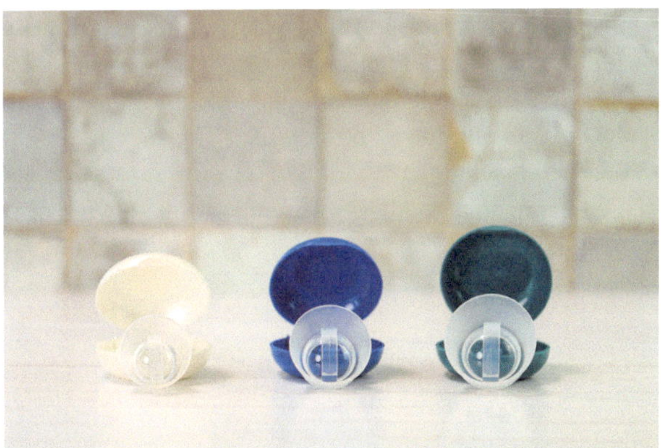

Fig. 11.11 FemCap cervical cap

Indications for Cervical Cap Placement

- Nonhormonal, immediately reversible, female-controlled method of birth control.
- Comfortable with insertion and removal of the device and willing to use the device with every act of coitus.
- Cervical caps are most appropriately chosen for nulliparous patients due to the higher rate of failure in women with vaginal birth prior to fitting.
- Cervical caps are less likely to be associated with an increased frequency of urinary tract infections.
- The size of a cervical cap is unaffected by weight changes [18].

Contraindications to the Cervical Cap

- History of toxic shock syndrome
- Immediate postpartum (<6 weeks) or postabortion (<2 weeks) use
- Anatomic barriers, such as cervical polyps
- Abnormal cervical cell cytology
- Patient's inability to insert or use properly
- Patient's inability to clean, store, or transport the device to the location of use
- Should not be used during menses
- Presence of sexually transmitted disease, history of HIV, or high risk for HIV exposure

Complications and Risks, Cervical Cap

- Unintended pregnancy (not as effective)—particularly parous patients.
- Toxic shock syndrome (risk is 2.4 cases per 100,000 women, particularly when left in place more than 24 h) [8].
- Cervical or vaginal lacerations, ulcerations, or abrasions.
- Dislodgement during intercourse.
- Vaginal discharge or odor can develop if left in place too long.
- Female or male partner awareness of the device or pain with the device.
- Penile abrasions.

Equipment List, Cervical Cap

- Cervical caps in three sizes to be provided to the patients
- Vaginal speculum
- Nonsterile gloves
- Water based lubricant
- Informational materials and video for patient review

1. The patient should have known normal cervical cytology before proceeding and be at least 2 weeks post abortion or 6 weeks post-birth.
2. Have the patient empty their bladder.
3. Place the patient in the dorsal lithotomy position and insert the vaginal speculum.
4. Examine the cervix for lacerations, polyps, or other structural abnormalities.
5. Perform pelvic exam to check cervical size (Table 11.1).
6. Choose cervical cap size based on exam and obstetrical history using the above chart.
7. Allow the patient to insert her own FemCap™ based on the manufacturer's instructions.
8. Check placement by digital exam to ensure cervix is completely covered and that the cap is not dislodged easily by movement or with a Valsalva maneuver (Fig. 11.12).
9. Ensure the patient can remove the FemCap™ on her own.
10. Instruct the patient on how to use one-half to three-fourths teaspoon spermicide in the groove facing the vaginal vault prior to use.

Table 11.1 Cervical cap fitting

Cervical cap size	Patient characteristics
22 mm	Patient has never been pregnant
26 mm	Patient has been pregnant, but no vaginal delivery
30 mm	Patient has had a vaginal delivery

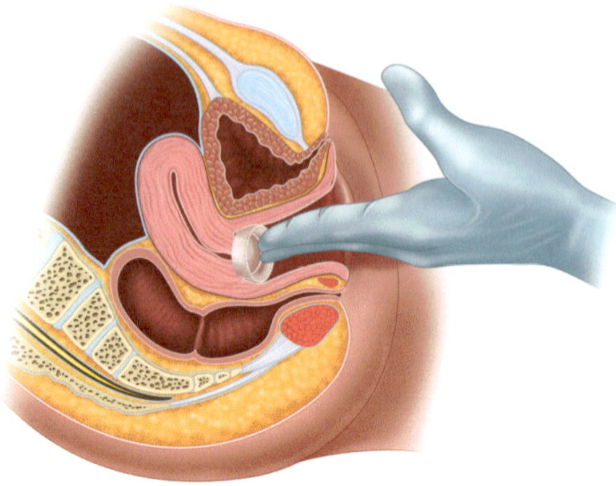

Fig. 11.12 Proper cervical cap placement on the cervix

Tricks and Helpful Hints, Cervical Cap

- Consider a prescription for emergency contraception given the higher failure rates of barrier devices.
- Women with a long, short, or anterior cervix may not be amenable to fitting with a cervical cap and will need to use another method.
- The FemCap™ should always be inserted prior to any sexual arousal.
- Removal can be facilitated by squatting and bearing down.

Procedure Note

Diaphragm

The patient was placed in the dorsal lithotomy position. Vaginal speculum was inserted, and the cervix and vagina were visually inspected and found to be normal. Diaphragm size was estimated by manual exam measurement. Fitting diaphragm was inserted to ensure proper size selection and #_______ was prescribed. Patient was instructed about insertion, care, use, and removal and demonstrated the ability to independently insert and remove the diaphragm. The patient tolerated the procedure well.

Cervical Cap

The patient was placed in the dorsal lithotomy position. Vaginal speculum was inserted, and the cervix and vagina were visually inspected and found to be normal. Manual vaginal examination was performed to estimate the size of the cervix. The patient's FemCap™ size was selected based on obstetrical history and examination and a size #_____ was selected. The patient viewed the instructional materials and was able to adequately insert her own FemCap™ with the provided instructions. FemCap™ placement was checked by manual exam, and the size was found to be appropriate. Patient demonstrated the ability to independently remove the device. Patient tolerated the procedure well.

Coding

Diaphragm

CPT Diaphragm or cervical cap fitting with instructions	57170
HCPCS code for Supply of Diaphragm	A4266
Procedure ICD-10 for insertion of the diaphragm	Z30.018

Cervical Cap

CPT fitting a diaphragm or cervical cap for contraception	57170
Procedure ICD-10 for cervical cap fitting	Z30.018
HCPCS code for the supply of a cervical cap	A4261

Postprocedure Patient Instructions

Diaphragm

Ensure that the patient receives proper training regarding the insertion and removal of the device while in the office.

Patient should insert the device 2 h prior to intercourse.

Patient can insert up to 6 h prior to intercourse, but if so, an applicator of spermicide should be added at the time of intercourse.

Device should be left in place for a minimum of 6 h after intercourse but can stay in place up to 24 h.

The patient should check for dislodgement after intercourse and reposition if it occurs with the insertion of an additional applicator of spermicide.

If additional episodes of intercourse take place, the device should be left in place and an additional applicator of spermicide should be inserted prior.

Instruct the patient to inspect the diaphragm for holes or tears prior to each use by holding it up to the light.

The diaphragm should be cleaned after each use with mild soap and water, wiped dry, and kept in its case avoiding extremes of temperature during storage.

Cervical Cap

The patient should return in 2 weeks for a follow-up visit with the cap in place to ensure correct usage.

Pap smear must be performed within 3 months of initiation of use and treated as indicated. If cytology is normal, the patient can resume yearly exams.

Instruct the patient not to use during menstruation.

Instruct the patient to check the position after intercourse to ensure it has not dislodged.

FemCap should be washed with antibacterial hand soap and water, dried, and stored in its container.

The FemCap should be replaced yearly or sooner if worn or damaged.

Case Study Outcome

After discussing the specifics of the diaphragm barrier method, Kara was willing to try it. She felt that the risk of pregnancy was acceptable and was willing to use emergency contraception in the event of device failure. Kara was examined and found to be approximately 65 mm. Review of her gynecological and obstetrical history revealed no contraindications to diaphragm usage. She was tested for fit and appropriateness with the Caya® test kit and was able to independently place and remove it. The patient was instructed in its use and care and provided with a prescription and a follow-up appointment.

References

1. Trussell J, Aiken ARA, Nelson AL, et al. Contraceptive efficacy. In: Contraceptive technology. 2nd ed. New York: Ayer Company Publishers; 2018. p. 844.
2. Obiero J, Mwethera PG, Hussey GD, Wiysonge CS. Vaginal microbicidal for reducing the risk of HIV infection in women: systematic review and meta-analysis. BMC Infect Dis. 2012;12:289. https://doi.org/10.1186/1471-2334-12-289.
3. Black A, Guilbert E, et al. Canadian contraceptive consensus (part 2 of 4). J Obstet Gynaecol Can. 2015;37(11):s1–s39. https://doi.org/10.1016/j.jogc.2016.10.005.
4. MzF G, Grimes DA, Lopez LM, Schulz KF. Non-latex versus latex male condoms for contraception. Cochrane Database Syst Rev. 2006; https://doi.org/10.1002/14651858.CD003550.pub2.
5. Handley MA, Reingold AL, Shiboski S, Padian NS. Incidence of acute urinary tract infection in young women and use of male condoms with and without nonoxynol-9 spermicides. Epidemiology. 2002;13:431–6.

6. Male (External) Condom Use. https://www.cdc.gov/condomeffectiveness/external-condom-use.html. 2022.
7. Gallo MF, Kilbourne-Brook M, Coffey PS. A review of the effectiveness and acceptability of the female condom for dual protection. Sex Health. 2012;9:18–26. https://doi.org/10.1097/00001648-200207000-00011.
8. Trussel J. Contraceptive failure in the United States. Contraception. 2011;83:397–404. https://doi.org/10.1016/j.contraception.2011.01.021.
9. Beksinka M, Smit J, Joanis C, Usher-Patel M, Potter W. Female condom technology: new products and regulatory issues. Contraception. 2011;83:316–21. https://doi.org/10.1016/j.contraception.2010.07.022.
10. Hatcher RA, Trussel J, Nelson A, Cates W, Kowal D, Policar M. Contraceptive technology. 20th ed. New York: Ardent Media; 2011.
11. Van Damme L, Ramjee G, Alary M, Vuylsteke B, Chandeying V, Rees H, et al. Effectiveness of COL-1492, a nonoxynol-9 vaginal gel, on HIV-1 transmission in female sex workers: a randomized controlled trial. Lancet. 360:971–7. https://doi.org/10.1097/AOG.0000000000000721.
12. Schwartz JL, Weiner DH, Lai JJ, et al. Contraceptive efficacy, safety, fit and acceptability of a single-size diaphragm developed with end-user input. Obstet Gynecol. 2015;125:895–903.
13. Cook L, Nanda K, Grimes D. Diaphragm versus diaphragm with spermicides for contraception (review). Cochrane Library. 2007;1 https://doi.org/10.1097/01.AOG.0000278078.45640.13.
14. Barnhart KT, Rosenberg MJ, MacKay HT, Blithe DL, Higgins J, Walsh T, et al. Contraceptive efficacy of a novel spermicidal microbicide used with a diaphragm: a randomized controlled trial. Obstet Gynecol. 2007;110:577–86.
15. d'Oro LC, Parazzini F, Naldi L, LaVecchia C. Barrier methods of contraception, spermicides and sexually transmitted diseases: a review. Genitourin Med. 1994;70:410–7. https://doi.org/10.1136/sti.70.6.410.
16. Gallo MF, Grimes DA, Shulz KF. Cervical cap versus diaphragm for contraception. Cochrane Database Syst Rev. 2003;1 https://doi.org/10.1002/14651858.CD003551.
17. FDA summary of safety and effectiveness data. FemCapTM. 2003.
18. Alfred S, Brody SA, Julia Barrett-Mitchell J. The Renaissance of Hormone-Free Barrier Contraception and Development of FemCap™: Hormone-Free Contraception. Gynecol Reprod Health. 2020;4(4):1–6.

Additional Resources

Caya®: www.hpsrx.com
FC2: https://fc2.us.com
FemCap™: www.femcap.com
Milex®: www.coopersurgical.com

Chapter 12
Fertility Awareness-Based Method/Natural Family Planning

Dawn Brink-Cymerman

Introduction

Fertility awareness-based method (FABM) or natural family planning (NFP) is one of the oldest practiced methods of birth control. Also known as periodic abstinence, rhythm method, and fertility awareness method, it can be used for either pregnancy prevention or planning and is acceptable to all major religious groups. Although it is not a common method of birth control, there are couples who still choose to practice natural family planning and may request the assistance and support of their health care provider. In motivated patients with appropriate instruction, FABM may be an effective method of preventing or spacing pregnancies. Eighty-five percent of patients will get pregnant within a year of having intercourse without contraception. With perfect use, 3–5% of US women aged 15–45 who have been instructed and use FABM will become pregnant [1]. However, perfect use is uncommon, with typical use rates of pregnancy ranging from 2–23% of US FABM users. FABM users learn fertility awareness, which is particular appealing to those who wish space pregnancies and avoid side effects and risks of other contraceptive methods. FABM methods avoid penile-vaginal intercourse or use additional methods of contraception during the days of the menstrual cycle more likely to lead to pregnancy. Inconsistent use of FABM is more likely to cause pregnancy to occur [2].

There are many methods of FABM, including the calendar method, the lactational amenorrhea method, the basal temperature method, the Billings method or cervical mucus method, the Creighton method, the symptothermal method, and the standard days method/two-day method, the Marquette method, and two apps that are now FDA approved as birth control devices.

D. Brink-Cymerman (✉)
Faculty, St. Joseph's Family Medicine Residency, Syracuse, NY, USA
e-mail: dawn.brink-cymerman@sjhsyr.org

S. M. Sulik, C. B. Heath (eds.), *Primary Care Procedures in Women's Health*,
https://doi.org/10.1007/978-3-032-07061-6_12

The calendar method is based solely on the calculation of the days of a patient's cycle. This method is based on the theory that a patient ovulates approximately 14 days prior to menses. Most patients have variations of one to several days in their cycle; therefore, predicting the day of menses is difficult. This is even more difficult in patients with irregular cycles. Although the calendar method may be appropriate for patients with regular cycles, additional means of assessing ovulation may be necessary for patients with irregular cycles.

The lactational amenorrhea method (LAM) can be used by breastfeeding patients in the postpartum period. This method should only be considered by patients who are exclusively breastfeeding eight to ten times per day and at least one time during the night. This assures prolactin levels remain high enough to suppress ovulation [3]. LAM should not be used after the initial 6 months postpartum as fertility can return prior to the onset of menses.

The basal temperature method is based on the change in the early morning basal temperature at the time of ovulation when the cycle comes under the influence of progesterone. Intercourse is avoided from the onset of menses through the ovulation period. This lengthy period of abstinence may be unacceptable to some couples. The basal body temperature rises under the influence of progesterone, with most ovulatory cycles having a lower temperature in the first half of the cycle and a higher temperature with the onset of ovulation. At the time of ovulation, the temperature usually rises by 0.4 °F and remains elevated until menses. Patients should be instructed that their fertile period lasts until the temperature is elevated for at least 3 days.

The cervical mucus method (also called the ovulation method or Billings ovulation method) is a method that instructs a patient to check her cervical mucus pattern daily to determine the time of ovulation. She learns to recognize patterns of mucus by sensations on the vulva and visual inspection and avoids intercourse during the ovulation period. Probabilities of pregnancy are 3.1% in the first year with perfect use and 86.4% during imperfect use. It is crucial that couples who choose this method follow some very important rules, which include no intercourse during mucus days, no intercourse during times of stress, and no intercourse within 3 days after the peak of fecundity [1].

The different types of mucus are based on glucose composition. Changes in cervical mucus occur at the beginning and end of the fertile period even in irregular cycles. Secretions should be observed by how they look, by touch, and by feel. Patients chart their mucus changes to be aware of their fertile period. There is variation in mucus composition patient to patient, but each individual has a pattern that remains fairly stable. Ultrasound studies have confirmed that these symptoms accurately identify the timing of ovulation [4]. A study supported by the World Health Organization (WHO) found that 93% of women were able to determine the state of the cervical mucus regardless of educational level and cultural influences [5]. The Creighton model of birth control is a modification of the cervical mucus method and was developed at the Pope Paul VI Institute by Dr. Thomas Hilgers in 1980. It was intended as a natural procreativity education method that allowed a couple to know when their fertile periods occurred. When a couple uses this method, they meet with an instructor over a period of approximately 1 year to accurately learn to recognize the changes in cervical mucus and body changes that indicate fertility. The vulvar mucus is observed and intercourse is avoided during the 3 days prior to until 2 days after the peak vulvar mucus [6]. Proponents of the method quote studies that state the failure rate is less than 1% per year; however, some couples who became pregnant during the study were deliberately not counted as failures as investigators believed the couples intended pregnancy [7].

The symptothermal method is a combination of monitoring symptoms that indicate fertility, using the basal body temperature to assess for ovulation and using calendar calculations to assess peak fertility. In this method, patients assess cervical mucus and observe symptoms of fertility, such as midcycle cramping and breast tenderness, to help determine the period prior to ovulation that they may engage in intercourse. Patients also use calendar calculations to monitor fertile periods and also monitor basal body temperatures to indicate when ovulation has occurred and that they have passed through the fertile period of the menstrual cycle. By combining these methods, couples may avoid the prolonged periods of abstinence required by other FBAM; however, a higher level of instruction is necessary for its appropriate use. Monitoring cervical mucus and observing symptoms of fertility such as midcycle cramping and breast tenderness aid a woman in determining the time prior to ovulation during which she may engage in intercourse without risking pregnancy. By combining symptom observation and basal body temperature monitoring, couples can avoid the prolonged period of abstinence recommended with the use of the basal body temperature method alone.

The standard days method [8] is based on the probability of pregnancy and the timing of ovulation. Studies have shown that a patient's fertile period is approximately 6 days: 5 days before ovulation and for 24 h after ovulation. After 24 h, there is decreased probability of pregnancy. Thus, the fertile window in a patient's cycle is 6 days. Data have also shown that ovulation occurs in the middle of the cycle when the cycles last between 26 and 32 days. Couples avoid intercourse on days 8–19 of every cycle to avoid pregnancy. With correct use, the failure rate is approximately 4% with actual rates that approach 9% [9]. The standard days method may be used for multiple years in those who were successful in the first year [10]. CycleBeads® (Cycle Technologies, Inc., Washington, DC) is a color-coded string of beads to help women keep track of their cycles. To use the beads, a rubber ring is moved over the beads each day of the cycle to track where she is in the cycle. The colors of the beads indicate fertile and nonfertile days.

The Marquette method is one that is taught to the patient by a health care provider who has taken an online course to become knowledgeable about the method and then train patients. The advancement in this method is that while it does use basal body temperature and cervical mucus, it also incorporates an electronic monitoring system. The system is used at home to check urine for metabolites of estrogen, leutinizing hormone, and/or progesterone. This is to enhance the accuracy of predicting the fertile period of the cycle. This method has the advantage of being able to be used with increased accuracy in patients with irregular periods and those who are breastfeeding [11].

The first app to be approved by the FDA as a birth control device was Natural Cycles®. It uses dates of cycles and basal body temperature to identify periods of ovulation. One can also use urine metabolites of LH to enhance the accuracy. An algorithm is created that will predict the fertile time period. It is only approved for users over 18 years of age, there is a cost, and as the other methods discussed, it must be used properly to attain the predicted 93% effectiveness. The second app is Clue and only uses dates and not any additional information such as temperature or hormonal information [12].

There are several systematic reviews that have looked at the efficacy and pregnancy rates of the various methods. Perfect use pregnancy rates reported in Urrutia et al. ranged between 0 and 12.1%, with typical use pregnancy rates between 3 and 33% [13].

There are now multiple websites, downloadable apps, and electronic hormone fertility monitors (EFMH) available that may improve the success rates of use as they incorporate more information to determine the fertile period. Some of these methodologies may be expensive, requiring one to use test strips and other purchased equipment which may become cost-prohibitive for the average consumer.

Case Study

A 22-year-old patient and her partner present at the office to discuss birth control. They have not been sexually active prior to this time and are planning to be married in 3 months. They would like to put off pregnancy for 1–2 years yet and would like to have a method that is consistent with their religious beliefs. In their premarital counseling sessions, there was a discussion of natural family planning methods.

Diagnosis (Algorithm 12.1)

Request for natural family planning methods.

Indications (Algorithm 12.1)

- Patients who prefer a nonhormonal contraceptive method due to religious, personal preference or financial reasons
- Patients who have contraindications due to concomitant diseases or side effects to hormonal birth control
- Patients requesting immediately reversible contraception
- Patients who wish an increased awareness of their own body's hormonal cycles, including fertility and infertility

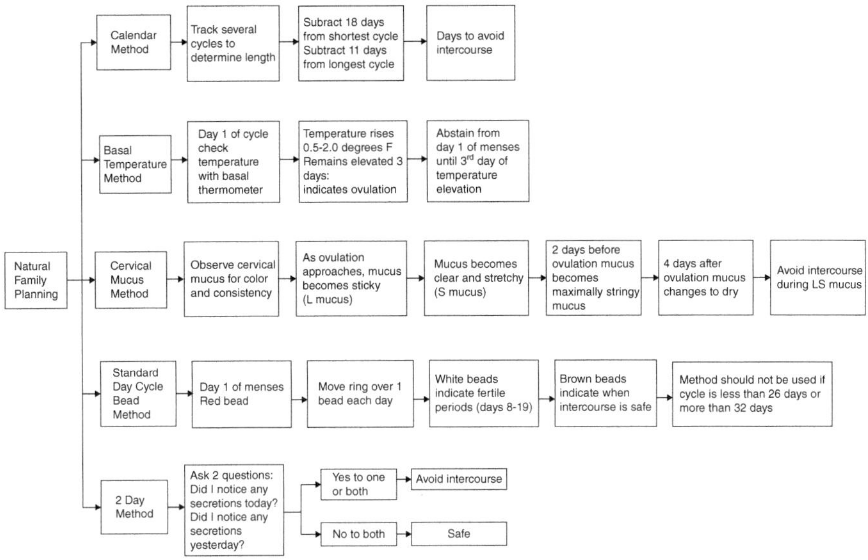

Algorithm 12.1 Decision tree for choosing a method of family planning

Contraindications, Complications, and Risks (Algorithm 12.1)

- High failure rate in couples who are not highly motivated.
- Requires periods of abstinence from intercourse.
- Less effective for patients with irregular menstrual cycles.
- No protection against sexually transmitted infections.
- Interference in charting the correct temperature can be caused by illness, alcohol use, travel, or interrupted sleep (at least 3 h of sleep must occur). These events should be noted on the chart.
- Monitoring of cervical mucus may be inaccurate if a vaginal infection is present, with the use of douches, vaginal creams, or gels, or if there is an illness or use of medication.

Equipment

- Basal body temperature thermometer (Fig. 12.1)
- Chart for temperature and recording consistency of cervical mucus
- Mucus and menstrual bleeding chart (Fig. 12.2)

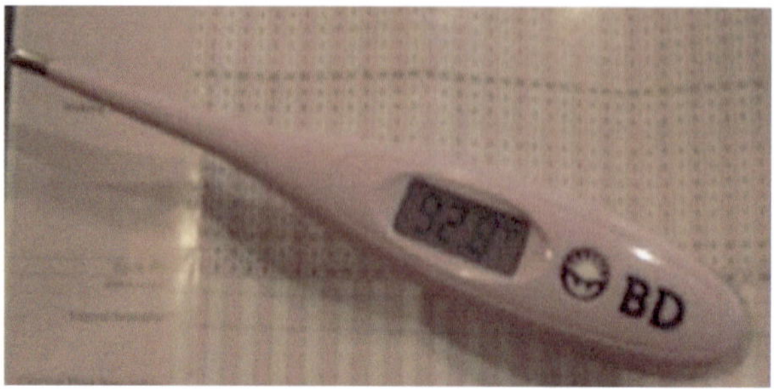

Fig. 12.1 Sample digital basal body temperature thermometer (Becton Dickinson & Co., Franklin Lakes, NJ)

Basal Body Temperature Chart

Name: ____________________ Age: ________

Cycle Day:	1	2	3	4	5	6	7	8	9	10	11	12	13	14	15	16	17	18	19	20	21	22	23	24	25	26	27	28	29	30	31	32
Date:																																
99.0																																
98.9																																
98.8																																
98.7																																
98.6																																
98.5																																
98.4																																
98.3																																
98.2																																
98.1																																
98.0																																
97.9																																
97.8																																
97.7																																
97.6																																
97.5																																
97.4																																
97.3																																
97.2																																
97.1																																
97.0																																

Take your temperature before getting out of bed. Record the temperature by placing a mark in the box that correlates to your temperature for the day of cycle. A lasting elevation in temperature indicates ovulation occurred two or three days prior. Cycle day one is the first day of menses.

Fig. 12.2 Basal body temperature and cervical mucus chart

Procedure and Patient Instructions (Algorithm 12.1)

Calendar Method

1. Track several menstrual cycles to determine length. (Cycle determination is based on the first day of menses as day 1 of the cycle.)
2. Subtract 18 days from the shortest cycle.
3. Subtract 11 days from the longest cycle.
4. This determines the range of days to avoid intercourse.

Example

- Month 1 cycle 30 days.
- Month 2 cycle 28 days.
- Month 3 cycle 32 days.
- Month 4 cycle 28 days.

- Patient subtracts 28–18 = 10.
- Patient subtracts 32–11 = 21.
- Patient would avoid intercourse between days 10 and 21.

Basal Temperature Method

1. Day 1 of cycle (menses) begins charting basal body temperature with a basal thermometer marked to detect small fluctuations in body temperature.
2. Temperature must be checked prior to getting out of bed at the same time each morning.
3. A rise in temperature of 0.5–2.0 °F that remains elevated for 3 days indicates ovulation. Ovulation occurs just prior to the temperature elevation.
4. A true postovulatory rise lasts 10 days.
5. The period of abstinence should be from the first day of menses through the third day of temperature elevation to completely cover the fertile period.
6. Interference in charting the correct temperature can be caused by illness, alcohol use, travel, or interrupted sleep (at least 3 h of sleep must occur). These events should be noted on the chart.

Cervical Mucus Method

1. Patients should be instructed to observe their cervical mucus:

   Observe the mucus for color and consistency on undergarments or toilet paper. Highly fertile secretions are wet, slippery, clear, and stretchy. Ovulation can occur the day before, during, or after the day of the clear stretchy mucus.

2. At the end of menses: G mucus forms a plug in the cervix causing the patient to be dry or without cervical mucus discharge.
3. As ovulation approaches, G mucus decreases and L mucus increases. L mucus has a sticky, cloudy nature.
4. With increasing estrogen: S mucus increases and peaks on the day of peak estrogen during the cycle. The combination of S and L mucus causes clear, stretchy mucus that aids the survival of sperm and transport through the female genital tract.
5. Two days prior to ovulation, the stringy sensation is at a maximum.
6. Two hours prior to ovulation, the slippery sensation or wetness is at its most noticeable.
7. Four days after ovulation, the mucus pattern reverts back to dry or unchanging as the G mucus again develops under the influence of progesterone.

Monitoring of cervical mucus may be inaccurate if there is vaginal infection; use of douches, vaginal creams, or gels; illness; or use of medication.

The Standard Day (CycleBead® Method, Cycle Technologies, Inc., Washington, DC) (Fig. 12.3)

1. Patients are considered fertile on days 8–19 of their cycle.
2. Patients start on the first day of their menstrual cycle with the red bead.
3. Move the ring over one bead each day.
4. White beads indicate fertile periods.
5. Brown beads indicate nonfertile periods when intercourse is safe.
6. The dark brown bead indicates a cycle shorter than 26 days, and this method should not be used.
7. If the menses does not start by the end of the brown beads, the cycle is longer than 32 days, and this method should not be used.

Two-Day Method

- Uses cervical secretions to determine fertility.
- Patient asks herself two questions:
  - "Did I notice any secretions today?"
  - "Did I notice any secretions yesterday?"
- If the patient noticed secretions, either day she is potentially fertile and should avoid intercourse.

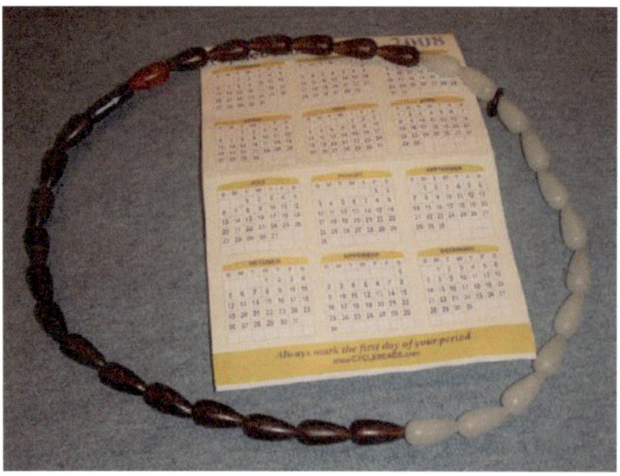

Fig. 12.3 CycleBeads® (Cycle Technologies, Inc., Washington, DC)

- If the answer is no to both questions, then the probability of pregnancy is low and intercourse is safe.

  Fertility rates are similar to the standard day method.

Marquette Method

- Patient measures six cycles using monitor and mucus.
- The estimated fertile window begins on day six and ends 3 full days after the last peak reading.
- After 6 cycles, the fertility period is based on the earliest high reading of the last 6 cycles.
- Method must be taught by a trained health professional.

Procedure Note (Provider to Customize as Needed)

The patient and her partner were counselled on the different methods of Natural Family Planning and made aware of the advantages and disadvantages of each, including the risk of pregnancy. The patient was instructed to chart her menstrual bleeding and symptoms throughout the month and to bring the chart with her to future visits so that the chart could be evaluated with the patient to aid in understanding of cyclic periods of fertility. The patient and partner will decide whether they want to include basal temperature monitoring as a part of their daily monitoring. They are encouraged to hire a natural family planning coach to give further instruction and training in the method they choose.

Coding

CPT® Codes (Current Procedural Terminology, AMA, Chicago, IL)	
Preventive Medicine Counselling:	
99401–15 min	
99402–30 min	
99403–45 min	
99404–60 min	
ICD 10-CM-Diagnostic Codes (International Classification of Diseases, 9th Revision, Clinical Modification, Centers for Disease Control and Prevention)	
Z30.02	Counselling and instruction in Natural Family Planning to avoid pregnancy

Case Study Outcome

After 1 year of use of natural family planning, the couple continues to be satisfied with their choice of birth planning method. The patient has discontinued the use of basal temperature as her comfort level with the use of cervical mucus to determine that fertility has increased. She also considers it an added benefit that she has increased understanding of her fertility cycles and will be able to use that information to her advantage when she does desire pregnancy.

References

1. Bradley S, Polis C, Micks E et al. Effectiveness, Safety & Comparative Side Effects In: Carson P, et al, editor. Contraceptive Technology. 22 rev ed. Burlington MA: Jones & Bartlett Learning; 2023. p. 189–227.
2. Grimes DA, Gallo MF, Grigorieva V, Nanda K, Schulz K. Fertility awareness-based methods for contraception: systematic review of randomized controlled trials. Contraception. 2005;72:85–90.
3. Tommaselli GA, Guida M, Palomba S, Barbato M, Nappi C. Using complete breastfeeding and lactational amenorrhoea as birth spacing methods. Contraception. 2000;61(4):253–7.
4. Frank-Herrmann P, Gnoth C, Baur S, Strowitzki T, Freundl G. Determination of the fertile window: reproductive competence of women – European cycle databases. Gynecol Endocrinol. 2005;20(6):305–12.
5. Ryder RE. Natural family planning: effective birth control supported by the Catholic Church. BMJ. 1993;307:723–76.
6. Stanford JB, Smith KR, Dunson DB. Vulvar mucus observations and the probability of pregnancy. Obstet Gynecol. 2003;101(6):1285–93.
7. Hilgers TW, Stanford JB. Creighton model NaProEducation technology for avoiding pregnancy. Use effectiveness. J Reprod Med. 1998;43:495–501.
8. Germano E, Jennings V. New approaches to fertility awareness-based methods: incorporating the standard days and 2Day methods into practice. J Midwifery Womens Health. 2006;51:471–7.
9. Smoley BA, Robinson CM. Natural family planning. Am Fam Phys. 2012;86(10):924–8.
10. Sinai I, Lundgren RI, Gribble JN. Continued use of the standard days' method. J Fam Plann Reprod Health Care. 2012;38(3):150–6.
11. Mu Q, Fehring RJ, Bouchard T. Multisite effectiveness study of the Marquette method of natural family planning program. Linacre Q. 2022;89(1):64–72. https://doi.org/10.1177/0024363920957515. Epub 2020 Sep 27. PMID: 35321484; PMCID: PMC8935430
12. Scherwitzl EB, Danielsson KG, Sellberg JA, Scherwitzl R. Fertility awareness-based mobile application for contraception. Eur J Contracept Reprod Health Care. 2016;21(3):234–41. https://doi.org/10.3109/13625187.2016.1154143.
13. Urrutia RP, Polis CB, Jensen ET, et al. Effectiveness for fertility awareness-based methods for pregnancy prevention: a systematic review. Obstet Gynecol. 2018;132(3):591–604. https://doi.org/10.1097/AOG.0000000000002784.

Web Sites

An in-depth explanation of the method and assistance in finding an instructor can be found at the web site: www.CreightonModel.com.
Couple to Couple League: http://www.ccli.org/
http://www.familyplanning.net
http://www.popepaulvi.com
http://www.irh.org
http://www.fertaware.com
http://www.woomb.org
https://www.mmnfp.com/marquettenfp

Chapter 13
Copper Intrauterine Device

Elizabeth H. McNany and Meghan E. Boshart

Introduction

The intrauterine device (IUD) is a popular and reliable form of reversible contraception, accounting for 16.8% of contraception in patients of reproductive age worldwide [1]. In the United States, 17% of patients have IUDs as their chosen contraceptive method; three percent of these IUDs are non-hormonal copper IUDs [2]. Modern IUDs are recognized as a safe and effective form of birth control when prescribed to appropriate candidates.

There are currently five types of IUDs in use in the United States. Four of these devices contain varying doses of the progestin hormone levonorgestrel and are effective for 3 to 8 years, depending on the device. The fifth IUD is the copper device, first approved by the FDA in 1984 for use under the brand name ParaGard®. It is the only nonhormonal LARC in use [3]. It can remain in place effectively for up to 10 years, with evidence-based research supporting 12 years of use although not yet FDA approved for the longer use [4]. Both hormonal and nonhormonal IUDs are extremely effective forms of birth control, with rates of unintentional pregnancy of 0.1–0.4% and 0.8%, respectively. [5].

The copper IUD (Cu-IUD) is thought to provide contraception by interfering with several steps of the reproductive process and ultimately preventing fertilization. Insertion of the IUD creates a localized foreign body response within the endometrium, recruiting inflammatory products that are released into the luminal fluid. These products, along with the copper ions released from the IUD, are toxic to spermatozoa and oocytes, and their presence in the luminal fluid impairs sperm and

E. H. McNany (✉)
Faculty, St. Joseph's Family Medicine Residency, Syracuse, NY, USA
e-mail: Elizabeth.McNany@sjhsyr.org

M. E. Boshart (✉)
PGY2, Boston Medical Center Family Medicine Residency, Boston, MA, USA

S. M. Sulik, C. B. Heath (eds.), *Primary Care Procedures in Women's Health*,
https://doi.org/10.1007/978-3-032-07061-6_13

ovum migration. This prevents the meeting of healthy gametes and thus the formation of viable embryos [6]. Because this effect is so rapid at its onset, Cu-IUDs can also serve as an effective form of emergency contraception (EC) when inserted within five days of unprotected intercourse. Unlike hormonal forms of EC, its effectiveness does not decrease with larger body habitus. Over 99% of patients who opt for Cu-IUD as EC do not become pregnant, establishing it as the most reliable form of emergency contraception [7].

Determining which IUD is most appropriate for a patient depends on multiple elements including individual characteristics, accessibility, affordability, patient preferences, and medical comorbidities. The provider should obtain a detailed history and ensure the patient has a thorough understanding of the benefits and risks associated with the copper IUD as well as when to seek emergency care. The clinician should emphasize this, and a patient handout may be given to the patient for reference.

Case Study

A 27-year-old female patient presents to the office requesting an IUD. She has been on oral contraceptives for the past 10 years. She often forgets to take them and would like something more permanent. She has had a stable male partner for the past 10 years, and they do not wish to have a child within the next few years. Her periods are regular, she has never had a sexually transmitted infection, and her pap smears have all been normal. She is interested in a copper IUD, as she prefers a nonhormonal method.

Indications (Algorithm 13.1) [7, 8]

- Patients who desire long-term reversible contraception
- Failure of a previous birth control method due to noncompliance
- Previous uncomplicated use of IUD
- Contraindications to hormonal contraception
- Transgender males with a uterus who wish to have a hormone-free LARC
- Emergency contraception within 5 days of intercourse
- Patients with the following medical conditions have no contraindications to Cu-IUD use:
  - Breastfeeding
  - Breast cancer
  - Prior ectopic pregnancy
  - Past PID
  - HIV infection
  - Obesity
  - Poorly controlled diabetes mellitus, hypertension, or liver disease

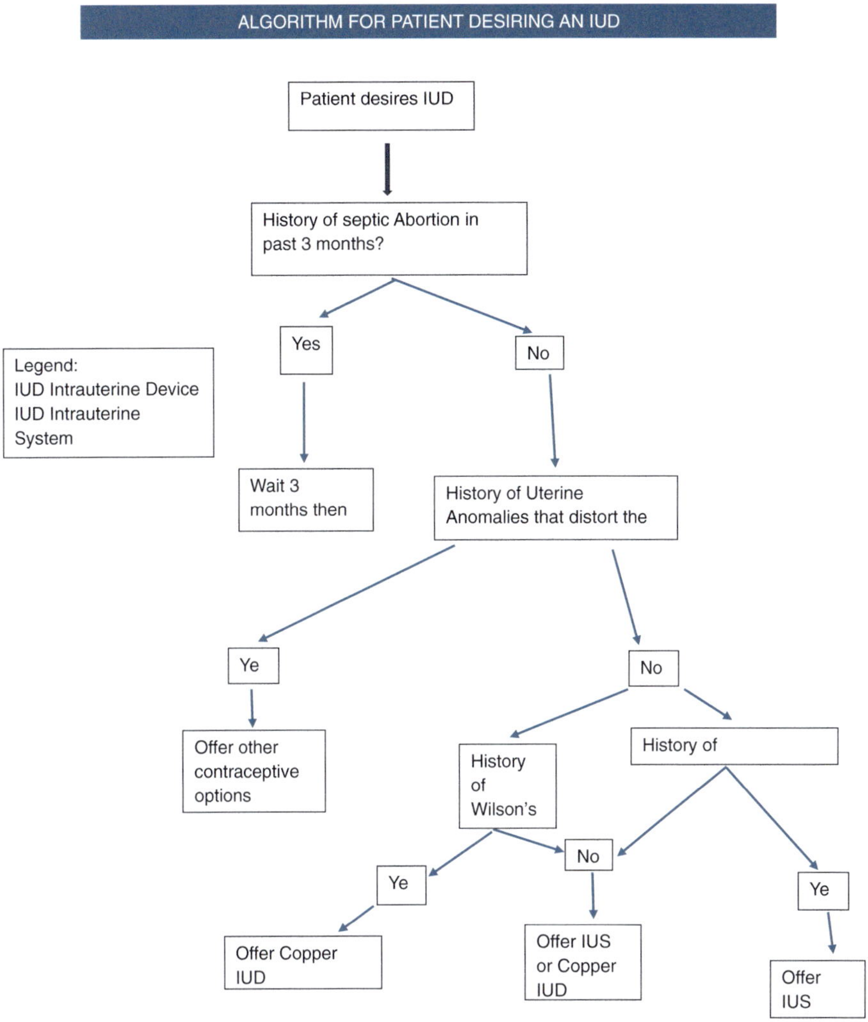

Algorithm 13.1 Decision tree for determining a long-acting reversible contraceptive method. *IUD* intrauterine device, *LNG-IUD* levonorgestrel IUD, *Cu IUD* copper IUD. Cu IUD Duramed Pharmaceuticals, Cincinnati, OH; LNG-IUD Bayer Pharmaceuticals Inc., Wayne, NJ; Nexplanon®, NV Organon, Schering Corporation, Kenilworth, NJ; Essured®, Conceptus Inc, San Carles, CO; Depo-Provera®

Contraindications [8–11] (Algorithm 13.1)

Absolute Contraindications

- Current pregnancy
- Postpartum endometritis or postabortal endometritis within the past 3 months
- Anatomical abnormalities of the uterus resulting in distortion of the uterine cavity
- Current pelvic inflammatory disease

- Confirmed gestational trophoblastic disease with persistently elevated β-Hcg levels or malignant disease
- Known or suspected uterine or cervical malignancy
- Vaginal bleeding of unknown etiology
- Active purulent cervicitis, chlamydial infection, or gonococcal infection
- Pelvic tuberculosis
- Wilson's disease
- Allergy to any component of Paragard®
- A previously placed IUD that has not been removed.

Relative Contraindications (Algorithm 13.1)

- Excessively heavy periods or marked dysmenorrhea
- Severe thrombocytopenia
- Small uterine cavity (higher risk of expulsion if uterus <6 cm)

Equipment (Fig. 13.1)

- Paragard® T 380A (Duramed Pharmaceuticals, Cincinnati, OH)
- Speculum
- Basin with cotton balls moistened with antiseptic solution
- Cervical tenaculum
- Uterine sound
- Sterile gloves
- Nonsterile gloves
- Sterile towel for tray top
- Long suture scissors
- Topical anesthetic (Hurricane®, Beutlich LP Pharmaceuticals, Waukegan, IL)
- Ring forceps

Procedure

1. Recommended timing of device insertion
    - Device may be inserted at any time during the menstrual cycle for patients not currently using contraception or patients switching from oral, transdermal, or vaginal form of hormonal contraception or an injectable progestin contraceptive. Previous method should be discontinued at this time.

- If switching from a contraceptive implant or other intrauterine system, the device should be inserted on the same day the previous method is removed.
- Device should be inserted immediately following abortion or miscarriage.
- Device may be inserted immediately postpartum.

2. Prior to placement:

- Discuss thoroughly with the patient the risks, benefits, and expectations for follow-up after placement and obtain signed consent.
- Document negative pregnancy test.
- Screen patients based on CDC recommendations who have not undergone routine screening for sexually transmitted infection (STI). If the patient requires screening due to increased risk of STIs or previous lack of screening, IUD insertion should not be delayed. STI screening and IUD insertion should occur at the same visit. Placement of the IUD should not be delayed for the results of the screen. Treatment of a positive screen can occur without the removal of the IUD. The American College of Obstetricians and Gynecologists (ACOG) does not recommend screening the low-risk patient [10].
- Pain management should be discussed with the patient prior to the procedure. There is good evidence that use of topical lidocaine or paracervical block are both effective for pain management with IUD insertion. While NSAIDs are commonly recommended there is no evidence that they reduce the pain with IUD insertion unlike endometrial biopsy [12].

3. Perform a bimanual exam to check for the position of the uterus.
4. Insert a warm vaginal speculum (large enough to easily visualize the cervix)

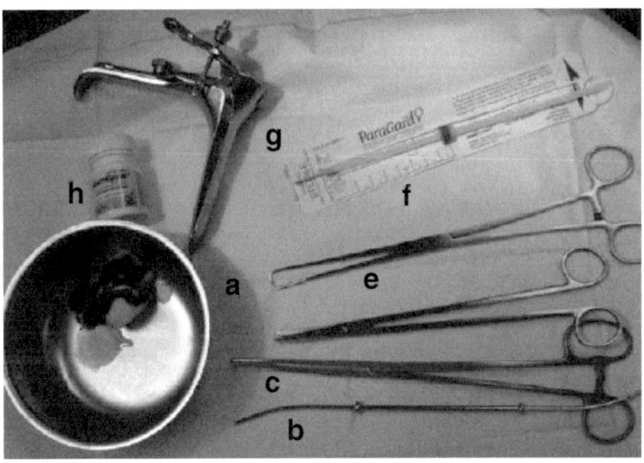

Fig. 13.1 Equipment setup for copper IUD. (**a**) Metal basin with cotton balls soaked in iodine; (**b**) sterile uterine sound; (**c**) sterile long Kelly forceps; (**d**) long scissors; (**e**) sterile cervical tenaculum; (**f**) sterile Paragard® (Duramed Pharmaceuticals, Cincinnati, OH) IUD Contraceptive; (**g**) Graves speculum; (**h**) topical cervical anesthetic (Hurricane®, Beutlich LP Pharmaceuticals, Waukegan, IL)

5. Clean the cervix with an antiseptic solution.
6. Apply a topical anesthetic to the cervix (if a tenaculum is going to be used).
7. Remove nonsterile gloves and put on sterile gloves.

Steps 8–18 should be done using sterile technique.

8. Use a sterile uterine sound to determine the depth of the uterus. The uterus should be between 6 and 9 cm to continue with the placement of an IUD.
9. Stabilize cervix, if needed, by the application of a single-tooth tenaculum to the anterior lip of the cervix.
10. Have the assistant place the contents of the IUD package on a sterile towel. Alternatively, do this step prior to changing into sterile gloves, making sure the contents of the package drop onto the sterile towel in a manner that maintains the sterile field.
11. Insert the solid white inserter rod so that it just touches the tip of the vertical arm of the IUD (Fig. 13.2).
12. Fold the horizontal arms down and place them inside the tube. (Do not do this step more than 5 min prior to placement.) Insert the arms no further than necessary to ensure retention.
13. Adjust the blue flange on the inserter rod to the depth of the uterus as determined by sounding, measuring from the top of the folded IUD to the blue flange. Be sure that the horizontal arms of the T of the IUD are parallel to the horizontal orientation of the long axis of the blue flange to ensure the arms open in the correct direction (Fig. 13.3).
14. If needed, use the tenaculum to stabilize the cervix.
15. Next, pass the insertion tube through the cervical canal and into the uterus up until the blue flange reaches the level of the cervix (Fig. 13.4).
16. Ask an assistant to hold the tenaculum in place (if using) and hold the solid white rod steady in the nondominant hand.
17. Using the dominant hand, pull back on the clear insertion tube 1 cm to release the arms of the IUD. The solid-colored rod should *not* move (Fig. 13.5).

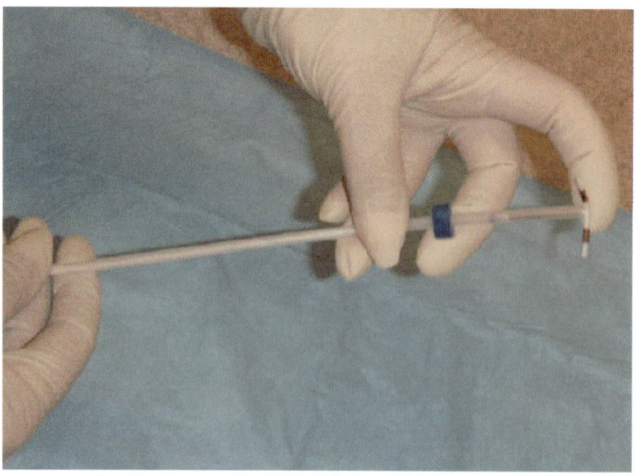

Fig. 13.2 Insert the white rod into the insertion tube and move up to the tip of the IUD. Keep a finger on the IUD to prevent it from falling out of the insertion tube

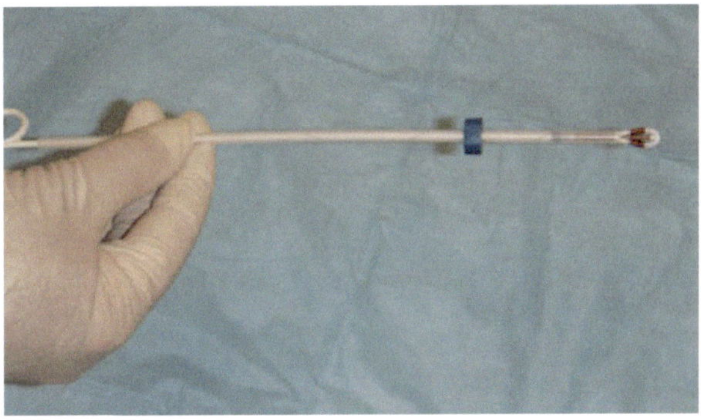

Fig. 13.3 Fold down the arms into the insertion tube just enough to hold in place. Adjust the blue flange to the measured uterine length

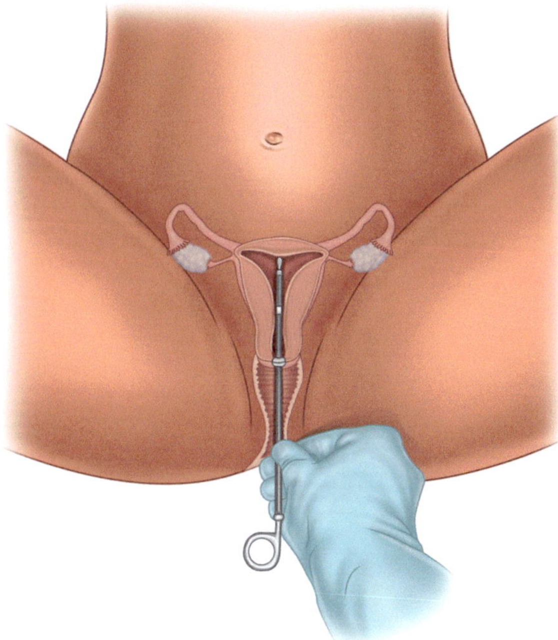

Fig. 13.4 Insert the IUD into the uterus until it meets the fundus (measured by the blue flange)

18. Once the IUD is released, gently push the tube inserter toward the fundus until slight resistance is felt to ensure the highest placement of the IUD.
    - Hold the insertion tube steady and withdraw the solid white rod.
    - Slowly and gently withdraw the insertion device, leaving only threads protruding from the cervix.
19. Cut the threads protruding from the cervical os to 3–5 cm in length (Fig. 13.6) and document length in records.
    - It is best to leave threads longer because they can be shortened at the follow-up visit if necessary.

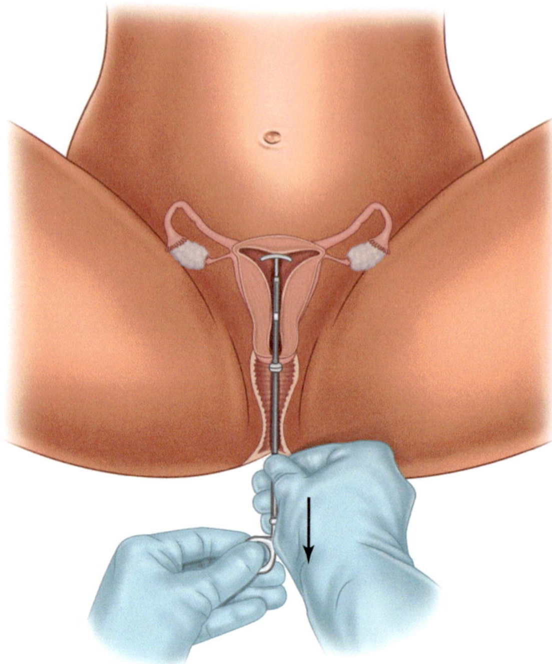

Fig. 13.5 Holding the white rod steady, pull the insertion tube toward the clinician. Once the IUD is released, push the insertion tube back up to the blue flange to anchor the IUD in the fundus of the uterus. Then, remove the rod and the insertion tube

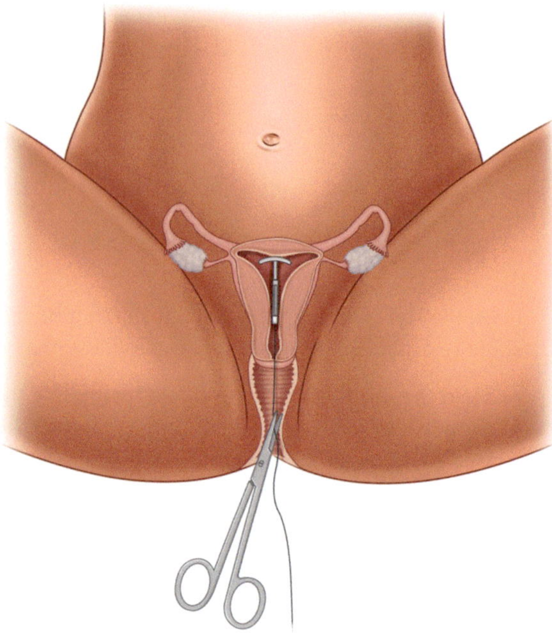

Fig. 13.6 Cut the strings 3–5 cm from the os and give the strings to the patient so she knows what they feel like on self-examination

20. Instruct the patient on how to check for strings after each menstrual period and prior to intercourse. Be sure to give the patient the handout provided by the company that gives information about when to contact a healthcare provider.
21. Schedule a follow-up appointment with the patient after the first menstrual period to assess placement. If there is any concern about whether the IUD is properly placed, an ultrasound can be done to assess placement (this is rarely needed).

Complications and Risks

- Cramping and bleeding:
  - This is the most common reason that women request removal within the first year at rates of approximately 12% [10]. The cramping can be treated with nonsteroidal anti-inflammatory drugs (NSAIDs), but if bleeding symptoms persist for more than three to four cycles, consider prescribing a short course of estrogen or oral contraceptive pills. If the bleeding persists, removal may be considered.
- Expulsion:
  - Expulsion rates of 2.3% were seen in clinical trials [10]. Expulsion typically occurs during menses, and if the uterine cavity is greater than 9 cm. Remind the patient to check for the strings on a regular basis [5, 10]. If the location of the device is uncertain, an ultrasound can determine the location of the IUD.
  - When the IUD is inserted later in the menstrual cycle, the expulsion rates are lower.
  - Risk of expulsion is elevated with immediate postpartum insertion as the uterus is not completely involuted at this time [10].
- Pelvic inflammatory disease (PID):
  - Risk immediately after IUD placement is 0.5% [11]. Patients who are at low risk for STIs have little risk of PID with IUD use after the initial 20 days post-insertion. There is no indication for prophylactic antibiotics at the time of insertion to reduce PID. A meta-analysis confirmed that prior antibiotic use conferred little benefit [13].
- Uterine perforation.
  - Partial or complete uterine perforation is a rare complication (occurring in 0.1–0.3% of placements). The device should be located and removed once perforation has occurred, and surgical correction may be required. Delay in identifying perforation may allow for device migration outside of the uterine cavity resulting in further complications [10]. Proper technique and uterine sounding are important to help prevent this from occurring.

- Pregnancy.
  - If pregnancy is confirmed and the IUD is in place, the IUD should be removed as soon as possible. There is a higher rate of ectopic pregnancy in patients who become pregnant while using an IUD. However, pregnancy is rare due to its high rate of effectiveness.

Tricks and Helpful Hints

- Advance a large cotton-tipped applicator (Scopette®, Birchwood Laboratories, Eden Prairie, MN) in with the uterine sound. The applicator's cotton swab will stop at the cervix; continue to advance the sound to the fundus of the uterus. Then remove the applicator and the sound simultaneously with the same hand. The distance from the top of the cotton applicator to the top of the sound is a clear indication of the uterine depth.
- Disposable uterine sounds are smaller and more comfortable for the patient than traditional metal sounds. They are typically the same size as the IUD applicator.
- Show the device through the packaging to the patient prior to insertion to reassure her of the small size and configuration of the device.
- If the IUD is contaminated or dropped, call the manufacturer who will replace it free of charge or contact the manufacturer through their website. Be sure to keep both the IUD and the box to give to the manufacturer's representative.

Procedure Note (Provider to Customize as Needed)

Complications, risks, and benefits of IUD discussed. Consent signed by patient and provider. Pregnancy test performed, and patient is not pregnant. Bimanual examination performed; speculum applied, and cervix visualized without difficulty. Cervix washed with antiseptic three times. Tenaculum placed under local anesthetic. Uterus sounded to 6–9 cm in size. IUD inserted without difficulty. Strings cut to appropriate length. Strings given to the patient to feel, and instructions given on how to check for the strings. Patient tolerated the procedure well.

Coding

CPT® Codes (Current Procedural Terminology, AMA, Chicago, IL)

58,300 Insertion of IUD
J7300 Charge for the cost of copper IUD

ICD 10-CM-Diagnostic Codes (International Classification of Diseases, 10th Revision, Clinical Modification, Centers for Disease Control and Prevention)

Z30.430 Encounter for insertion of intrauterine contraceptive device
Z30.431 Encounter for routine checking of intrauterine contraceptive device

Postprocedure Patient Instructions [10]

- Educate the patient on how to check for strings once a month.
- Be sure to give the patient the handout provided by the company that gives information about when to contact a healthcare provider. Emphasize the following major concerns:
  - The patient should check for the strings of the IUD after each menstrual period. If not palpable, she should contact her healthcare provider.
  - Remind the patient to report any of the following: excessive pain, malodorous discharge, excessive bleeding, fever, prolonged pelvic discomfort or pain during intercourse, genital lesions, suspicion of STIs, missed period, or any other concerns she may have.
- Schedule a follow-up appointment with the patient after the first menstrual period to assess placement.

Case Study Outcome

The patient had an IUD inserted without difficulty in her provider's office. She was delighted to discontinue her oral contraceptive pills and reported no difficulty with her IUD.

Postprocedure Patient Handout (Provider to Customize as Needed)

- Check for the strings from the IUD after each menstrual period, and if you cannot feel them, contact your provider immediately.
- You may have increased bleeding during your periods and spotting between periods during the first 2–3 months after placement. Typically, these symptoms improve with time, but if they persist, contact your provider.
- You may have cramping associated with the placement of the IUD, but if the pain is severe, let your provider know.
- When to contact your provider:

– If you think you are pregnant.
– If you cannot feel the strings from the device or the length has changed.—If you have severe menstrual bleeding.
– If you have pelvic pain during sex.
– If you have unusual vaginal discharge or genital sores.
– If you have an unexplained fever.
– If you may have been exposed to any STI.
– If you or your partner becomes HIV positive.
– Continued cramping pain, particularly within the first month after insertion.

References

1. United Nations Department of Economic and Social Affairs, Population Division (2022). World Family Planning 2022: Meeting the changing needs for family planning: Contraceptive use by age and method. UN DESA/POP/2022/TR/NO. 4.
2. Gomez AM, Bennett AH, Arcara J, et al. Estimates of use of preferred contraceptive method in the United States: a population-based study. Lancet Reg Health Am. 2024;30:100662. https://doi.org/10.1016/j.lana.2023.100662.
3. Howard SA, Benhabbour SR. Non-hormonal contraception. J Clin Med. 2023;12:4791. https://doi.org/10.3390/jcm12144791.
4. Wu JP, Pickle SA. Extended use of the intrauterine device: a literature review and recommendations for clinical practice. Contraception. 2014;89(6):495–9.
5. Trussell J, Aiken ARA, Micks E, Guthrie KA. Efficacy, safety, and personal considerations. In: Hatcher RA, Nelson AL, Trussell J, Cwiak C, Cason P, Policar MS, Edelman A, Aiken ARA, Marrazzo J, Kowal D, editors. Contraceptive technology. 21st ed. New York: Ayer Company Publishers; 2018.
6. Ortiz ME, Croxatto HB. Copper-T intrauterine device and levonorgestrel intrauterine system: biological bases of their mechanism of action. Contraception. 2007;75(6 Suppl):S16–30. https://doi.org/10.1016/j.contraception.2007.01.020.
7. Goldstuck ND, Cheung TS. The efficacy of intrauterine devices for emergency contraception and beyond: a systematic review update. Int J Womens Health. 2019;11:471–9. https://doi.org/10.2147/IJWH.S213815. PMID: 31686919; PMCID: PMC6709799
8. Curtis KM, Tepper NK, Jatlaoui TC, et al. U.S. Medical Eligibility Criteria for contraceptive use, 2016. MMWR Recomm Rep. 2016;65(No. RR-3):1–104. https://doi.org/10.15585/mmwr.rr6503a1externalicon.
9. ACOG practice bulletin, long-acting reversible contraception: implants and intrauterine devices, Number 186, November 2017.
10. Paragard package insert, FEI Products LLC, Last revision February 2020.
11. Wu JP, Moniz MH, Ursu AN. Long-acting reversible contraception-highly efficacious, safe, and underutilized. JAMA. 2018;320(4):397–8. https://doi.org/10.1001/jama.2018.8877.
12. Pain Management for In-office Uterine and Cervical Procedures: ACOG Clinical Consensus No 9, Obstetrics and Gynecology 146(1): p. 161–177, July, 2025.
13. Grimes DA, Schulz FK. Antibiotic prophylaxis for intrauterine contraceptive device insertion. Cochrane Database Syst Rev. 1999;3:CD001327. https://doi.org/10.1002/14651858.CD001327.

Additional Resources

Website

Supplier: Duramed Pharmaceuticals: www.paragard.com

Chapter 14
Levonorgestrel Intrauterine System Insertion

Meghan E. Boshart

Introduction

The levonorgestrel-releasing intrauterine system (LNG IUS) is one of the most effective, safe, and convenient reversible contraceptive methods. Current rates of all long-acting reversible contraceptive (LARC) methods have increased fivefold from 2005 to 2015 [1]. Women are choosing LARCs at a higher rate than previously with 14% of patients in the United States choosing an intrauterine device (IUD) and 4% choosing a subdermal implant [2].

These increasing rates are seen alongside decreasing rates of unintended pregnancy in the United States indicating that LNG IUS usage is likely a contributing factor [2]. These increases can be seen worldwide and are likely due to the variety of advantages that this method provides. The LNG IUS can be used in fertile patients irrespective of age or parity, and its localized release of hormones results in relatively low systemic blood levels making its side effects less severe for many patients. The LNG IUS also provides noncontraceptive health benefits including treatment of menorrhagia, uterine fibroids, and, potentially anemia as often the patient has little or no menses while using LNG IUS. LNG IUS is an excellent LARC whose user-effective rates are equal to its method-effective rates [3].

LNG IUS insertion is a relatively simple procedure that can be performed in the office setting by trained providers. The LNG IUS consists of a polyethylene T-shaped device with a hormone reservoir, which releases small amounts of levonorgestrel at a constant rate into the uterine cavity over time. Mirena® was the first LNG IUS introduced in the United States, and several additional LNG IUS have been added to the marketplace within the last several years [4].

M. E. Boshart (✉)
PGY2, Boston Medical Center Family Medicine Residency, Boston, MA, USA
e-mail: boshartm@upstate.edu

S. M. Sulik, C. B. Heath (eds.), *Primary Care Procedures in Women's Health*,
https://doi.org/10.1007/978-3-032-07061-6_14

All LNG IUS have similar mechanisms of action. The major effect is by thickening the cervical mucus and suppressing the formation of the endometrial lining of the uterus. The thick mucus prevents sperm passage through the uterus, while the progestin effects on the endometrium allow it to remain thin and nonproliferative [5]. A localized foreign body reaction is also observed in the uterine cavity upon insertion of the IUD, making the environment hostile for spermatozoa survival [6]. Contrary to older beliefs that LNG IUDs act as an abortifacient, recent tubal washing studies have demonstrated that these combined mechanisms provide contraception through prevention of fertilization [6].

Currently, there are four Food and Drug Administration (FDA)-approved LNG IUS available in the United States, each with varying levonorgestrel doses, lengths of efficacy, and device sizes. The currently approved devices are LNG-20 (Mirena®), LNG-19.5 (Kyleena®), LNG-18.6 (Liletta®), and LNG-13.5 (Skyla®). Mirena® and Liletta® each contain a total of 52 mg of levonorgestrel, and release 20 mcg/day and 18.6 mcg/day, respectively. Kyleena® contains a total of 19.5 mg of levonorgestrel and releases 17.5 mcg/day; Skyla® contains a total of 13.5 mg of levonorgestrel and releases 14 mcg/day of levonorgestrel (see Fig. 14.2).

Mirena® and Liletta® have both been FDA approved for 8 years of contraceptive prevention and are the only LNG IUSs that have been FDA approved for treatment of menorrhagia, each for a duration of up to 5 years. These devices were found to have comparable effects in reducing blood loss and improving the quality of life in users with heavy menstrual bleeding [7]. Kyleena® and Skyla® have been FDA-approved for contraception for up to 5 years and 3 years, respectively. All LNG IUS have similar side effect profiles and comparable efficacy rates (>99%). Bleeding pattern changes including decreased menstrual bleeding and amenorrhea are less severe with LNG IUS with lower hormone concentration [4].

Mirena®, Kyleena®, and Skyla® have a similar inserter design and use the same technique for insertion. All three are nonreloadable. The newer single-handed Liletta® inserter with a double slider mechanism is slightly different from the other LNG IUS in terms of design and technique. Liletta®'s inserter tube is 2 cm longer than the other LNG IUS and has the capacity to be reloaded. Kyleena® and Skyla® are smaller in size (28X30 mm) with narrow inserters, which allows easier insertion.

Interval placement of LNG IUS (insertion at 4 plus weeks postpregnancy) is the current most common postpartum practice decreasing the risk of expulsion. However, numerous studies have been conducted evaluating the safety and efficacy of immediate postplacental (IPP) placement, placement at the time of medication abortion, and placement immediately after early pregnancy manual vacuum aspiration (MVA) abortion. All of these methods have been determined to be safe and effective at reducing pregnancy rates within the first year. Contrary to initial concerns, IPP placement has been shown to have no effect on breastfeeding initiation, continuation, or infant growth. Decision on placement timing should involve shared decision-making with the patient [8].

The cost of IUDs in the United States ranges between $600 and $1400 in 2024, not including the insertion fee; cost has been a major limiting factor for both providers and patients. Some insurance companies have a buy-and-bill policy for LNG IUS, which limits some providers due to the high cost of stocking LNG IUS in the office. Other insurances allow the patient or provider to order the LNG IUS on an individual basis. Most private insurance companies cover one type of LNG IUS, with an additional standard fee for the insertion. Liletta® was developed to be a low-cost option available to public health clinics.

Case Study

A 26-year-old, who is now G2P1011, returns to your office 6 months postpartum requesting birth control. She has been together with the father of the baby for 3 years, and they do not have any partners outside this relationship. Her Pap smear was normal. She has no history of CIN or HPV, and screening for other infections during pregnancy was negative.

Indications (Algorithm 14.1)

- Long-term reversible contraception
- Monogamous
- Prefers continuous contraception

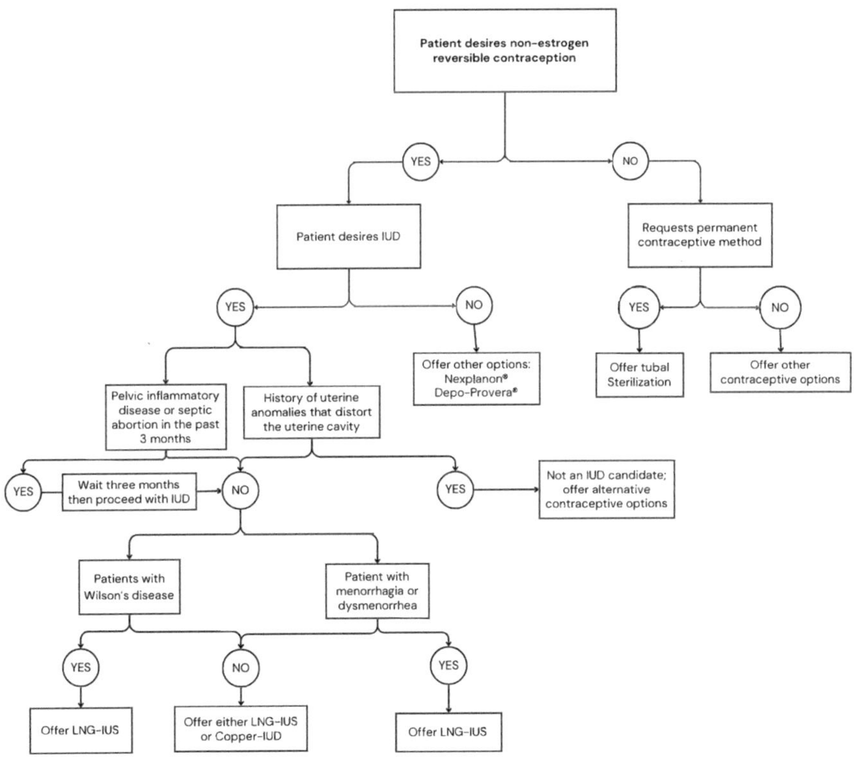

Algorithm 14.1 Candidates for IUD placement

Contraindications (Algorithm 14.1)

Relative Contraindications [9]

- Past diagnosis of breast cancer without evidence of current disease for the past 5 years
- Systemic lupus erythematosus
- Decompensated cirrhosis
- •Hepatocellular adenoma or carcinoma

Absolute Contraindications [9]

- Pregnancy
- Postpartum sepsis or immediate postseptic abortion
- Unexplained vaginal bleeding
- Suspected or known endometrial, breast, or uterine neoplasia or any progestin-sensitive cancer
- Confirmed malignant gestational trophoblastic disease
- Abnormal uterine anatomy (some patients with fibroids may be candidates)
- Current pelvic inflammatory disease (PID)
- Current purulent cervicitis or chlamydial infection or gonococcal infection
- Uterine cavity less than 6 cm or greater than 9 cm depth (associated with higher expulsion rates)
- Sensitivity to prior exposure to systemic levonorgestrel

Time of Insertion

- LNG IUS can be inserted at any time during the menstrual cycle if reasonably certain that there is no pregnancy. If inserted in the first 7 days of the menstrual cycle, then no backup contraception is needed. If switching from other forms of hormonal contraception, discontinue use of prior method 7 days after IUD insertion. LNG IUS can be used immediately after childbirth or abortion. Insertion can be delayed up to 4 weeks postpartum to decrease the risk of device expulsion. If the provider and patient choose to place LNG IUS immediately postpartum, the patient needs to be counseled about the higher possibility of expulsion or malposition. LNG IUS is not approved for the use of emergency contraception [2, 4, 8].

Equipment (Fig. 14.1)

- Levonorgestrel intrauterine system (Fig. 14.2)
- Nonsterile exam gloves
- Sterile gloves
- Urine pregnancy test
- Speculum
- Light source
- Iodine/povidine solution
- Tenaculum

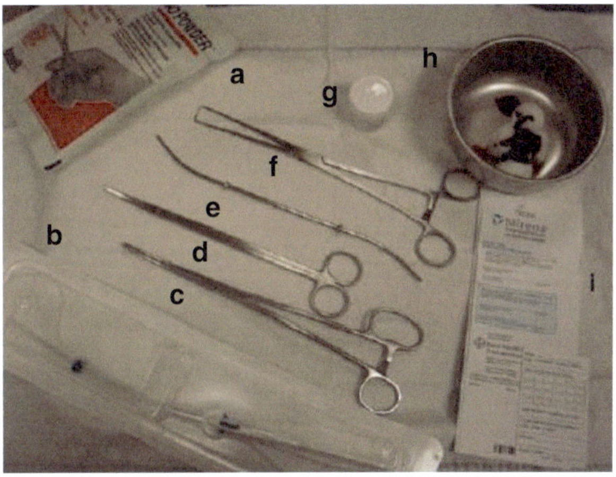

Fig. 14.1 Sterile tray for Levonorgestrel IntraUterine System insertion: (**a**) sterile nonlatex gloves; (**b**) LNG IUS in sterile package; (**c**) long Kelly forceps; (**d**) long scissors; (**e**) sterile uterine sound; (**f**) sterile cervical tenaculum; (**g**) specimen jar (if needed for Pap); (**h**) metal basin with sterile cotton balls soaked in iodine; (**i**) Mirena® permit and patient card

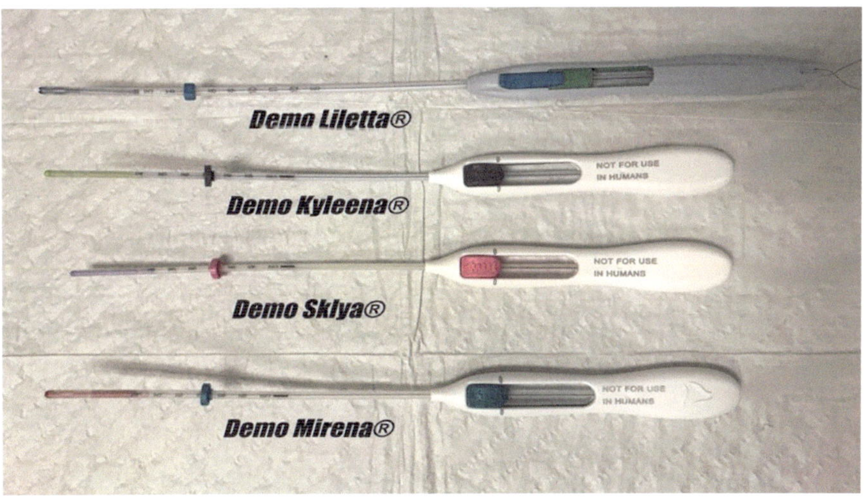

Fig. 14.2 Different LNG intrauterine systems available in the United States

- Uterine sound
- Ring forceps
- Gauze
- Large cotton swabs (with a long shaft for use in a speculum). Scopettes®(Birchwood Labs, Eden Prairie, MN)
- Long-handled scissors
- Instruments and anesthesia for paracervical block

Insertion Procedure (Figs. 14.3, 14.4, 14.5, 14.6, 14.7, 14.8, 14.9, 14.10, 14.11, and 14.12)

1. Patients should receive the LNG IUS manufacturer's patient education to review before the procedure. Pamphlets and a video are also available. Review the patient's STI risk and any screening for STIs. Review risks, benefits, and side effects with the patient. Ask if she has any questions about LNG IUS use.

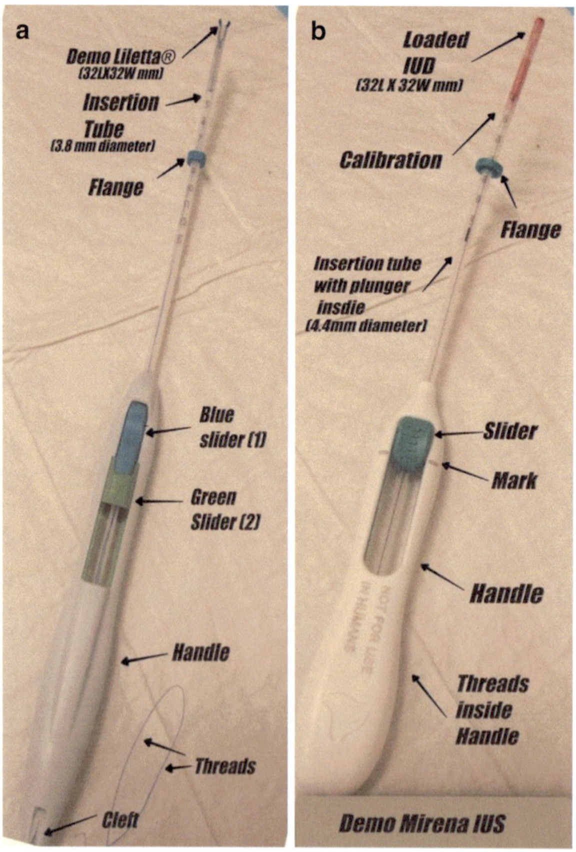

Fig. 14.3 Terminology for (**a**) Liletta® and (**b**) Mirena® IUS insertion system

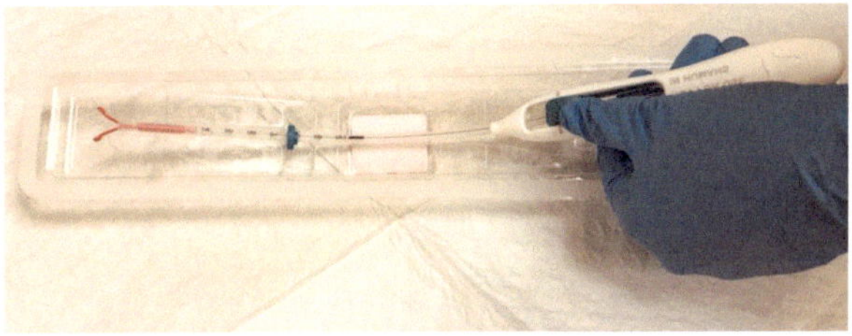

Fig. 14.4 Remove IUS from sterile packaging using a sterile technique

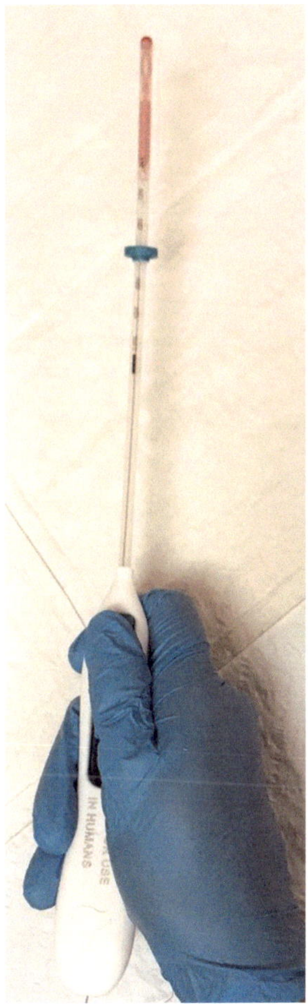

Fig. 14.5 Advance the slider to the furthest away position which causes the IUS device to be folded into the insertion tube

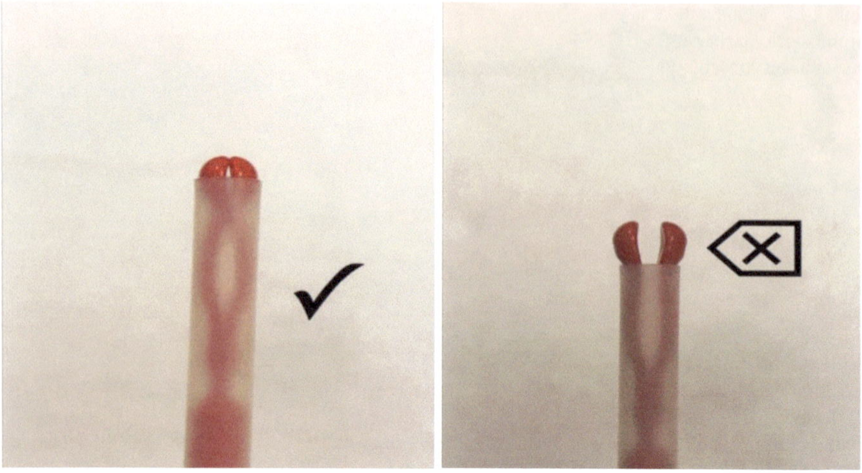

Fig. 14.6 Horizontal arm tips fold superiorly into the insertion tube

Fig. 14.7 Adjust flange to the depth of the uterine sound using the sterile side of the packaging as a counterpressure

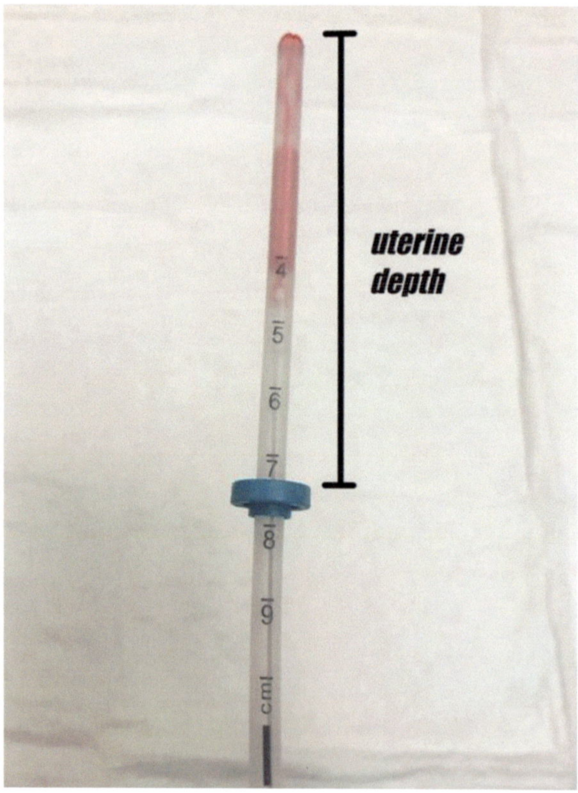

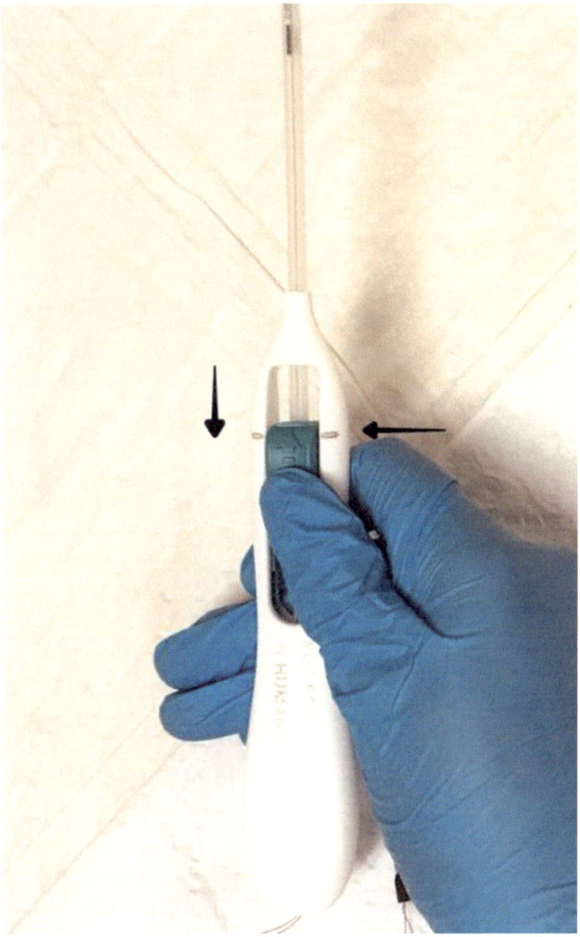

Fig. 14.8 Close-up of mark on handle

2. Confirm that the patient is not pregnant with a urine pregnancy test. Sign the consent form and ask the patient to sign the consent form with a witness present.
3. Place the patient in the dorsal lithotomy position. Perform a bimanual exam to estimate the uterine size and to confirm the position and direction of the uterine cavity.
4. Place a speculum and visualize the cervix.
5. Replace your exam gloves with a new pair of sterile gloves.
6. Swab the cervix with an antiseptic. Use large swabs or gauze folded in the ring forceps, and paint the cervix with the iodine solution to sterilize the outer cervix.
7. Grasp the anterior lip of the cervix with the tenaculum about 1.5 cm from the os. Close the tenaculum slowly until one tooth is engaged.

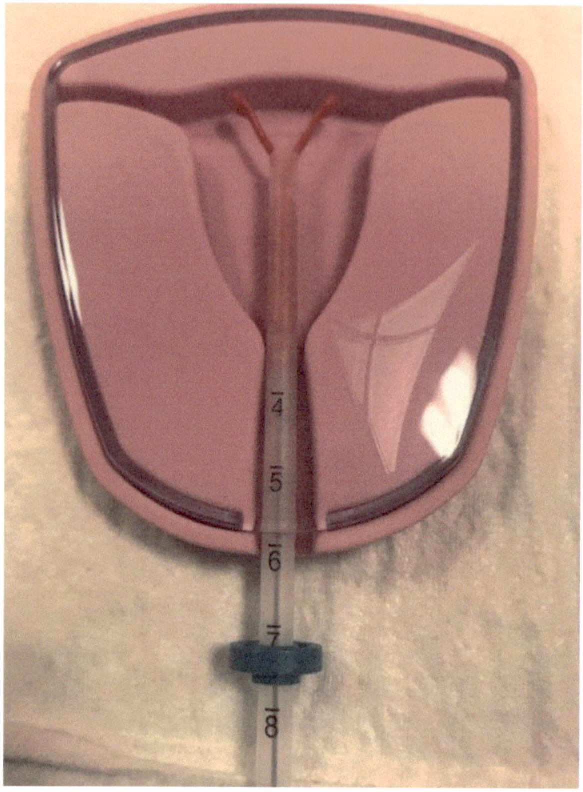

Fig. 14.9 Extend arms horizontally by pressing the slider to mark on the handle

8. Gently pull on the tenaculum to straighten the endometrial cavity before sounding the uterus. Maintain this traction when inserting the sound. Determine the endometrial cavity size with the uterine sound.
9. Open the IUS package and maintain the IUS in a sterile state (Fig. 14.4).
10. Remove the LNG IUS from the package by grasping the handle below the slider. Do not attempt to remove the IUS by pulling on the inserter tube (Fig. 14.4).
11. Push the slider on the inserter to the limit away from you. Confirm that the arms of the IUS are horizontal (Figs. 14.5 and 14.6).
12. Set the marker/flange on the inserter to the uterine depth measured with the uterine sound (Fig. 14.7).
13. Insert the IUS into the uterine cavity. Stop when the flange is 1.5–2 cm away from the cervix (Fig. 14.14).

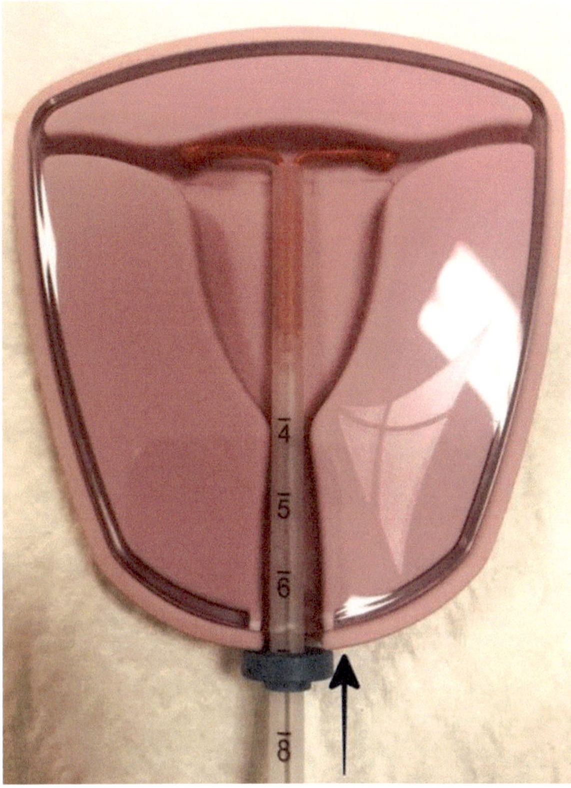

Fig. 14.10 Advance the handle so that the flange touches the endocervical os

14. Pull the slider 1 cm to allow the arms of the IUS to open. There is a mark on the inserter indicating that it has been pulled 1 cm back (Figs. 14.8 and 14.9). Allow 10–15 s so the IUS arms fully open.
15. Advance the whole inserter until the flange is at the os. This will place the open arms at the top of the uterine fundus (Fig. 14.10).
16. Pull the slider switch back to the limit toward you, releasing the IUD in the uterus (Fig. 14.11).
17. Remove the IUD inserter.
18. Trim the strings with the scissors so that 3–5 cm will remain (Fig. 14.12).
19. Remove the tenaculum and inspect for bleeding. Apply gentle pressure with a swab to achieve hemostasis.
20. Complete the removal date reminder card and give it to the patient.

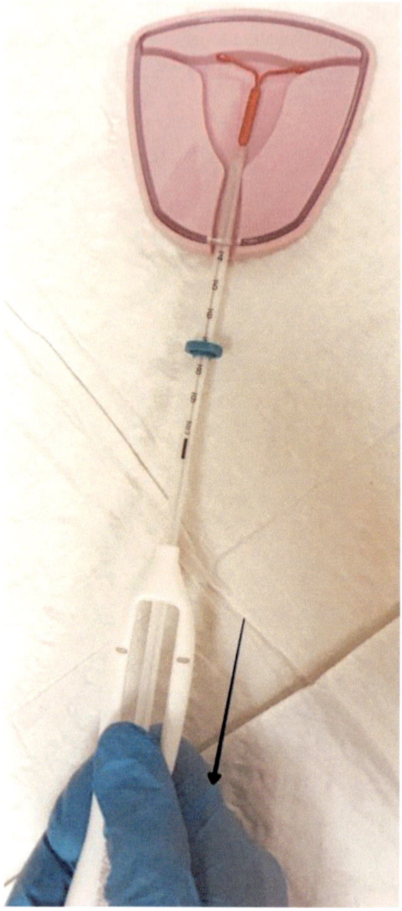

Fig. 14.11 Pull the slider fully toward the inserter, releasing the IUD in the uterine cavity

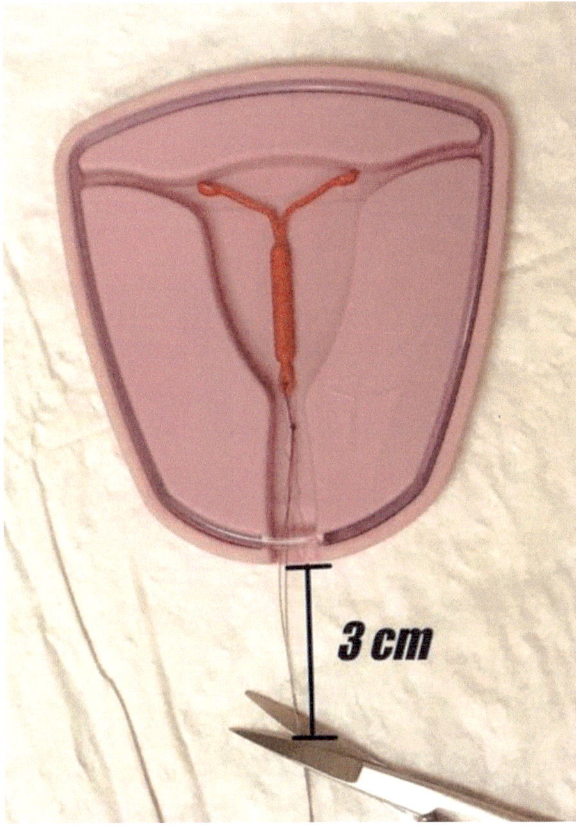

Fig. 14.12 Cut string 3–5 cm beyond the os

Liletta Insertion

1. Follow steps 1–10 above.
2. For Liletta®, push your thumb on the blue slider keeping the green slider steady as shown in Fig. 14.5.
3. For loading Liletta® IUD in the inserter tube, pull the strings at the base of the inserter until the LNG IUS system is drawn into the inserter. Lock the strings into the handle of the inserter (Figs. 14.13).
4. Insert the IUD into the uterine cavity. Stop when the flange is 1.5–2 cm away from the cervix. For Liletta®, maintain forward pressure on the blue slider while inserting the IUD (Fig. 14.14).
5. Pull the slider 1 cm to allow the arms of the IUD to open. There is a mark on the inserter indicating that it has been pulled 1 cm back (Figs. 14.8 and

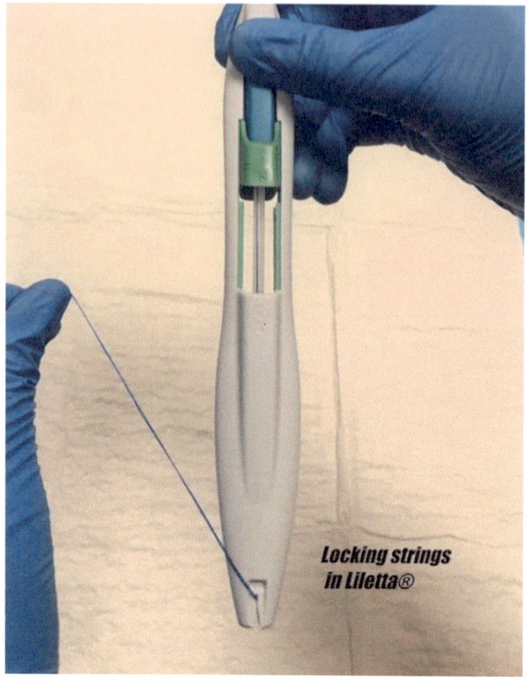

Fig. 14.13 For Liletta®, lock strings into place maintaining forward pressure on the blue slider to load the IUD

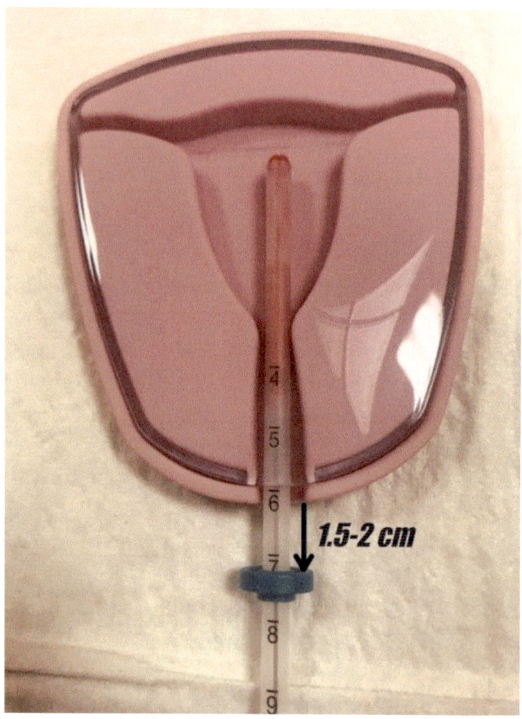

Fig. 14.14 Insert system to within 1–2 cm of flange marker

14.9). For Liletta®, move the blue slider toward the green slider so that both sliders merge (Figs. 14.15 and 14.9). Allow 10–15 s so the IUD arms fully open.

6. Advance the whole inserter until the flange is at the os. This will place the open arms at the top of the uterine fundus (Fig. 14.10).
7. Pull the slider all the way to the limit toward you, releasing the IUD in the uterus (Fig. 14.11). For Liletta®, pull both the sliders (green and blue) toward you to release the IUD and confirm that this has released the strings (Fig. 14.16).
8. Remove the IUD inserter.
9. Trim the strings with the scissors so that 3–5 cm will remain (Fig. 14.12).
10. Remove the tenaculum and inspect for bleeding. Apply gentle pressure with a swab to achieve hemostasis.
11. Complete the removal date reminder card and give it to the patient

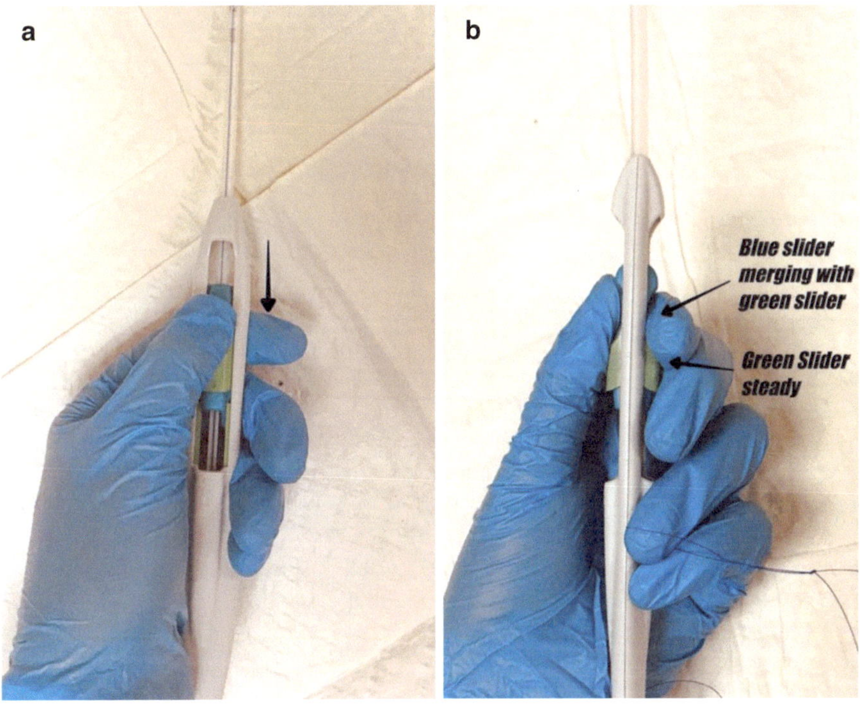

Fig. 14.15 Releasing arms in the uterine cavity (Liletta®)

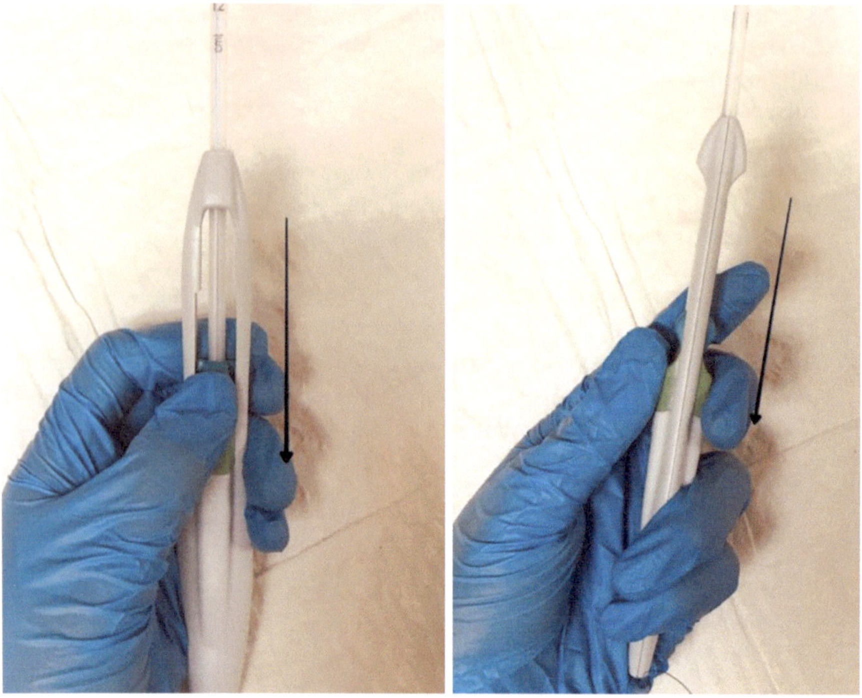

Fig. 14.16 Pull the slider toward the inserter, allowing the strings to release

Complications and Risks [10]

- Uterine perforation (rare)
- Expulsion (increased risk with immediate postpartum placement)
- Pelvic infection (greatest in the first month after insertion)
- Functional ovarian cysts
- Pain during placement
- Bleeding and cramping (common up to a week postprocedure)
- Spotting and irregular bleeding during the first 6 months
- Eventual amenorrhea

Tricks and Helpful Hints

- Show patients a nonsterile IUS and let them hold it when counseling them. Seeing how small and flexible an IUD is may reduce patient fear.

- Some providers prefer to do IUS insertions when patients are menstruating. This may be inconvenient but somewhat helpful with nulliparous and adolescent women with a narrower cervical canal.
- Before gripping the cervix with the tenaculum, you may want to pause the procedure and use lidocaine or Hurricane to anesthetize the anterior cervix or to perform a paracervical block. A 1% lidocaine paracervical block decreases pain during IUS insertions [11].
- If the uterus is retroverted, placing the tenaculum on the lower lip of the cervix and maintaining traction will help straighten the endometrial cavity.
- When maintaining traction on the tenaculum, you may need to monitor the speculum to ensure that it is not displaced.
- When advancing the sound, use torque to advance the tip. Put a very gentle bend in the sound and twist the tip from side to side to advance it. This is safer than pushing the tip in. If you meet resistance at the level of 3–4 cm, consider that you may be at the endocervix or at the fold near where the cervix joins the uterine body. Check to see if more traction is needed to straighten the uterus. In case of suspected cervical stenosis, the use of a dilator would be beneficial to overcome resistance [12]. Alternatively, use disposable plastic sounds which are of a similar diameter to the insertion device.
- Marking the maximum advance of the sound visually is difficult. Insert the long end of a swab adjacent to the sound and align the tip of this with the exocervix. Then, pull the sound and the swab out together. The tip should line up with the sound mark that corresponds to the uterine depth.
- Rinse the cut end of the IUS string and allow the patient to hold it so she can see what it feels like on her fingertip. This may facilitate finding the strings when the IUD is in place.
- Complete the reminder card from the LNG IUS package insert and give it to the patient.

Procedure Note

(Provider to fill in blanks/circle applicable choice when given multiple choices and customize as needed.)

- *Recent Pap shows no dysplasia, and cultures show no signs of sexually transmitted infections.*
- *Patient has no history of recent STIs.*
- *Patient understands the risk of bleeding, infection, pain/cramping, and the patient knows alternatives. She consented to IUD placement in writing after having an opportunity to ask questions.*
- *Bimanual exam performed.*
- *Speculum placed, cervix normal looking and midline.*
- *Cervix visualized and swabbed three times with Betadine.*

- *Tenaculum clamped onto anterior lip of cervix; uterus sounded to _____cm.*
- *Levonorgestrel IUS placed without complications per package insert.*
- *Arms deployed in a high fundal position.*
- *String trimmed and string palpation described to the patient. Bimanual exam after placement demonstrates no/minimal uterine tenderness.*

Coding

CPT® Codes (Current Procedural Terminology, AMA, Chicago, IL)
58,300 IUD insertion
58,301 IUD removal

HCPCS codes (healthcare common procedure coding system, level II)
J7298 Mirena, LNG-20 system
J7297 Liletta, LNG-18.6 system
J7296 Kyleena, LNG-19.5 system
J7301 Skyla, LNG-13.5 system
Skyla, LNG-13.5 system

ICD10-CM-diagnostic codes (international classification of diseases, tenth revision, clinical modification, Centers for Disease Control and Prevention)
Z30.430 IUD insertion
Z30.431 IUD surveillance
Z30.432 IUD removal
Z97.5 Presence of an IUD

Postprocedure Patient Instructions

Instruct the patient to return in 4–6 weeks for IUS string check. If the IUS is inserted after the first 7 days of the menstrual cycle, then a backup method (condoms or spermicide) should be used for 1 week postinsertion. Tell the patient to check the IUS string after each period. Instruct the patient to use ibuprofen after the insertion, as needed for cramping, and to call the office if she develops purulent discharge, fever, chills, nausea, vomiting, or excessive bleeding.

Case Study Outcome

The patient selected the levonorgestrel intrauterine system, which was inserted without difficulty in the office. She tolerated the procedure well and remarked at her follow-up visit that she was very satisfied with her selection.

Postprocedure Patient Handout

(Provider to fill in blanks/circle applicable choice when given multiple choices.) You have just had a Levonorgestrel Intrauterine System (LNG IUS) inserted on___________ (insert date). This contraceptive system is effective for ___ (insert years). Your levonorgestrel intrauterine system should be removed prior to__________________ (insert date/years from date of insertion).

Please remember to check for the LNG IUS string after every period.

Most women have no side effects from the LNG IUS, but common side effects include:

- Uterine cramping, which usually goes away within the first 3 months. Consider taking two 600 mg ibuprofen for pain up to every 6 h as needed.
- Change in bleeding pattern, including spotting and between-period bleeding. Most women eventually have little or no period.
- Acne, breast tenderness, weight gain, and back pain occur rarely (less than 3.5% of the time).

Please call your clinician's office if:

- You develop a smelly discharge or have a fever.
- Develop severe abdominal pain not relieved by ibuprofen.
- If the bleeding becomes excessive (more than one pad per hour or more than ten pads per day).
- You are interested in getting pregnant and wish for your provider to remove the LNG IUS. Please be aware that fertility returns immediately upon removal.

Please make a follow-up appointment in the office in 1 month.

References

1. Branum AM, Jones J. Trends in long-acting reversible contraception use among U.S. women aged 15–44. NCHS data brief, no 188. National Center for Health Statistics: Hyattsville; 2015.
2. Baker C, Creinin M. Long-acting reversible contraception. Obstet Gynecol. 2022;140(5):883–97. https://doi.org/10.1097/AOG.0000000000004967.
3. Rademacher KH, Sripipatana T, Pfitzer A, Mackay A, Thurston S, Jackson A, Menotti E, Traeger H. A global learning agenda for the Levonorgestrel intrauterine system (LNG IUS): addressing challenges and opportunities to increase access. Glob Health Sci Pract. 2018;6(4):635–43. https://doi.org/10.9745/GHSP-D-18-00383.
4. Long-Acting Reversible Contraception: Implants and Intrauterine Devices. ACOG practice bulletin no. 186. American College of Obstetricians and Gynecologists. Obstet Gyenocol. 2017;130:e251–69.
5. Bahamondes L, Fernandes A, Monteiro I, Bahamondes MV. Long-acting reversible contraceptive (LARCs) methods. Best Pract Res Clin Obstet Gynaecol. 2020;66:28–40. https://doi.org/10.1016/j.bpobgyn.2019.12.002.

6. Ortiz ME, Croxatto HB. Copper-T intrauterine device and levonorgestrel intrauterine system: biological bases of their mechanism of action. Contraception. 2007;75(6 Suppl):S16–30. https://doi.org/10.1016/j.contraception.2007.01.020.
7. Creinin MD, Barnhart KT, Gawron LM, Eisenberg D, Mabey RG Jr, Jensen JT. Heavy menstrual bleeding treatment with a Levonorgestrel 52-mg intrauterine device. Obstet Gynecol. 2023;141(5):971–8. https://doi.org/10.1097/AOG.0000000000005137. Epub 2023 Apr 5. PMID: 37023455; PMCID: PMC10108838.
8. Goldthwaite LM, Cahill EP, Voedisch AJ, Blumenthal PD. Postpartum intrauterine devices: clinical and programmatic review. Am J Obstet Gynecol. 2018;219(3):235–41. https://doi.org/10.1016/j.ajog.2018.07.013.
9. Curtis KM, Tepper NK, Jatlaoui TC, et al. U.S. medical eligibility criteria for contraceptive use, 2016. MMWR Recomm Rep. 2016;65(RR-3):1–104. https://doi.org/10.15585/mmwr.rr6503a1externalicon.
10. Mansour D. The benefits and risks of using a levonorgestrel-releasing intrauterine system for contraception. Contraception. 2012;85(3):224–34. https://doi.org/10.1016/j.contraception.2011.08.003.
11. Akers AY, Steinway C, Sonalkar S, Perriera LK, Schreiber C, Harding J, Garcia-Espana JF. Reducing pain during intrauterine device insertion: a randomized controlled trial in adolescents and young women. Obstet Gynecol. 2017;130(4):795–802.
12. Prine L, Shah M. Long-acting reversible contraception: difficult insertions and removals. Am Fam Physician. 2018;98(5):304–9.

Websites

https://hcp.mirena-us.com/mirena-insertion-removal-video/.
https://www.lilettahcp.com/.
https://hcp.kyleena-us.com/insertion-removal/.
http://hcp.skyla-us.com/insertion-and-removal/skyla-insertion-and-removal-video.php.

Chapter 15
Intrauterine Device Removal

Jennifer Amico and Cathryn B. Heath

Introduction

One of the many benefits of utilizing intrauterine contraception is the ease of use after insertion [1, 2]. However, while the intrauterine device (IUD) removal procedure is a short and straightforward procedure [1], needing a clinician to discontinue the method can be a downside to its use [3], and health care providers should strive to remove barriers to IUD removal whenever possible in order to support reproductive autonomy for IUD users [4, 5]. Following a request for removal and informed consent, retrieval of the apparatus can typically be accomplished in a short office visit.

There are currently five options for intrauterine contraception available for use in the United States. The T380A intrauterine copper contraceptive (Paragard®, CooperSurgical, Inc., Trumbull, CT) is licensed for use up to 10 years [6]. The hormonal intrauterine devices available in 2025 in the United States include Mirena [7] (Bayer, Whippany, NJ) and Liletta [8] (Abbvie Inc, North Chicago, IL), which are licensed for 8 years of use; Kyleena [9] (Bayer), which is licensed for 5 years of use, and Skyla [10] (Bayer), which is licensed for up to 3 years of use. Patients seek to have their IUD removed for a variety of reasons, including when they desire pregnancy, when they have reached the maximum recommended time for utilization of the apparatus, when they prefer a different method, or when they experience side

J. Amico
Department of Family Medicine and Community Health, Rutgers, Robert Wood Johnson Medical School, New Brunswick, NJ, USA
e-mail: jennifer.amico@rutgers.edu

C. B. Heath (✉)
Rutgers University Student Health, New Brunswick, NJ, USA
e-mail: heathcb@scarletmail.rutgers.edu

S. M. Sulik, C. B. Heath (eds.), *Primary Care Procedures in Women's Health*,
https://doi.org/10.1007/978-3-032-07061-6_15

effects such as pelvic cramping, irregular vaginal bleeding, hormonal effects from the progestin-containing devices (e.g. mood changes, ovarian cyst formation), or partner discomfort during intercourse [2, 11, 12]. While providers may be hesitant to remove an IUD for side effects that are likely to resolve or for side effects they feel are not due to the IUD, it is essential that the user be able to make an informed decision for removal regardless of the reason [4, 13].

While patients are typically advised to make an appointment with a clinician when they want the IUD removed, some users can successfully remove the IUD themselves [14, 15]. Since the start of the Covid-19 pandemic, more providers and organizations are counselling users about IUD self-removal [16, 17] and some organizations have created guides to assist IUD users in removing their own devices [18, 19]. However, current evidence demonstrates that only approximately 20% of users will be successful in removing their own IUDs [14], and many turn to self-removal only when removal by a provider is difficult for them to access [20]. Clinicians and organizations should strive to reduce barriers to IUD removal by a clinician when the patient desires the removal.

Case Study

A 27-year-old female, gravida 2 para 1011, presents to the office concerned about irregular bleeding since the insertion of her hormonal IUD 7 months ago. She reports that she was aware that cramping and irregular bleeding could occur, but her symptoms are more disruptive than she anticipated. She has also noted mood changes and weight gain of 15 pounds in the last 7 months. The patient originally tried to bear with it because she appreciates not having to worry about using birth control, and she and her partner are not ready for another child right now. The patient and her husband have unprotected sex regularly, and they remain mutually monogamous. She is otherwise healthy. Prior to the IUD, she had light regular periods and rarely needed nonsteroidal antiinflammatory medications (NSAIDs) for cramping.

She reports that she had a visit to see one of your colleagues and requested IUD removal 2 months ago, but your colleague instead told her to get more exercise and referred her for an ultrasound. She completed the ultrasound last month and tells you that she had difficulty making time to go to both radiology and this follow-up appointment today due to needing child care and arranging transportation for these visits. She is frustrated that her IUD was not removed 2 months ago when she requested it, especially because she was told it could be removed whenever she wanted.

You review her pelvic ultrasound images (Figs. 15.1 and 15.2) which confirm the presence of the IUD at the uterine fundus without abnormalities noted. You reassure the patient that you can take out the IUD today if she wants and regardless of whether she'd like to discuss another method today. She reports that she would like to switch to another highly effective method that doesn't cause irregular

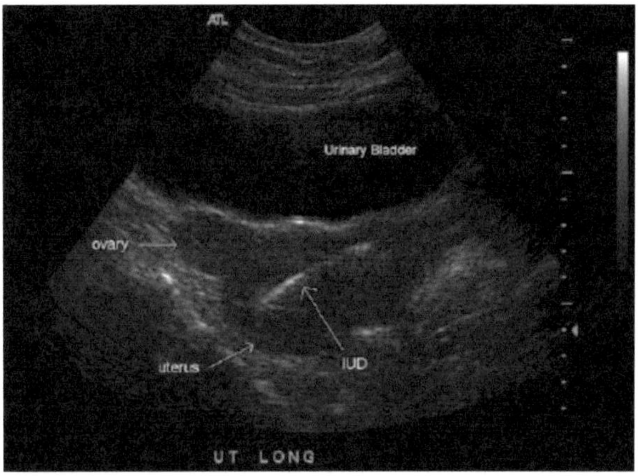

Fig. 15.1 Longitudinal view of an intrauterine device in the uterus

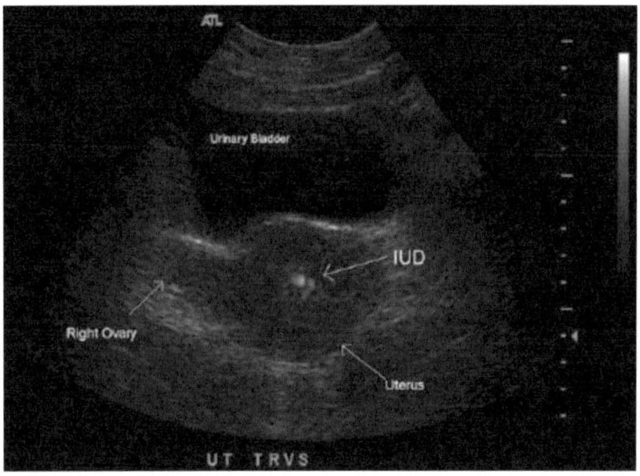

Fig. 15.2 Cross-sectional view of an IUD in the uterus

periods and that she doesn't have to remember every day or every week. Using her preferences as a guide, you discuss the copper IUD and the vaginal ring, and she prefers the copper IUD, but she is concerned about having difficulty accessing IUD removal again. You assure her that you will always be willing to remove her IUD given the strings are visible, and offer to discuss with her about how she can remove her IUD herself in the future if she desires, with the caveat that IUD self-removal is successful about 20% of the time. She appreciates having the potential to remove the IUD herself in the future if she desires, and you give her a resource that reviews how to self-remove an IUD. You discuss leaving the strings longer (4–5 cm) in order to aid in self-removal in the future and decrease the chances of missing strings in the future. She consents to IUD removal and replacement today and has appropriate insurance coverage verified for a copper IUD. A urine pregnancy test is negative.

On pelvic exam, a normal appearing cervix is identified, and IUD strings are noted passing through the external os approximately 2 cm long, with no abnormalities identified on bimanual exam. You easily remove the IUD with ring forceps prior to placing the copper IUD using the manufacturer's guidelines. The patient was given anticipatory guidance about IUD insertion (see Chap. 12).

Diagnosis and Indications

- Patient request for any reason
- Patient side effects and adverse reaction:
  - Pelvic pain
  - Back pain
  - Dysmenorrhea
  - Heavy menstrual bleeding, amenorrhea
  - Hormonal side effects including breast tenderness, mood changes, nausea, headaches, and ovarian cyst formation
  - Partial IUD expulsion
- Patient desires pregnancy
- Patient has reached the maximum recommended time for use
- Patient no longer has need for contraception (e.g., menopause, same-sex monogamous relationship, partner with vasectomy)
- Patient dissatisfaction
- Partner discomfort with intercourse
- Method failure: current intrauterine pregnancy

Contraindications

IUD removal in the presence of pregnancy should be performed by an experienced clinician following appropriate patient counseling and review of informed consent [21]. In the case of a rare IUD migration, embedment into the myometrium or cervical stroma, the IUD should be removed by an experienced clinician which may or may not require hysteroscopy. Perforation of the IUD through the uterine wall must be removed via referral for laparoscopic removal [21].

Equipment (Fig. 15.3)

Equipment for Straightforward IUD Removal

- Vaginal speculum
- Nonsterile gloves
- Ring forceps

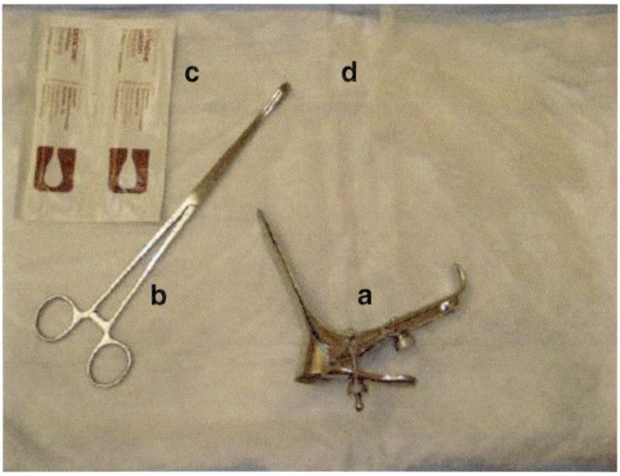

Fig. 15.3 Setup for IUD removal: (**a**) Pederson speculum; (**b**) ring forceps; (**c**) Betadine® Solution Swabsticks (Purdue Pharma, Stamford, CT); (**d**) gloves

Equipment for Potentially Complicated IUD Removal Including Evaluation of Absent Strings [21, 22]

- Vaginal speculum
- Nonsterile gloves
- Cytobrush, cytobroom, or two sterile cotton swabs
- Antiseptic solution
- Single-toothed tenaculum
- Alligator forceps or IUD hook
- Endocervical speculum
- Ring forceps
- Uterine sound or cervical dilators

Optional Equipment

- Colposcope
- Monsel's solution
- Silver nitrate sticks
- Topical or injectable anesthetic
- Ultrasound

Procedure

When IUD Strings Are Visualized [1]

1. Insert a speculum into the vagina to bring the cervix into view. Note that the IUD strings are visualized (Fig. 15.4).

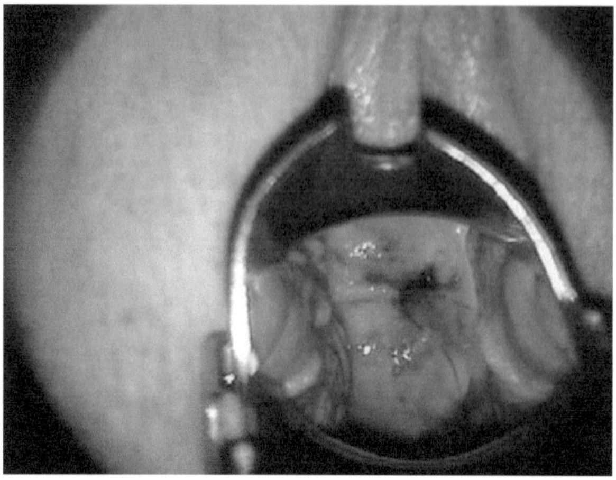

Fig. 15.4 Vaginal view of IUD string prior to removal

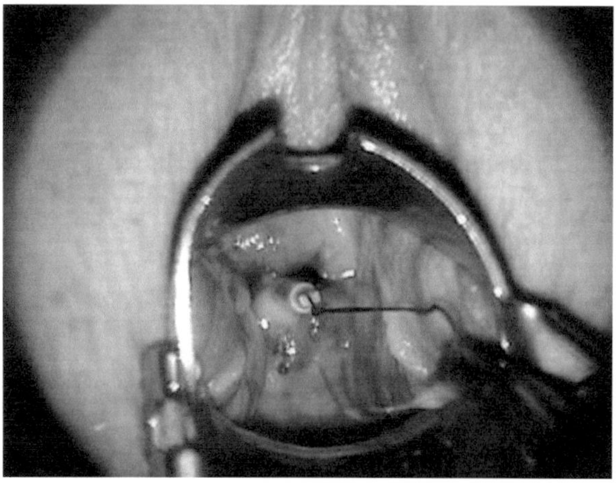

Fig. 15.5 Vaginal view of IUD during removal

2. Grasp the IUD strings with ring forceps and gently apply steady traction.
3. Encourage the patient to take a deep breath and exhale slowly, allowing for enhanced relaxation of the pelvic floor musculature as the IUD is withdrawn through the cervix (Fig. 15.5).

When IUD Strings Are Absent (Algorithm 15.1) [21, 22]

1. Perform a pregnancy test.
2. Perform a bimanual examination to determine the size and position of the uterus.
3. Insert a speculum into the vagina to bring the cervix into view. Cleanse the cervix with an antiseptic solution prior to instrumentation.

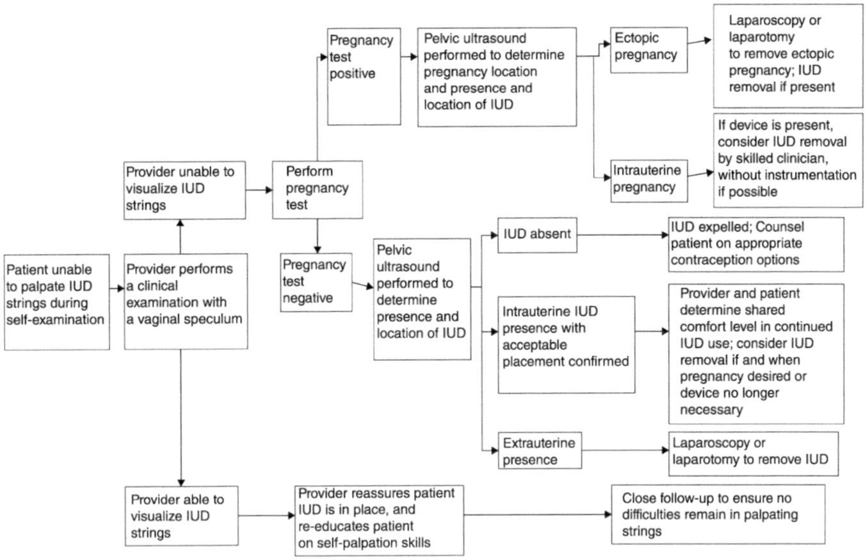

Algorithm 15.1 Decision tree for absent IUD strings. Note that some IUDs available outside the United States do not have strings

4. Consider a paracervical block with 10–20 cc of 0.5–1% lidocaine with or without epinephrine, particularly if cervical dilation is anticipated or if initial maneuvers (e.g., cytobrush) are unsuccessful.
5. Grasp the anterior lip of the cervix with a single-toothed tenaculum in order to maintain gentle traction to facilitate instrumentation.
6. Insert a cytobrush into the os, twirling as it is withdrawn, in the hopes of snagging the strings to permit removal of the device.
   - Alternatively, two sterile cotton swabs may be inserted and then twirled as they are withdrawn, in an attempt to snag the strings.
   - The cervix may be dilated with a uterine sound or cervical dilators, and an endocervical speculum may be inserted to facilitate visualization of the strings; alligator forceps or an IUD hook may then be passed to attempt grasping the strings.
7. Visualization of the uterus with an ultrasound may aid in more difficult removals but is not necessary for simple removals.
8. When retrieval has been attempted unsuccessfully, the patient may then require having the IUD removal performed with hysteroscopy in the operating room under anesthesia.

Tricks and Helpful Hints

- Advising a patient to take NSAIDs such as ibuprofen or naproxen prior to her appointment may help limit discomfort experienced during and following the procedure.
- Although less commonly utilized, specially designed instruments for IUD removal are commercially available, including the IUD hook and IUD thread retriever.
- It may be necessary to apply a single-toothed tenaculum to the anterior lip of the cervix in order to stabilize the cervix and uterus prior to instrumentation. Once the tenaculum has been removed, pressure can be applied to the puncture sites with a large swab to control any oozing of blood; silver nitrate or Monsel's solution can be used to treat any excessive bleeding.

Interpretation of Results

See Algorithm 15.1, which illustrates possible options for proceeding when IUD strings are absent [7].

Procedure Note: IUD Strings Visualized

(Clinician to customize as needed)

The patient was placed in the lithotomy position, a speculum was inserted into the vagina, and the cervix was identified. The IUD strings were noted to be passing through the external os. The strings were grasped with a ring forceps, and gentle traction was applied. The IUD was retrieved without incident. The patient tolerated the procedure without difficulty.

Procedure Note: IUD Strings Not Visualized

(Clinician to customize as needed)

The patient was placed in the lithotomy position, a speculum was inserted into the vagina, and the cervix was identified. The IUD strings were not visualized passing through the external os. Cytobrush was placed into the cervix to retrieve the strings with/without success. Paracervical block with [10–20 ml] of 1% lidocaine with/without epinephrine was administered. Single-tooth tenaculum was applied to the anterior lip of the cervix. Cervical dilation was achieved with cervical dilators (type, size)/uterine sound. Alligator forceps/IUD hook was utilized to grasp/retrieve

IUD strings with/without ultrasound guidance. Gentle traction was applied to remove the IUD intact. The patient tolerated the procedure without difficulty.

Coding

CPT® Codes (Current Procedural Terminology, AMA, Chicago, IL)
58301 Removal of intrauterine device
–22 modifier additional time needed for procedure
–52 modifier Failed procedure due to physical factors
–53 modifier Discontinued procedure due to patient well-being (e.g., vaso-vagal syncope)
76998 Ultrasonic guidance, intraoperative

ICD 10-CM-Diagnostic Codes (International Classification of Diseases, 10th Revision, Clinical Modification, Centers for Disease Control and Prevention)
Z30.432 Encounter for removal of an intrauterine device
Z30.433 Encounter for removal and reinsertion of an intrauterine device
Z 32.02 Pregnancy test-negative

Postprocedure Patient Instructions

The patient should be advised that she may experience mild cramping and minimal vaginal spotting and/or discharge in the first 12–24 h following removal. Although no further follow-up is usually necessary, any excessive bleeding should be reported immediately and the patient re-evaluated. Patients should be reminded of the subsequent rapid return to fertility once the apparatus has been removed [23].

Case Study Outcome

The patient presented to the office 15 months later for removal of her IUD, as she and her partner had decided that they were now emotionally and financially prepared to conceive again. The patient's periods had become regular, and her hormonal symptoms resolved after replacement of her hormonal IUD with a copper IUD last year, and she had no continued weight gain. She was considering removing her own IUD, but your office was able to offer a timely appointment that worked for her schedule, and she wanted to talk with you about planning for pregnancy. Upon repeat examination, the IUD strings were visualized and easily removed with ring forceps. You provided anticipatory guidance about IUD removal and pre-conception counselling prior to the end of the visit.

Postprocedure Patient Handout

(Provider to customize as needed)

- Today, your clinician removed your intrauterine device. You may expect minimal vaginal spotting or discharge and possibly mild abdominal cramping. You may have bleeding similar to a period or delayed irregular bleeding after removal of a hormonal IUD.
- If you experience heavier bleeding, foul-smelling vaginal discharge, persistent abdominal pain, or fevers, please call your clinician right away.
- Abdominal cramping is usually temporary. You may wish to take three ibuprofen 200 mg tablets every 6 hours (h) or two acetaminophen 325 mg tablets every 4–6 h, as needed.
- As a reminder, immediately following removal of your intrauterine device (IUD), you are now able to get pregnant if you have vaginal sex without the use of a condom or other barrier method. In fact, the majority of people trying to conceive are able to successfully become pregnant in the first year after removal of their IUD.
- Please call the office if you have any problems or questions.

References

1. Curtis KM, Jatlaoui TC, Tepper NK, et al. U.S. selected practice recommendations for contraceptive use, 2016. MMWR Recomm Rep. 2016;65(RR-4):1–66. https://doi.org/10.15585/mmwr.rr6504a1.
2. Long-Acting Reversible Contraception: Implants and Intrauterine Devices. ACOG practice bulletin no. 186. American College of Obstetricians and Gynecologists. Obstet Gynecol. 2017;130:e251–69.
3. Asker C, Stokes-Lampard H, Beavan J, Wilson S. What is it about intrauterine devices that IUD-users find unacceptable? Factors that make IUD-users non-users: a qualitative study. J Fam Plann Reprod Health Care. 2006;32(2):89–94.
4. Strasser J, Borkowski L, Couillard M, Allina A, Wood SF. Access to removal of long-acting reversible contraceptive methods is an essential component of high-quality contraceptive care. Womens Health Issues. 2017;3:253–5.
5. Gomez AM, Fuentes L, Allina A. Women or LARC first? Reproductive autonomy and the promotion of long-acting reversible contraceptive methods. Perspect Sex Reprod Health. 2014;46(3):171–5.
6. Cooper Surgical, Inc. ParaGard® prescribing information. February, 2020.
7. Bayer, Healthcare Pharmaceuticals: Inc Mirena® prescribing information. August, 2022.
8. Abbvie; Liletta:levonorgestrel releasing intrauterine system. Prescribing information. June, 2023.
9. Bayer Healthcare Pharmaceuticals Inc. Kyleena prescribing information. March, 2023.
10. Bayer Healthcare Pharmaceuticals Inc. Skyla prescribing information. March, 2023.
11. Diedrich JT, Madden T, Zhao Q, et al. Long-term utilization and continuation of intrauterine devices. Am J Obstet Gynecol. 2015;213(822):e1–6.

12. Cohen R, Sheeder J, Teal SB. Predictors of discontinuation of long-acting reversible contraception before 30 months of use by adolescents and young women. J Adolesc Health. 2019;65:295–302.
13. Manzer JL, Bell AV. The limitations of patient-centered care: the case of early long-acting reversible contraception (LARC) removal. Soc Sci Med. 2022;292(114362):1–8.
14. Foster DG, Grossman D, Turok DK, Peipert JF, Prine L, Schreiber CA, Jackson AV, Barar RE, Schwarz EB. Interest in and experience with IUD self-removal. Contraception. 2014;90(1):54–9.
15. Stimmel S, Hudson S, Gold M, Amico JR. Exploring the experience of IUD self-removal in the United States through posts on internet forums. Contraception. 2022;106:34–8.
16. Stifani BM, Madden T, Micks E, Moayedi G, Tarleton J, Benson LS. Society of Family Planning Clinical Recommendations: contraceptive care in the context of pandemic response. Contraception. 2022;113:1–12.
17. Fay KE, Traore F, Amico JR. Intrauterine device self-removal practices during the COVID-19 pandemic among family planning clinics. Contraception. 2023;118(109889):1–4.
18. Fact sheet: IUD Self-removal. https://www.reproductiveaccess.org/wp-content/uploads/2021/03/IUD-self-removal.pdf. Accessed 3/1/24.
19. How to Remove Your Intrauterine Device (IUD) by Yourself. https://picck.org/wp-content/uploads/2022/08/. PICCK-How-to-Remove-Your-Intrauterine-Device-IUD-By-Yourself.pdf. Accessed 3/1/24.
20. Amico JR, Stimmel S, Hudson S, Gold M. "$231 … to pull a string!!!" American IUD-users' reasons for IUD self-removal: an analysis of internet forums. Contraception. 2020;101(6):393–8.
21. Clinical Challenges of Long-Acting Reversible Contraceptive Methods. ACOG committee opinion no. 672. American College of Obstetricians and Gynecologists. Obstet Gyenocol. 2016;128:e69–77.
22. Prine L, Shah M. Long-acting reversible contraception: difficult insertions and removals. Am Fam Physician. 2018;98(5):304–9.
23. Stoddard AM, Xu H, Madden T, Allsworth JE, Peipert JF. Fertility after intrauterine device removal: a pilot study. Eur J Contracept Reprod Health Care. 2015;20:223–30.

Additional Resources

Web Sites

https://www.paragard.com/.
http://www.skyla-us.com/index.php.
https://www.liletta.com/.
https://www.mirena-us.com.
https://www.kyleena-us.com.

Chapter 16
Etonogestrel Subdermal Contraceptive Implant: Insertion

Jeffrey P. Levine and Joshua A. Mleczko

Introduction

The progestin-only, etonogestrel implant, Nexplanon®, is a sterile 4-cm × 2-mm single flexible rod that is implanted subdermally in a pregnancy-capable patient's upper arm and can provide up to 3–5 years of continuous highly effective contraception. Each rod contains 68 mg of the progestin etonogestrel and 15 mg of barium sulfate, encased in an ethylene vinyl acetate copolymer core and rate-controlling membrane [1]. It is supplied in a sterile, preloaded disposable applicator that prevents non-insertion, facilitates proper insertion in a superficial plane, reduces the risk of infection via contamination of the sterile rod, and allows insertion without the need for incision and concomitant risk of scarring.

Nexplanon® (FDA-approved 2011) replaced the original etonogestrel subdermal contraceptive implant, Implanon® (FDA-approved 2006), due to cases of incorrect insertions with the Implanon® applicator device. The changes from Implanon® to Nexplanon® include the addition of barium sulfate to the implant to allow for visibility on X-ray and CT scan and redesign of the applicator to facilitate single-handed insertion in the superficial plane of the skin.

The Implanon® and Nexplanon® rods look identical and contain the exact same amount of etonogestrel and ethylene vinyl acetate (EVA) copolymer. In a 3-year clinical trial, Nexplanon® and Implanon® yielded comparable exposure to

J. P. Levine (✉)
Department of Family Medicine and Community Health, Rutgers Robert Wood Johnson Medical School, New Brunswick, NJ, USA
e-mail: jeff.levine@rutgers.edu

J. A. Mleczko
Capital Health Primary Care – Bordentown, Bordentown, NJ, USA
e-mail: jmleczko@capitalhealth.org

S. M. Sulik, C. B. Heath (eds.), *Primary Care Procedures in Women's Health*,
https://doi.org/10.1007/978-3-032-07061-6_16

etonogestrel with the same pharmacokinetic, efficacy, and side effect data from earlier clinical trials utilizing Implanon®.

All physicians and advanced practice clinicians should participate in the FDA-mandated 2-hr live Nexplanon® Clinical Training Program to certify their ability to properly insert, localize, and remove the etonogestrel implant prior to performing these procedures on patients (www.nexplanontraining.com) [2]. In addition, they should review the insertion and removal instructions and package insert information prior to each related patient visit [1].

The Etonogestrel Implant (EI) is FDA-approved for patients seeking safe, convenient, highly effective, continuous, long-acting, and rapidly reversible contraception. Once inserted, EI offers patient convenience since its effectiveness is not user-dependent [3]. The implant can be removed at any time, with a rapid return to fertility. In particular, EI is a consideration for patients who do not want or cannot/should not use estrogen-containing contraceptives (e.g. uncontrolled hypertensive patients or cigarette smokers over 35 years old), and those willing to tolerate irregular menses, possibly for the full duration of use [4].

EI does not protect against sexually transmitted infections (STIs). While EI was not initially evaluated in patients >130% of their ideal body weight, several post marketing studies have not shown decreased efficacy with an increased body mass index (BMI) [5, 6]. Thus, there is no weight or BMI limit for EI use.

The etonogestrel implant is the most highly effective reversible contraceptive method, with a contraceptive failure rate of only 0.05% for both perfect and typical use, comparable to Intrauterine Devices (IUDs) (0.2–0.8%) and female sterilization (0.5%) [7]. Newer data demonstrate even higher EI contraceptive efficacy in real-world users (Pearl index 0.02–0.04) [8].

Efficacy depends on proper insertion. Expulsion may also occur if the full length of the needle is not inserted by the clinician when placing the implant. Failure to insert the implant completely and correctly can lead to unintended pregnancy. Too deep an insertion can hinder removal, and failure to remove the implant within the recommended time can also result in an unintended pregnancy.

Several studies have demonstrated the contraceptive efficacy of the etonogestrel implant up to 5 years, with 0 pregnancies occurring during the 2-year extension beyond the FDA-approved 3-year indication [9, 10]. Offering patients the option of continuing the same etonogestrel implant for up to 5 years has been offered in some practices. Patients should be informed that extended use of the same EI beyond 3 years is off-label, and this discussion should also be documented in the patient's medical record.

Unexpected changes to menstrual bleeding patterns are the most common side effect of hormonal contraceptives and the most common reason for patient discontinuation. Nexplanon® is no exception. Bleeding irregularities are the most common adverse events contributing to the discontinuation of EI use in clinical trials (11%) [11]. However, the typical bleeding changes that occur with etonogestrel implant use differ from other hormonal contraceptive methods. After the initial 3 months of EI use, approximately 50% of women will revert to their previous menstrual patterns prior to insertion, 20% will have decreased menses or amenorrhea, while 30%

Table 16.1 How to be reasonably certain that a woman is not pregnant [13]

A healthcare provider can be reasonably certain that a woman is not pregnant if she has no symptoms or signs of pregnancy and meets any one of the following criteria:
Is ≤7 days after the start of normal menses.
Has not had sexual intercourse since the start of the last normal menses.
Has been correctly and consistently using a reliable method of contraception.
Is ≤7 days after spontaneous or induced abortion.
Is within 4 weeks postpartum.
Is fully or nearly fully breastfeeding (exclusively breastfeeding or the vast majority [≥85%] of feeds are breastfeeds), amenorrheic, and <6 months postpartum.

will have irregular bleeding such as bleeding in between menses. These bleeding patterns may persist throughout the potential 3 years of implant use. Less common reasons for discontinuation (<3%) include emotional lability, weight gain, headache, acne, and depression at the same rate for the current EI as Implanon®. Advising patients about the potential bleeding changes and other possible side effects related to EI use is an essential part of the shared decision-making process regarding any contraceptive, including Nexplanon® [3].

Patients who are considering EI as their contraceptive method should undergo a focused history to assess for any potential contraindications. However, a physical exam (including gynecologic exam), Pap smear, or lab testing is unnecessary [12]. The clinician should document the counselling and patient consent process and provide a copy of the patient's labelling to the patient for reference [1]. A procedure consent form is included in each Nexplanon® package.

Nexplanon® can be inserted at *any time* provided the clinician is reasonably certain that the woman is not pregnant [13] (Table 16.1).

However, if EI is inserted >5 days after menses started, patients should use a backup method or abstain for at least 7 days following insertion [13].

A meta-analysis of six open studies and seven comparative trials found that etonogestrel implant insertions (average time: 0.5 min) and removals (average time: 3.6 min) are relatively short procedures [14] for experienced clinicians. Infection, expulsion, and local reactions are rare, especially when insertion is properly performed using the preloaded applicator.

Case Study

A 35-year-old patient, G3P3003, comes to your office for a routine gynecological exam. She is in a monogamous relationship with her husband, with no history of STIs. They use condoms as their only method of contraception, but she admits that they are not consistent with using them. She has smoked cigarettes (~1 ppd) for the past 12 years and is not ready to quit. She has three children and at this time does not want any more children. However, she is not ready to commit to sterilization, and she does not like the idea of having a foreign body in her uterus (IUD). She has no complaints and denies any chronic medical problems. Her physical exam is completely normal.

Indications

- Any pregnancy-capable patient desiring reversible contraception
- Smokers over age 35 who desire reversible contraception
- Pregnancy-capable patients who desire contraception but cannot utilize estrogen

Contraindications

Etonogestrel implant should not be used in women who have the following:

- Known or suspected pregnancy
- Current or past history of thrombotic disease*
- Hepatic tumors, active liver disease
- Undiagnosed abnormal genital bleeding
- Known, suspected, or history of breast cancer
- Hypersensitivity to any of the components of Nexplanon®

*While the Nexplanon® package insert lists the current and past history of thrombotic disease as a contraindication, evidence documented in the CDC (Centers for Disease Control and Prevention)2016 US Medical Eligibility Criteria shows that the benefit of the etonogestrel implant in preventing unintended pregnancy generally significantly outweighs any actual or theoretical risk of venous thromboembolism [15]. Clinicians should refer to the CDC 2016 US MEC to assess eligibility for various contraceptive methods in patients with chronic medical conditions. Clinicians can locate these criteria on the US Medical Eligibility Criteria (US MEC) for Contraceptive Use webpage at: Updated CDC Contraception Guidelines - Birth Control Pharmacist or download the "CDC Contraception 2024" Application for point of care access (Algorithm 16.1).

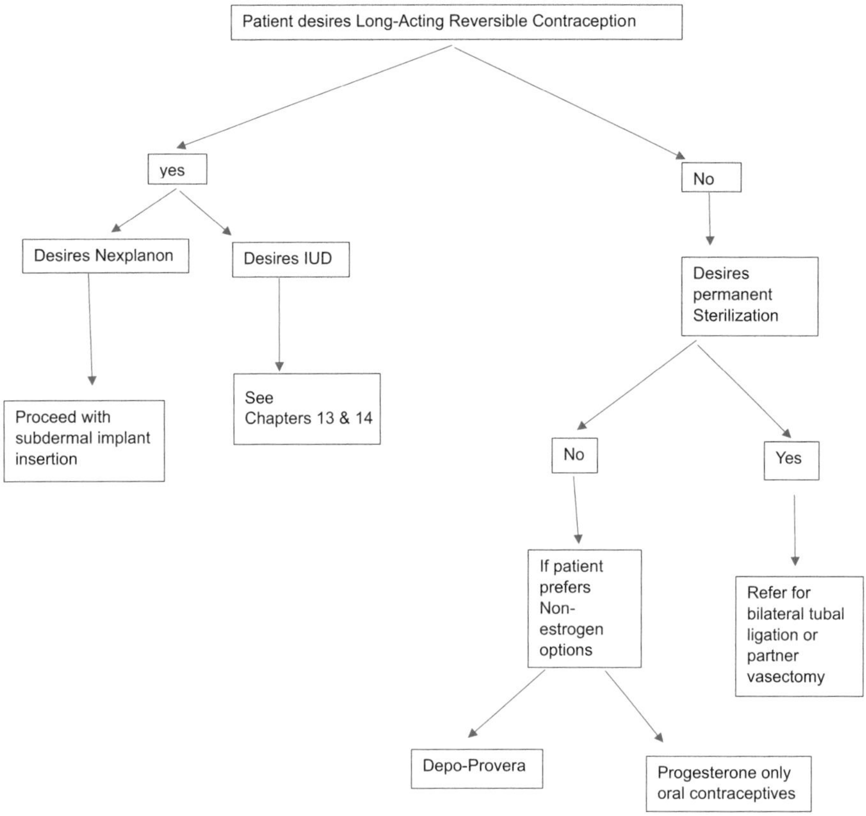

Algorithm 16.1 Flowchart illustrating decision-making for long acting reversible contraception

Insertion

Insertion Equipment (Fig. 16.1)

Before beginning, assemble everything needed for the insertion procedure. In addition to the sterile packing containing the Nexplanon® applicator, you will need the following:

- Sterile gloves (nonsterile gloves acceptable if utilizing appropriate "no-touch" technique)
- Sterile surgical drape
- Antiseptic solution (i.e., povidone-iodine or chlorhexidine swabs)

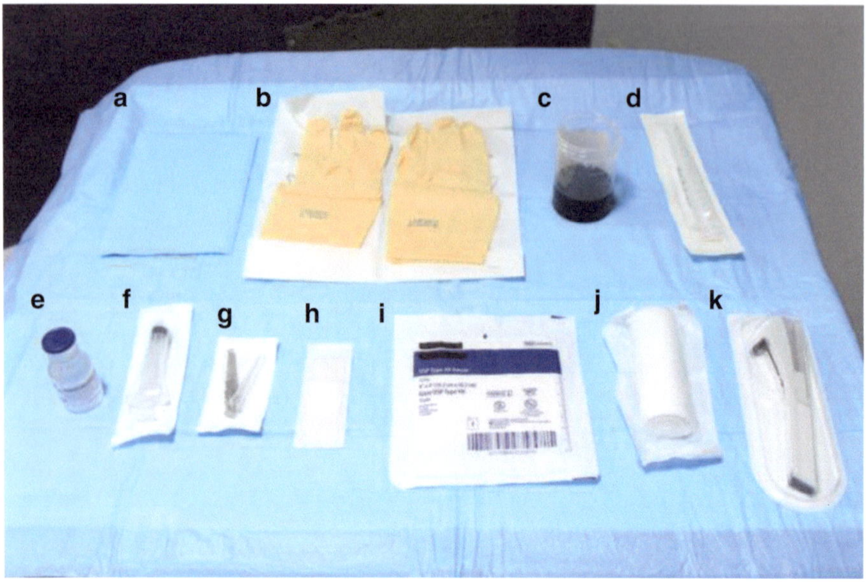

Fig. 16.1 Equipment list for insertion of Nexplanon®: (**a**) sterile drape; (**b**) sterile gloves; (**c**) antiseptic solution (i.e., povidone-iodine); (**d**) skin marking pen with paper ruler; (**e**) anesthetic (i.e., 1% lidocaine); (**f**) 3-cc syringe; (**g**) 25-gauge 1.5″ needle; (**h**) sterile bandage; (**i**) 4 × 4 cm cotton gauze; (**j**) 4″ cotton gauze bandage roll for arm; (**k**) Nexplanon® in applicator

- Local anesthetic (preferably 1% lidocaine), epinephrine is not needed
- Needles (preferably an 18-gauge to draw up lidocaine; a 1.5-in. 25-gauge to inject)
- Syringe (preferably 3 cc)
- Sterile gauze (4 × 4 cm)
- Adhesive bandage or wound closure strips
- 4″ Pressure bandage (gauze bandage rolls, elastic bandage wrap, or compression bandage)
- A sterile marker with a tape measure (optional)

Insertion Procedure

1. Schedule the patient at the appropriate time for insertion.
2. Obtain consent (procedure and anesthetic) and perform a urine pregnancy test, if indicated.
3. Place the patient in supine position on the exam table with the arm they selected for insertion (usually nondominant arm) rotated externally so that the elbow is flexed and the wrist is parallel to the ear, alongside the patient's head.

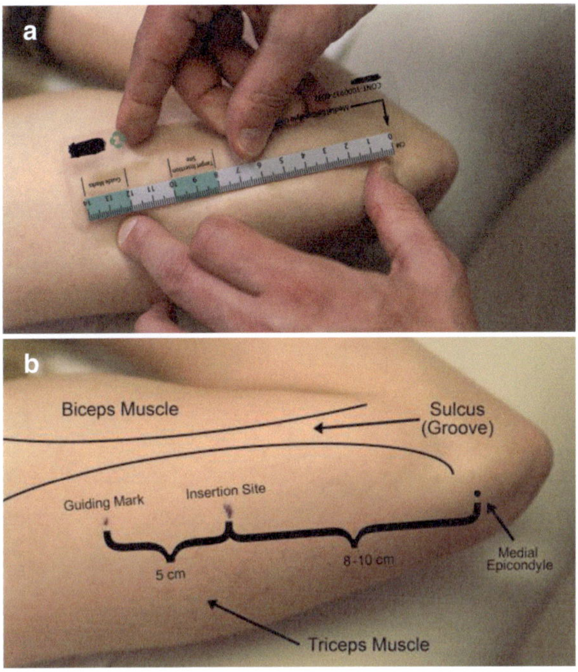

Fig. 16.2 (**a**, **b**) Identify insertion site, which is at the inner side of the selected upper arm about 8–10 cm (3–4 inches) proximal to the medial epicondyle of the humerus and 3–5 cm posterior to (below) the sulcus (groove) between the biceps and triceps muscles and the large blood vessels and nerves that lie there in the neurovascular bundle deeper in the subcutaneous tissue. When following these directions, it is expected that the implant will be inserted subdermally just under the skin over the triceps muscle. Use a sterile marker to make a dot where the implant will be inserted and then another about 5 cm proximal to the first, which serves as a direction guide

4. Identify the insertion site at the inner side of the selected upper arm approximately 8–10 cm proximal to the medial epicondyle of the humerus and at least 3–5 cm posterior to (below) the sulcus (groove) between the bicep and the tricep muscles. If it is not possible to insert at this location, the implant should be inserted as far posterior to the sulcus as possible. There have been a few documented cases in which the implant was inserted too deeply and into the neurovascular bundle within the sulcus/groove described above (Fig. 16.2a).
5. Use a sterile marker to make a dot where the implant will be inserted and then another about 5 cm proximal to the first, which serves as a direction guide (Fig. 16.2b).
6. Use an antiseptic solution to clean the insertion site and then anesthetize the area, preferably with 1% lidocaine along the insertion track prior to the insertion (1–2 mL should be sufficient) (Fig. 16.3).
7. Remove the applicator from its sterile packaging without removing the shield. It is helpful to grip the applicator with your thumb and forefinger of your dominant hand on the textured surface found on either side, adjacent to the insertion

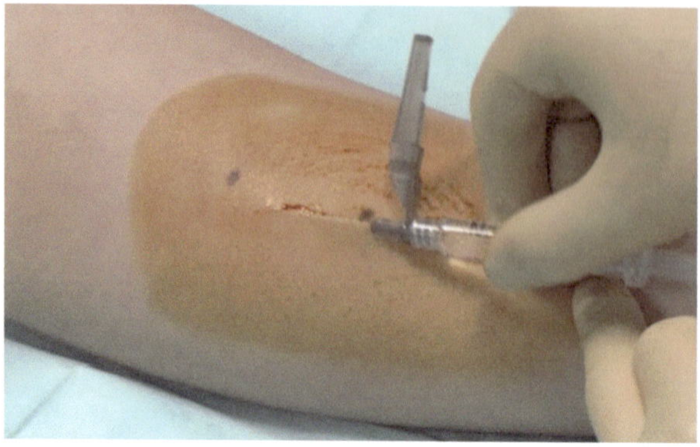

Fig. 16.3 Clean the insertion site with an antiseptic solution, and inject about 2 mL of 1% lidocaine or similar anesthetic (epinephrine is not necessary but can be used if desired) along the planned insertion tunnel. Test to make sure anesthetic is working ~2 minutes after insertion.

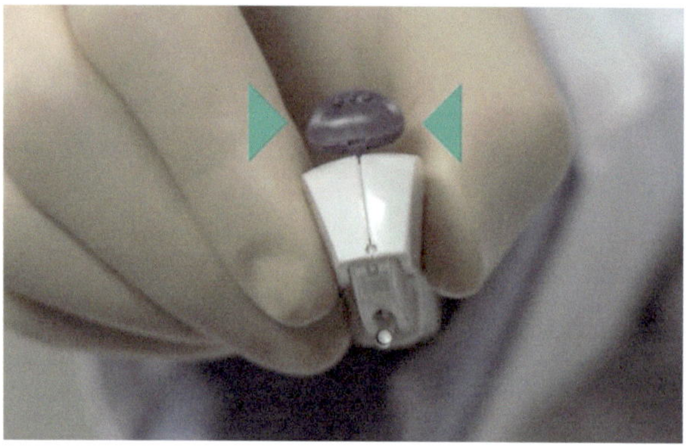

Fig. 16.4 Remove the sterile preloaded disposable Nexplanon® applicator carrying the implant from the blister package. Hold the applicator just above the needle at the textured surface area and remove the transparent protection cap by sliding horizontally away from the needle. Confirm the presence of the white implant inside the needle

slider. When ready, remove the needle shield to expose the needle containing the implant. You should be able to see the white implant (Fig. 16.4). *Do not move the purple slider until the needle is in the correct position under the skin.*

8. Applying counter-traction to the skin around the site, insert only the tip of the needle with the beveled side up at a slight (<30°) angle (Fig. 16.5a).
9. Next, lower the applicator until it is horizontal and parallel to the skin (Fig. 16.5b).
10. "Tent" the skin by lifting it with the tip of the needle, while still maintaining the needle in the subdermal connective tissue. In this position, gently and fully insert the entire needle, keeping it parallel to the skin surface in the superficial layer between the dermis and subdermal fat tissue (Fig. 16.6). Be sure that the entire length of the needle is buried in the subcutaneous layer before continuing. If the needle punctures through the other side of the skin during insertion, gently pull back and redirect in the desired direction.

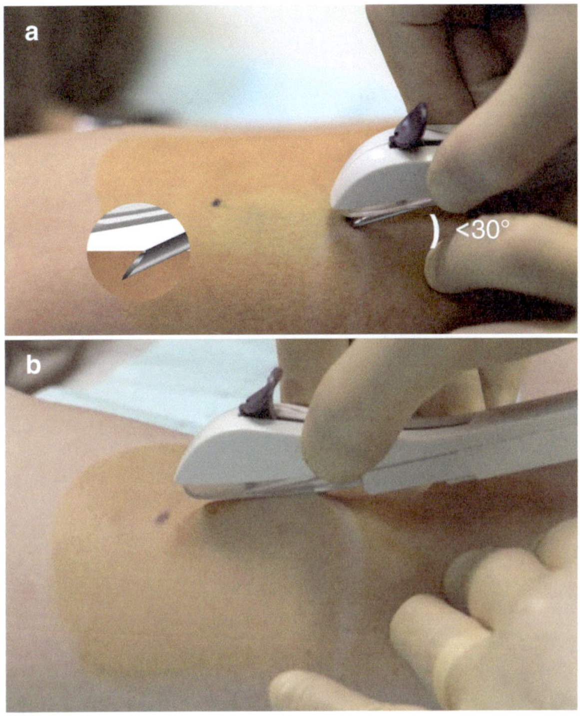

Fig. 16.5 (**a**) Stretch skin around the insertion site with fingers. Puncture the skin with the tip of the needle slightly angled less than 30°. (**b**) Lower the applicator to the horizontal position

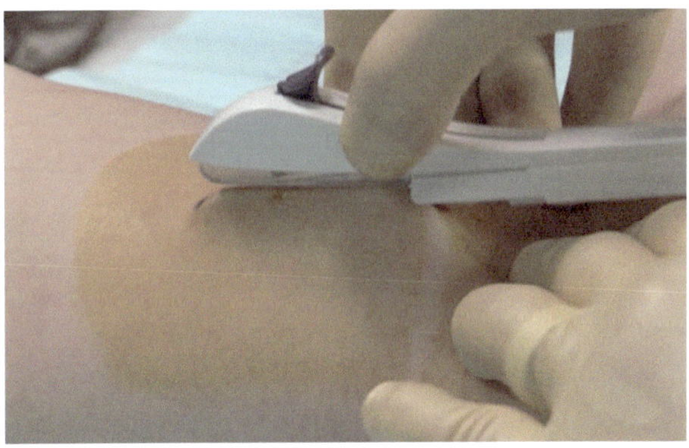

Fig. 16.6 While lifting (tenting) the skin with the tip of the needle, slide the needle to its full length. During the entire insertion procedure, you should be able to see the insertion site and the movement of the needle. You may feel slight resistance but *do not exert excessive force. If the needle is not inserted to its full length, the implant will not be inserted properly*

11. While keeping the applicator in the correct position, pull back on the purple insertion slider until it stops at the end of its track. There will be two audible clicks (one when the applicator is engaged and the other when the needle is fully retracted). When this procedure is performed as described, the rod will be left in the correct position (Fig. 16.7a, b).
12. Remove the applicator. Palpate the patient's arm immediately after insertion to verify the presence of both ends of the rod (Fig. 16.8).
13. Cover the site with a small adhesive bandage (Fig. 16.9).

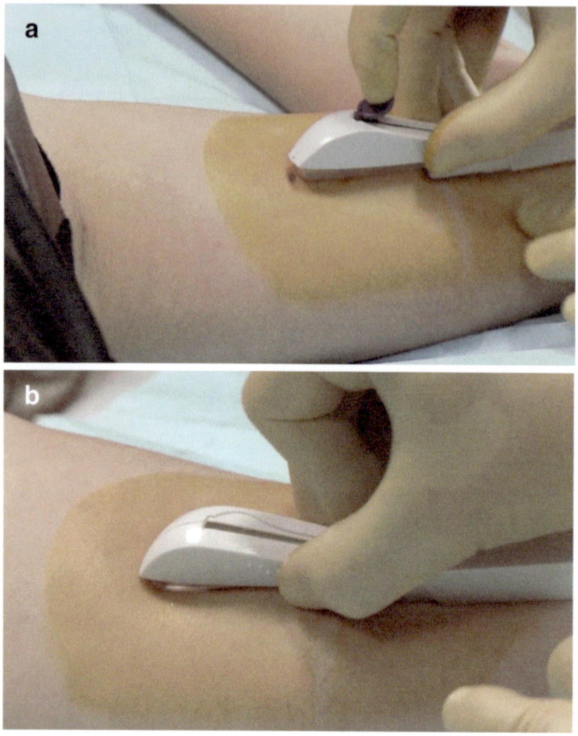

Fig. 16.7 (**a**, **b**) While keeping the applicator in the same position and the needle inserted to its full length, unlock the purple slider by pushing it slightly down. Move the slider fully back until it stops, leaving the implant now in its final subdermal position and locking the needle inside the body of the applicator. *If the applicator is not kept in the same position during the procedure or if the slider is not completely moved back, the needle will not be fully retracted and the implant will not be inserted properly*

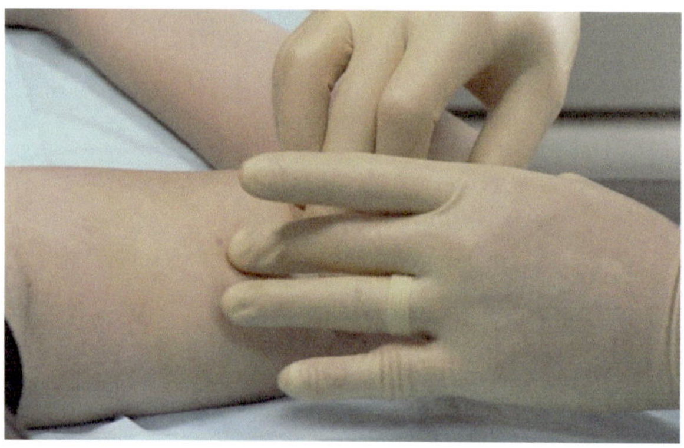

Fig. 16.8 Remove the applicator. Immediately after insertion, confirm the presence of the 4-cm implant by palpation

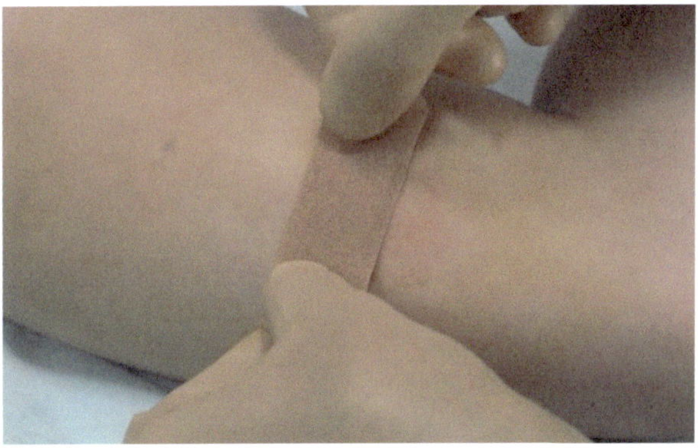

Fig. 16.9 Apply a small adhesive bandage over the insertion site

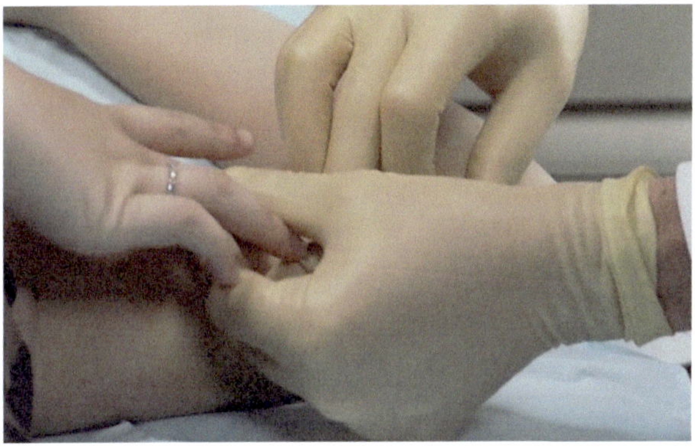

Fig. 16.10 Then have the patient palpate the rod as well

14. Then have the patient palpate the rod as well (Fig. 16.10).
15. Once the presence of the rod has been confirmed, apply a pressure bandage with sterile gauze to reduce the risk of bruising (Fig. 16.11). The implant should be palpated immediately after insertion by both the clinician and the patient. This is to both ensure that the Nexplanon® was inserted correctly and to teach the patient how to quickly localize it quickly. If the 4-cm rod is not palpable after insertion, during use or before removal, its presence should be verified using a two-dimensional X-ray. MRI, CT, and ultrasound can also be used to locate the implant.
16. Instruct the patient to keep the top bandage on for 24 hours and the small bandage on for 3–5 days. Use acetaminophen or NSAIDs if analgesics are needed.
17. Provide the patient with the completed User Card which contains the date their implant should be removed, and scan the completed Patient Chart Label to the patient's electronic medical record.
18. Provide the patient with written and verbal instructions on side effects and when to call the office for concerns/complications.
19. Dispose of the applicator in accordance with CDC guidelines for hazardous waste.

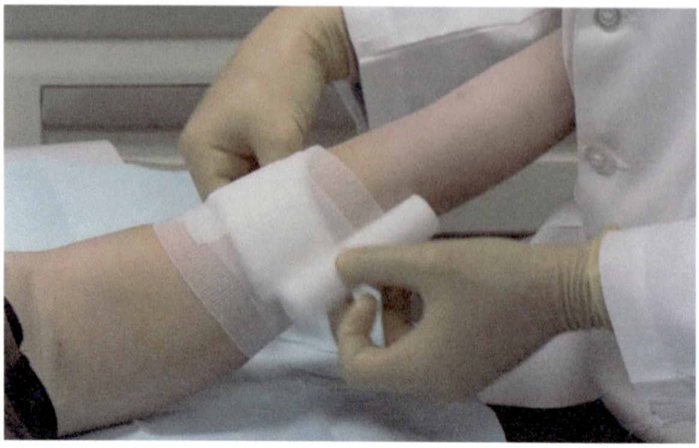

Fig. 16.11 Apply a pressure bandage with sterile gauze to minimize bruising

Complications and Risks

Complications are usually the result of deep intramuscular, fascial, or intravascular insertions and prolonged traumatic removal attempts.

- Pain
- Paraesthesia
- Hematoma
- Scarring
- Infection
- Migration of the implant
- Incomplete insertions or infections may lead to expulsion

Tricks and Helpful Hints

- #11 scalpel can be used to puncture the skin prior to using the applicator during insertion.
- May be helpful for the clinician to sit during the procedure to visualize the insertion fully and to ensure proper superficial insertion.

Procedure Note

(Provider to fill in blanks/circle applicable choice and customize as needed.)

Insertion

Age: ______ G: ______ P: ______ LMP: _______; Urine Pregnancy: +/−

BP____________ Pulse __________ Weight _________

Current Contraceptive Method: ____________________________________

Date of Last Delivery/Termination: __________________; Breastfeeding: Y/N

Informed Consent for Nexplanon® insertion (consent form provided with each device) has been signed and all questions answered. Patient has no contraindications to this method. Patient desires long-term protection against pregnancy. Patient has no pregnancy or risk of pregnancy at the time of insertion. Patient counselled about potential benefits, risks, side effects, and complications. Patient has no allergy to lidocaine, betadine, or tape.

Plans for backup contraception if needed:____________________________

Nexplanon® Lot #: __________ Expiration date: ___________

The ventromedial surface of the Left/Right arm was cleansed with antiseptic solution, and a sterile field created. Lidocaine 1% ____________ mL with/without epinephrine was injected intradermally into the planned insertion site, 8–10 cm proximal to the medial epicondyle of the humerus and 3–5 cm posterior to the sulcus between the bicep and tricep muscles. The implant was inserted according to the Nexplanon® system protocol. Both provider and patient were able to palpate the implant at the end of the procedure. Adhesive bandage/Wound closure strips and compression dressing applied to the insertion site.

Complications: None/______________________________________ __________

Post-insertion instructions were provided to the patient

Patient instructed to use backup method for 1 week if inserted outside the recommended timing.

Patient Labelling/Education booklet (provided with each device) given to the patient.

Follow-up appointment: ___________________

Patient advised to call ASAP if any symptoms/signs of infection.

Patient aware Nexplanon® must be removed on or before (mm/yyyy):______________

Signature/Title: ____________________________Date:_____________

Case Study Outcome

Given the patient's desire for long-term, reversible, non-daily or non-intrauterine contraception, and the fact that she is a 35-year-old 1 ppd smoker, she was counseled on Nexplanon® or Depo-Provera®. The patient chose Nexplanon® and it was inserted without difficulty. The patient returned the following year after Nexplanon® insertion for a recheck visit. She reports some occasional spotting but no other complaints. She is extremely satisfied with the method and has not smoked in over 3 months.

Coding

CPT® Codes (Current Procedural Terminology, AMA, Chicago, IL)	
11981	Insertion of a non-biodegradable drug delivery implant
11983	Removal with reinsertion of a non-biodegradable drug delivery implant
ICD-10-CM-Diagnostic Codes (International Classification of Diseases, 10th Revision, Clinical Modification, Centers for Disease Control and Prevention)	
Z30.01	Encounter for initial prescription of an implantable subdermal contraceptive
Z30.46	Encounter for surveillance of an implantable subdermal contraceptive

Postprocedure Patient Instructions

Patient labelling/education booklet is provided with each device.

Insertion

- Inform the patient of the need for a backup method for 1 week if inserted outside the recommended timing.
- Advise the patient to call ASAP if there are any symptoms/signs of infection.
- Ensure that the patient is aware that the Nexplanon® must be removed on or before 3 years (FDA-approved)/5 years (evidence-based) from the insertion date.
- Counsel patient to expect changes in their bleeding patterns that may be unpredictable and include changes in bleeding frequency, duration, and/or amenorrhea. Patients with persistent bleeding should be seen to rule out pregnancy or pathologic conditions.

Patient Handout

The contraceptive implant (Nexplanon®) is a very effective, convenient, and safe form of contraception. A small procedure under local anesthetic is needed to insert the implant under the skin in the office. Each implant lasts 3 years.

What Is Nexplanon®?

Nexplanon® is a contraceptive implant, a small flexible rod that is inserted under the skin. It contains a progestin hormone. Nexplanon® lasts for up to 3 years (based on current FDA approval) or 5 years (based on the latest research evidence). It is 99% effective.

How Does the Nexplanon® Work?

The progestin hormone in the implant is released slowly into the bloodstream at a steady rate. The progestin works mainly by stopping ovulation (the release of the egg from the ovary). It also thickens the mucus made by the cervix which forms a "mucus plug" in the cervix. This stops sperm from getting through to the uterus (womb) to fertilize an egg. It also makes the lining of the uterus thinner. This means that if an egg was to fertilize, it is not likely to be able to attach to the uterus.

How Effective Is Nexplanon®?

Nexplanon® is more than 99% effective. This means that less than 1 woman in 100 who uses this method of contraception will become pregnant each year. (Compare this to when no contraception is used. More than 80 in 100 sexually active women who do not use contraception become pregnant within 1 year).

What Are the Potential Advantages of Using Nexplanon®?

- You do not have to remember to take a pill every day.
- You only have to think about contraception every 3 years.
- It does not interfere with sex.
- It can be used when breastfeeding.
- Period pain is usually less than usual.

- It stops ovulation and thickens cervical mucus.
- It can be used by some women who cannot take pills that contain estrogen.
- It may help protect against Pelvic Inflammatory Disease (PID). (The mucus plug in the cervix may help to prevent bacteria from traveling into the uterus.)

What Are the Potential Disadvantages of Using Nexplanon®?

The release of progestin will usually cause changes to the pattern of periods. During the first year, it is common to have irregular bleeding. Sometimes, periods are heavier and longer than before. They usually settle back into a regular pattern after the first year but may remain irregular. In some women, the periods become infrequent and light or even stop altogether.

Some women worry about irregular or changed periods, but it does not mean anything is wrong and is of no consequence. However, unpredictable or irregular periods can be a nuisance.

It is not protective against sexually transmitted infections.

Who Cannot Use Nexplanon®?

Your healthcare provider will discuss any current and past illnesses. Some illnesses may mean that you cannot use progestin-based contraceptives such as Nexplanon®. However, the number of women this affects is small.

Are There Any Potential Side Effects with Nexplanon®?

Some women report side effects such as mood changes, breast discomfort, fluid retention, weight gain, headaches, and an increase in acne. These are uncommon, and, if they do occur, they tend to develop in the first few months only, and often resolve after 3–6 months if the implant remains. The area around the implant may be bruised and sore for a few days. You can apply an ice pack to the area and/or take some ibuprofen or acetaminophen to help with the discomfort.

How Is the Implant Put Under the Skin?

- It is put on the inner side of the upper arm.
- It is usually first inserted within 5 days of a period starting. (This ensures that you are not pregnant.) It is effective from insertion onward.

- An injection of local anesthetic is used to numb the skin. A small cut is made, and the implant is placed under the skin. The wound is dressed and will soon heal just like any other small cut.
- The area around the implant may be bruised and sore for a few days, but this soon goes away.

When Is the Implant Taken Out?

The implant is usually removed at the end of 3–5 years but may be removed sooner by patient request.

A replacement rod can be reinserted at the time of removal if so desired.

Once removed, the rod loses its effect immediately and another form of contraception should be used if pregnancy is not desired.

Further Information

Your healthcare provider and pharmacist are good sources of information if you have any questions. You may also call: (1-844-674-3200) or visit www.nexplanon.com

References

1. Nexplanon-etonogestrel implant. US Food and Drug Administration (FDA) approved product information. Revised 29 Sept 2023. US National Library of Medicine. Available online at https://dailymed.nlm.nih.gov/dailymed/drugInfo.cfm?setid=487f8a62-e142-457c-97cc-2e398fde7594. Accessed 19 Feb 2024.
2. Creinin MD, Kaunitz AM, Darney PD, et al. The US etonogestrel implant mandatory clinical training and active monitoring programs: 6-year experience. Contraception. 2017;95:205.
3. Long-acting reversible contraception: implants and intrauterine devices. Practice bulletin no. 186. American College of Obstetricians and Gynecologists. Obstet Gynecol. 2017;130:e251–69.
4. Diedrich JT, Zhao Q, Madden T, Secura GM, Peipert JF. Three-year continuation of reversible contraception. Am J Obstet Gynecol. 2015;213(662):e1–8.
5. Xu H, Wade JA, Peipert JF, Zhao Q, Madden T, Secura GM. Contraceptive failure rates of etonogestrel subdermal implants in overweight and obese women. Obstet Gynecol. 2012;120:21–6.
6. Morrell KM, Cremers S, Westhoff CL, Davis AR. Relationship between etonogestrel level and BMI in women using the contraceptive implant for more than 1 year. Contraception. 2016;93:263–5.
7. Trussell J. Contraceptive failure in the United States. Contraception. 2011;83:397–404.
8. Reed S, Minh TD, Lange JA, Koro C, Heinemann K. Pregnancy and pregnancy outcomes in a prospective cohort study: final results from the Nexplanon Observational Risk Assessment Study (NORA). Contraception. 2023 Apr;120:109920.

9. Ali M, Akin A, Bahamondes L, et al. WHO study group on subdermal contraceptive implants for women. Extended use up to 5 years of the etonogestrel-releasing subdermal contraceptive implant: comparison to levonorgestrel-releasing subdermal implant. Hum Reprod. 2016;31(11):2491–8.
10. McNicholas C, Swor E, Wan L, Peipert JF. Prolonged use of the etonogestrel implant and levonorgestrel intrauterine device: 2 years beyond the Food and Drug Administration-approved duration. Am J Obstet Gynecol. 2017;216(6):586.e1–6.
11. Mansour D, Korver T, Marintcheva-Petrova M, Fraser IS. The effects of Implanon on menstrual bleeding patterns. Eur J Contracept Reprod Health Care. 2008;13(Suppl 1):13–28.
12. Curtis KM, Jatlaoui TC, Tepper NK, et al. U.S. selected practice recommendations for contraceptive use, 2016. MMWR Recomm Rep. 2016;65:1.
13. CDC. U.S. selected practice recommendations for contraceptive use, 2013: adapted from the World Health Organization selected practice recommendations for contraceptive use, 2nd edition. MMWR Recomm Rep. 2013;62(RR-5):1–60.
14. Levine JP, Sinofsky FE, Christ MF, Implanon US Study Group. Assessment of Implanon insertion and removal. Contraception. 2008;78:409.
15. Curtis KM, Tepper NK, Jatlaoui TC, et al. U.S. medical eligibility criteria for contraceptive use, 2016. MMWR Recomm Rep. 2016;65(RR-3):1–104.

Web Sites

Information about insertion and removal of Nexplanon® is available from the manufacturer by contacting Organon at 1-844-674-3200 or www.nexplanon.com.

Nexplanon Questions and Answers: When should I call my healthcare provider? http://www.nexplanon.com/questions.

Chapter 17
Etonogestrel Subdermal Contraceptive Implant: Removal

Jeffrey P. Levine and Joshua A. Mleczko

Introduction

The progestin-only, etonogestrel implant, Nexplanon®, is a sterile 4-cm × 2-mm single flexible rod that is implanted subdermally in a pregnancy-capable patient's upper arm and can provide up from 3 years (FDA-approved) to 5 years (evidence-based) of continuous highly effective contraception [1]. Removal of the EI is a simple procedure that should be done by providers who have undergone the required training [2].

Unexpected changes to menstrual bleeding patterns are the most common side effect of hormonal contraceptives and the most common reason for patient discontinuation. Nexplanon® is no exception. Bleeding irregularities are the most common adverse events contributing to the discontinuation of EI use in clinical trials (11%) [3]. However, the typical bleeding changes that occur with etonogestrel implant use differ from other hormonal contraceptive methods. After the initial 3 months of EI use, approximately 50% of women will revert back to their previous menstrual patterns prior to insertion, 20% will have decreased menses or amenorrhea, while 30% will have irregular bleeding such as bleeding in between menses. These bleeding patterns may persist throughout the potential 3 years of implant use. Treatment of

J. P. Levine (✉)
Department of Family Medicine and Community Health, Rutgers Robert Wood Johnson Medical School, New Brunswick, NJ, USA
e-mail: jeff.levine@rutgers.edu

J. A. Mleczko
Capital Health Primary Care – Bordentown, Bordentown, NJ, USA
e-mail: jmleczko@capitalhealth.org

S. M. Sulik, C. B. Heath (eds.), *Primary Care Procedures in Women's Health*,
https://doi.org/10.1007/978-3-032-07061-6_17

bleeding irregularities can be addressed with the patient prior to removal if the patient desires. These include use of nonsteroidal anti-inflammatory drugs such as Mefenamic acid 500 mg orally three times a day or celecoxib 200 mg orally daily for 7 days, combined oral contraceptives, or supplemental estrogen including use of selective estrogen receptor modulators such as Tamoxifen 10 mg twice a day for 7 days [4].

Less common reasons for discontinuation (<3%) include emotional lability, weight gain, headache, acne, and depression, but none of these side effects were found to be significantly increased in clinical trials of Implanon®. Advising patients about the potential bleeding changes and other possible side effects related to EI use is an essential part of the shared decision-making process regarding any contraceptive, including Nexplanon® [5].

For a more detailed description of efficacy, evidence-based length of use versus FDA-approved length of use, please see the chapter on Etonogestrel Subdermal Contraceptive Implant: Insertion.

Case Study

A 31-year-old patient whose Nexplanon® has been in place for 2 years and 11 months presents to the office requesting the removal of her current device and a reinsertion of another one. The patient prefers to use the FDA-approved length of device removal after a shared decision-making discussion.

Indications for Removal (Algorithm 17.1)

- Device has performed to the full length of its effectiveness.
- Patient is interested in becoming pregnant.
- Patient finds side effects have outweighed the benefits of the device.
- Patient develops a contraindication to the device.
- Patient develops an allergy to one of the components of the device.

Contraindications for On-Site Removal

Clinicians who remove Nexplanon® need to have attended a Nexplanon® Clinical Training Program on removal. Consider referral to an experienced clinician if deep insertion or anticipated difficult removal.

Nonpalpable subdermal implants- use an X-ray to locate prior to any attempt at removal; consider referral to surgery.

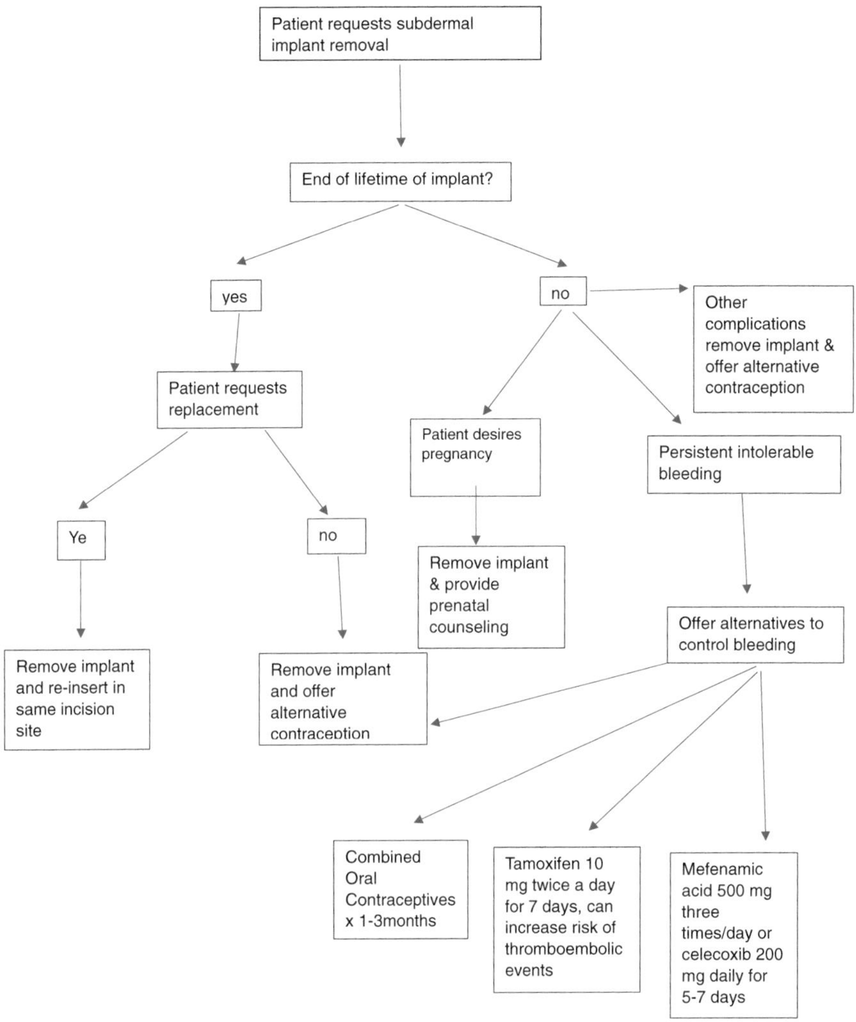

Algorithm 17.1 Subdermal Implant Removal

Causes for Discontinuation

- Bleeding (most common: accounts for 11% discontinuation rate)
- Emotional lability (<3%)
- Depression (<3%)
- Weight gain (<3%)
- Headache (<3%)
- Acne (<3%)

Removal of Equipment (Fig. 17.1)

The following equipment is needed for implant removal:

- Sterile gloves.
- Sterile surgical drape.
- Antiseptic solution (i.e., povidone-iodine or chlorhexidine swabs).
- Local anesthetic (preferably 1% lidocaine); epinephrine is not needed.
- Needles (preferably an 18-gauge to draw up lidocaine; a 1.5-in. 25 gauge to inject).
- Syringe (preferably 3 cc).
- #11 sterile scalpel.
- Mosquito clamps (straight and curved).
- Sterile gauze (4 × 4 cm).
- Wound closure strips.
- 4″ Pressure bandage (gauze bandage rolls, elastic bandage wrap, or compression bandage).
- A sterile marker (optional).

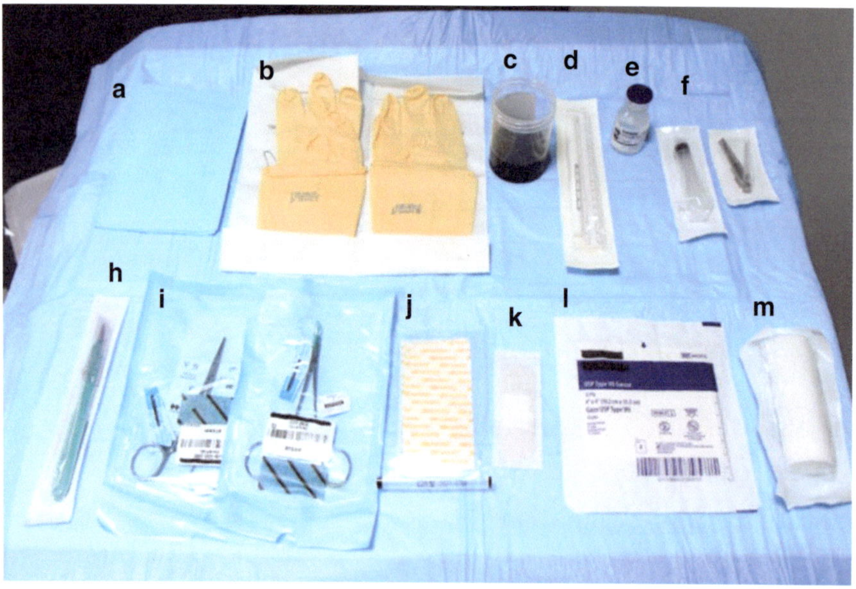

Fig. 17.1 Equipment list for removal of Nexplanon®: (**a**) sterile drape; (**b**) sterile gloves; (**c**) antiseptic solution (i.e., povidone-iodine); (**d**) skin marking pen with paper ruler; (**e**) anesthetic solution (i.e., 1% lidocaine); (**f**) 3-cc syringe; (**g**) 25-gauge 1.5″ needle; (**h**) #11 sterile scalpel; (**i**) straight and curved mosquito clamps; (**j**) wound closure strips; (**k**) sterile bandage; (**l**) 4 × 4 cm cotton gauze; (**m**) 4″ cotton bandage roll for arm

Removal Procedure

1. Check the patient's User Card or the Patient Chart Label to confirm which arm contains the implant and then locate the rod by palpation.
2. Clean the site where the incision will be made and apply an antiseptic solution.
3. Locate the implant by palpation and mark the distal end (end closest to the elbow) with a sterile marker. The incision for implant removal is performed at the same site/end as the insertion (Fig. 17.2a, b).
4. Anesthetize the arm with no more than 0.5–1 mL of 1% lidocaine at the marked site where the incision will be made. Be sure to inject the local anesthesia under the implant to keep it close to the skin surface.
5. Push down the proximal end of the implant to stabilize it; a bulge may appear, indicating the distal end of the implant. If the distal end does not easily pop up, removal of the implant may be more challenging and should only be performed by a provider experienced with difficult and deep removals. In this instance, refer to a provider experienced with difficult removals or call 1-844-674-3200 for more information about Centers of Experience. At the end of the implant closest to the elbow, make a 2–3 mm longitudinal incision with a #11 sterile scalpel blade, being careful to not bisect the tip of the implant (Fig. 17.3a, b).

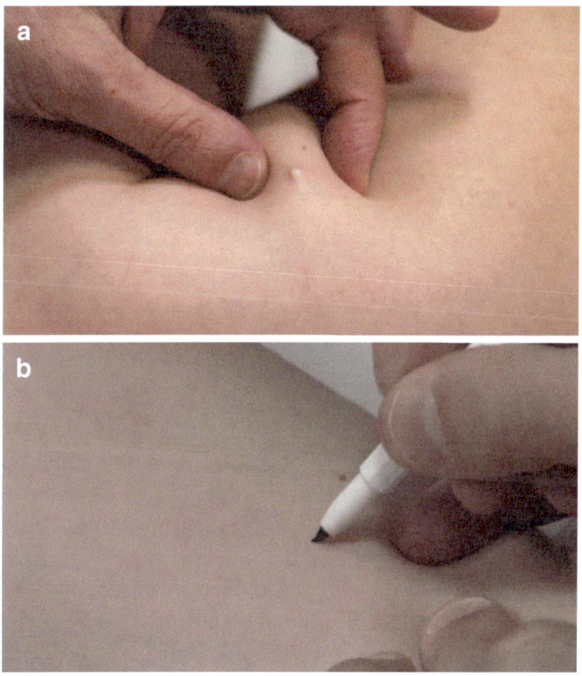

Fig. 17.2 (**a**, **b**) Locate the implant by palpation and mark the distal end (end closest to the elbow)

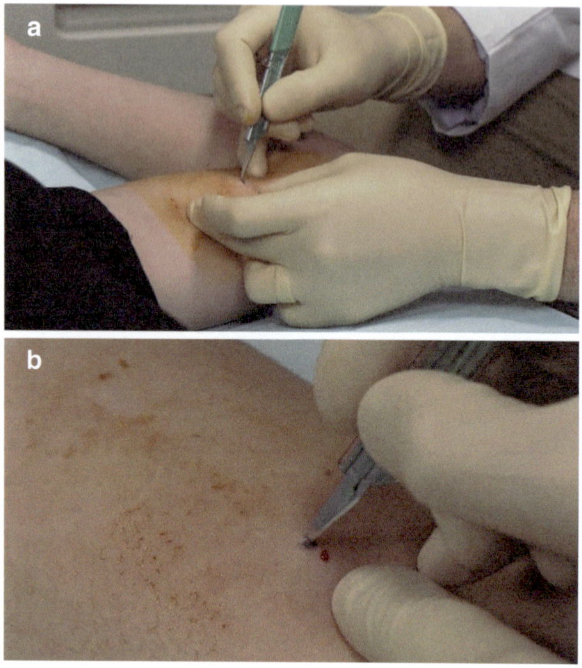

Fig. 17.3 (**a**, **b**) Push down the proximal end of the implant to stabilize it. Starting from the distal tip of the implant, make a longitudinal incision of 2 mm toward the elbow

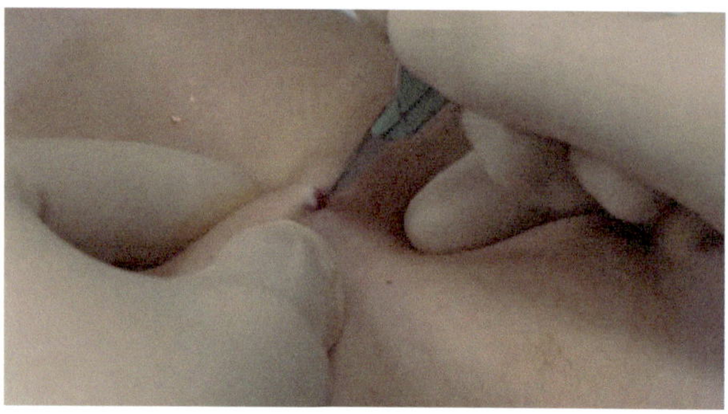

Fig. 17.4 Gently push the implant toward the incision until the tip is visible. If the implant is encapsulated, dissect the fibrous tissue sheath surrounding it

6. Gently push the implant toward the incision until you can see the tip (Fig. 17.4). Use a straight or curved mosquito clamp to grasp the distal tip and pull the implant out gently. If the tip is still not visible, but is able to be grasped, it may be necessary to dissect the fibrous tissue around it utilizing sterile gauze, the #11 blade tip, or a curved mosquito clamp (Fig. 17.5a). If the tip does not become visible at the incision site, insert forceps (preferably mosquito clamps with curved ends up) superficially into the incision. Gently grasp the distal end of the implant and flip your forceps to your other hand (Fig. 17.5b). With a second pair of forceps, carefully remove the surrounding tissue and grasp the

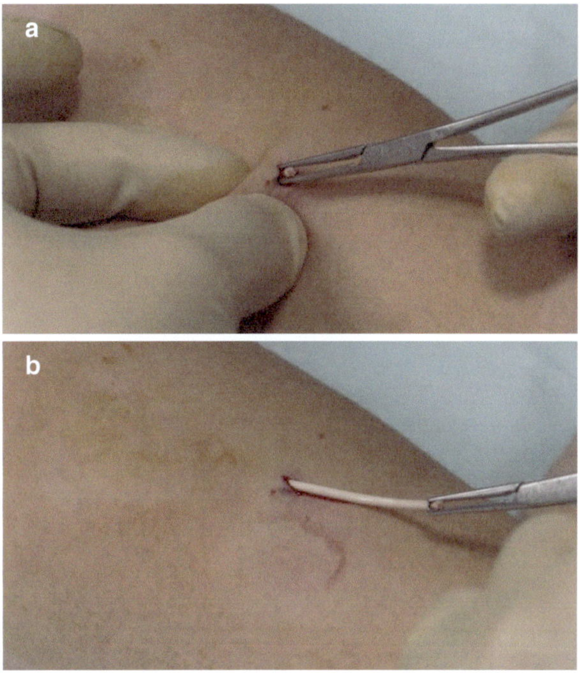

Fig. 17.5 (**a**, **b**) Grasp the implant with a curved or straight mosquito clamp, and gently remove it

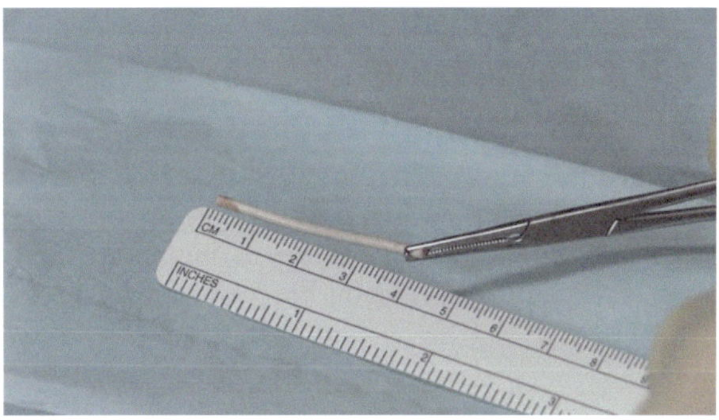

Fig. 17.6 Confirm that the entire 4 cm implant has been removed by measuring its length

implant. The implant should now be removed gently. Again, if there is difficulty with removal, stop the removal and refer to a provider experienced with difficult removals or call 1-844-674-3200.

7. Measure the rod to be sure that all of it (4 cm) has been removed (Fig. 17.6).
8. Approximate the incision edges with wound closure strips (Fig. 17.7).
9. Apply a pressure bandage with sterile gauze to reduce the risk of bruising (Fig. 17.8).
10. Instruct the patient to keep the top bandage on for 24 h, and the wound closure strips on for 3–5 days or until they fall off on their own. Use acetaminophen or NSAIDs if analgesics are needed.

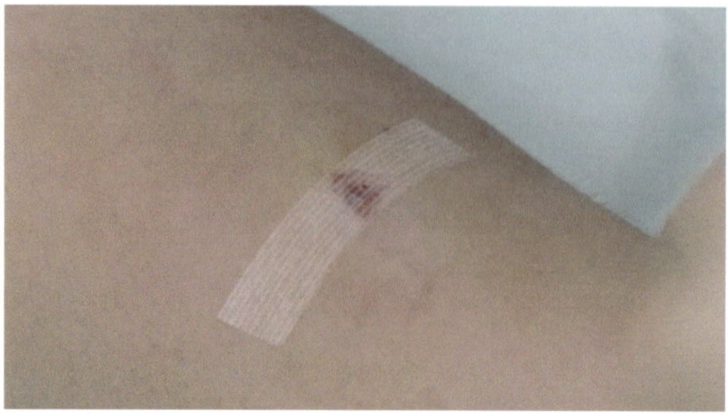

Fig. 17.7 Close the incision with wound closure strips

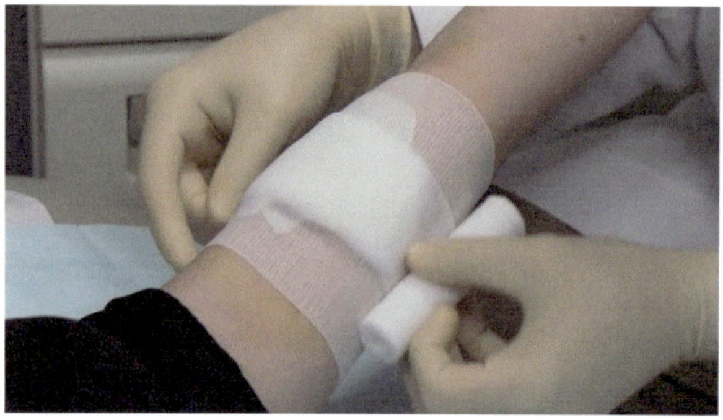

Fig. 17.8 Apply a pressure bandage with sterile gauze to minimize bruising

Complications and Risks

- Difficult removal: Deep insertion may lead to difficult or impossible removals, which require a surgical procedure in the operating room. Deep insertion may cause nerve or vascular damage or migration of the rod.
- Breakage of the implant during removal: may necessitate surgical removal.

Localization

The patient's card and chart should be checked for the correct arm where placement occurred. The Nexplanon® should be palpated in the patient's arm. Once localized, the implant removal procedure can take place. If the implant is not palpable, check the opposite arm for placement. If an implant cannot be palpated, its presence should be verified using a two-dimensional X-ray, MRI, CT, or ultrasound. The axilla should be investigated first if the implant is not palpable. The procedure should not be started until the implant is located.

If no rod is visible on imaging, contact the manufacturer at 1-844-674-3200 for specific instructions on obtaining an etonogestrel level [1].

Tricks and Helpful Hints

- Nexplanon® removals should be performed using sterile gloves.
- Injecting more lidocaine may interfere with localizing the distal rod tip.
- If the patient has chosen to continue Nexplanon®, the preferred method is to insert a new rod in the same location, using the same incision. Use an additional 1–2 ml of lidocaine anesthesia along the insertion track.
- Avoid the temptation to dissect the fibrous sheath with the scalpel since it is easy to inadvertently slice through the EI.

Procedure Note

(Provider to fill in blanks/circle applicable choice and customize as needed.)

Removal

Age:_______ BP____________ Pulse __________ Weight _________

Consent for Nexplanon® removal has been signed and all questions answered.

Reason for contraceptive implant removal: ___________________________

Plans for contraception after removal: _______________________________

Nexplanon® Lot #: __________ Expiration date: ___________

The ventromedial surface of ____________ arm was cleansed with antiseptic solution and a sterile field created. Lidocaine 1% ____________ mL with/without epinephrine was injected intradermally into the planned removal site. The implant was removed completely according to the Nexplanon® system protocol. Patient was shown the removed implant. Wound closure strips and compression dressing applied to the insertion site.

Removal Time: ____

Complications: None/____

Post-removal

Contraceptive method prescribed:_____________________________________

Follow-up appointment: ___________________________________

Patient advised to call ASAP if any symptoms/signs of infection.

Signature/Title:___________________________Date:____________________

Coding

CPT® Codes (Current Procedural Terminology, AMA, Chicago, IL)	
11982	Removal of a nonbiodegradable drug delivery implant
11983	Removal with reinsertion of a nonbiodegradable drug delivery implant
ICD-10-CM-Diagnostic Codes (International Classification of Diseases, 10th Revision, Clinical Modification, Centers for Disease Control and Prevention)	
Z30.46	Encounter for surveillance of an implantable subdermal contraceptive

Postprocedure Patient Instructions

- Advise the patient to call if any symptoms/signs of infection.
- Discuss other contraception needs or preconception counselling.

Case Study Outcome

Patient had Nexplanon® successfully removed and a new one inserted at the same site.

Patient Handout

The contraceptive implant (Nexplanon®) is a very effective, convenient, and safe form of contraception. A small procedure under local anesthetic is needed to insert the implant under the skin, and another small procedure under local anesthetic is needed to remove the implant.

What Is Nexplanon®?

Nexplanon® is a contraceptive implant, a small flexible rod that is inserted under the skin. It contains a progestin hormone. Nexplanon® lasts for up to 3 years (based on current FDA approval) or 5 years (based on the latest research evidence). It is 99% effective.

When Is the Implant Taken Out?

The implant is usually removed at the end of 3–5 years but may be removed sooner by patient request.

A replacement rod can be reinserted at the time of removal if so desired.

Once removed, the rod loses its effect immediately and another form of contraception should be used if pregnancy is not desired.

When to Call After Your Implant Is Removed

You may remove the pressure bandage in 6 h. Leave the Steri-strip on for another 2 days. Please call your provider for swelling and warmth at the incision.

Further Information

Your healthcare provider is a good source of information if you have any questions. You may also call: (1-844-674-3200) or visit www.nexplanon.com

References

1. Nexplanon-etonogestrel implant. US Food and Drug Administration (FDA) approved product information. Revised 29 Sept 2023. US National Library of Medicine. Available online at https://dailymed.nlm.nih.gov/dailymed/drugInfo.cfm?setid=487f8a62-e142-457c-97cc-2e398fde7594. Accessed 19 Feb 2024.
2. Creinin MD, Kaunitz AM, Darney PD, et al. The US etonogestrel implant mandatory clinical training and active monitoring programs: 6-year experience. Contraception. 2017;95:205.
3. Mansour D, Korver T, Marintcheva-Petrova M, Fraser IS. The effects of Implanon on menstrual bleeding patterns. Eur J Contracept Reprod Health Care. 2008;13(Suppl 1):13–28.
4. Edelman A. et al. Evaluation and management of unscheduled bleeding in individuals using hormonal contraception. in UpToDate, Connor RF (ed), Wolters Kluwer. (Accessed on October 22, 2025).
5. Long-acting reversible contraception: implants and intrauterine devices. Practice bulletin no. 186. American College of Obstetricians and Gynecologists. Obstet Gynecol. 2017;130:e251–69.

Web Sites

Information about insertion and removal of Nexplanon® is available from the manufacturer by contacting Organon at 1-844-674-3200 or www.nexplanon.com.

Nexplanon Questions and Answers: When should I call my healthcare provider? http://www.nexplanon.com/questions.

Chapter 18
Pessary

Catherine I. Keating

Introduction

A pessary is a device that allows for nonsurgical treatment of pelvic organ prolapse (POP) and/or stress urinary incontinence (SUI). One of the oldest known medical devices, the pessary dates back to Hippocrates' pessary design: a pomegranate soaked in vinegar. Other historical pessaries include other fruits, items of bronze, cotton wool, linen, wax-coated cork and wood, and rubber [1]. Today, the pessary is generally made of medical-grade silicone in many different styles. Recent innovations include custom-designed 3D-printed pessaries, including work with an estriol-eluting pessary, although these are not commonplace [2, 3]. There are two main types of pessaries: space-filling and support. Examples of space-filling pessaries are Cube, Inflatoball, and Donut. Support pessaries include Ring and Shaatz.

Indications for pessary use include uterine or vaginal prolapse, cystocele, rectocele, enterocele, and stress urinary incontinence. Less common indications include an incompetent cervix and the correction of a retroverted or incarcerated uterus. For the surgeon, the pessary can also be used for preoperative selection of patients with SUI, as correction of incontinence with the pessary can predict successful postoperative correction of incontinence. A pessary can allow for healing of prolapsed pelvic mucosa prior to surgery. The pessary was originally indicated for pregnant women, those wishing to have more children, or those who had contraindications to surgery. Today, however, a pessary is an excellent option for anyone who prefers nonsurgical treatment of their condition and should be offered to patients with POP as an alternative to surgery [4]. A patient's lifetime risk of undergoing surgery for urinary incontinence and/or prolapse by age 80 is between 11% and 20% [5, 6]. Despite the common use of surgery, a prospective study by Abdool et al. showed

C. I. Keating (✉)
Berkshire Family Practice Associates, North Adams, MA, USA
e-mail: ckeating@bhs1.org

S. M. Sulik, C. B. Heath (eds.), *Primary Care Procedures in Women's Health*,
https://doi.org/10.1007/978-3-032-07061-6_18

similar outcomes at 1 year in urinary, bowel, sexual function, and quality of life parameters between women treated with surgical repair and those treated with pessary placement for pelvic organ prolapse [7]. Successful reported continuation rates for pessary use for POP in studies range from 62% at 1 year to 75% at 5 years [8, 9].

One-third of premenopausal patients and up to 45% of postmenopausal patients experience POP and/or SUI [10]. While these symptoms are more common in parous women, nulliparity does not provide absolute protection against prolapse or SUI [11]. Different pessary styles are appropriate for different degrees, or stages, of prolapse. The pelvic organ Prolapse Quantification (POP-Q) defines Stage 1 as descent of the uterine cervix to above 2 cm from the hymen, Stage 2 as descent to within 1 cm of the hymen, either externally or internally, Stage 3 as descent 1–2 cm below the hymen, and Stage 4 as descent 2 cm past the hymen (Fig. 18.1) [12]. Reported successful use of pessaries ranges from 33.9% to 89% [13–15]. Although pessaries can successfully be used to treat most stages of prolapse, complete organ prolapse most often needs surgical repair. Studies have not shown an association between prolapse stage and outcome of a pessary trial [16, 17].

One study found that improvement in prolapse symptoms was limited to patients with anterior vaginal wall prolapse [14]. Patient characteristics associated with continued successful pessary use for pelvic organ prolapse are age greater than 65 years and being considered a high surgical risk [18]. Risk factors for unsuccessful pessary fittings and use are inconsistent across studies and include previous reconstructive surgery for prolapse or hysterectomy, obesity, increased parity, severe posterior vaginal wall prolapse, short vaginal length, menopause, and wide introitus [15, 16, 19–21]. One study demonstrated that weight was not a negative or positive predictor of successful fitting and use [15]. Another study among patients with pelvic floor dysfunction showed that pessary satisfaction was associated with improvements in sexual function and body image [22]. Patients who use vaginal estrogen had a higher incidence of continued pessary use and a lower incidence of vaginal discharge than patients who did not [23].

One complication of treating prolapse with a pessary is the unmasking of underlying urinary incontinence. One study showed that during treatment with a pessary

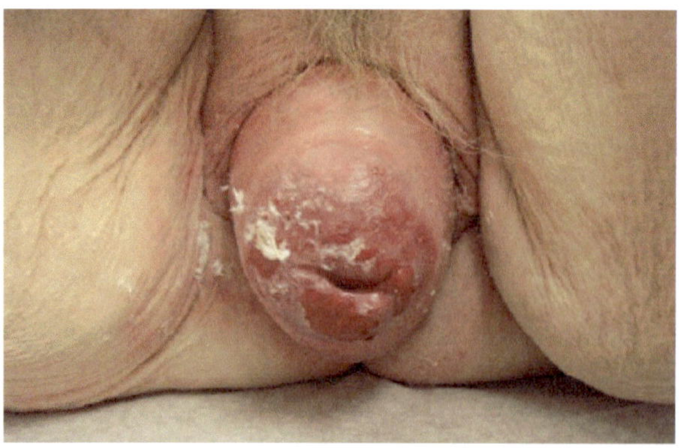

Fig. 18.1 Fourth-degree uterine prolapse

for prolapse, 21% of patients developed de novo stress incontinence, 6% urge incontinence, and 4% developed difficulty with voiding. Despite these findings, 67% of treated patients reported improvement in prolapse or incontinence symptoms with pessary use [17]. If a patient with POP develops stress incontinence once fitted with a pessary, switching to an incontinence pessary may be helpful [24].

Pessary treatment for stress urinary incontinence occurs by compressing the urethra against the upper posterior portion of the symphysis pubis and elevating the bladder neck. This results in an increase in outflow resistance and corrects the angle between the bladder and the urethra [21]. Patients who have undergone prior incontinence surgery have a higher failure rate of pessary use for their incontinence [13].

Pessary use should be individualized based on the patient's symptoms (Table 18.1; Figs. 18.2, 18.3, 18.4, and 18.5). Patients who are incontinent during daily activities can wear the pessary continually. For others who experience incontinence only during vigorous activities, the pessary can be worn as needed. One small study showed 5 of 14 subjects achieved complete continence during vigorous exercise [26]. A review showed a randomized controlled study of the use of pessaries which compared the effectiveness between Gellhorn and Ring pessaries. No significant differences in effectiveness (60%) were found between the two groups [27, 28]. For patients with pelvic organ prolapse, if the pessary fails to remain in place, a stiffer pessary such as a Shaatz or Gellhorn may be used. Cube pessaries may be better for severe prolapse but need close follow-up because of the higher risk of erosions and daily removal [29]. It is important for patients to follow up with their health care providers once fitted with any pessary. Major complications are more likely to occur in patients who are lost to follow-up.

Table 18.1 Pessary style choices based on symptom

First- and second-degree uterine prolapse	Ring, Donut, Milex® Inflatoball, Milex® Regula
Mild prolapse with cystocele	Ring with support, Shaatz
Third- and fourth-degree uterine prolapse	Cube, Donut, Milex® Inflatoball, Gellhorn
Third- and fourth-degree uterine prolapse with cystocele	Gehrung
Prolapse s/p hysterectomy	Ring with support
Mild cystocele	Ring with support, Dish with support, Hodge with support, Donut, Gehrung
Moderate cystocele	Gellhorn, Gehrung
Rectocele and enterocele	Gellhorn, Donut, Milex® Inflatoball, Cube, Gehrung
Stress incontinence	Incontinence Ring, Incontinence Dish
Incontinence during exercise	Ring, Ring with knob, Cube, Hodge, Inflatoball
Incontinence and cystocele	Hodge, Hodge with support

Data from Weber and Richter [11]; Viera and Larkins-Pettigrew [25]; http://milexproducts.com Milex®, CooperSurgical, Trumbull, CT

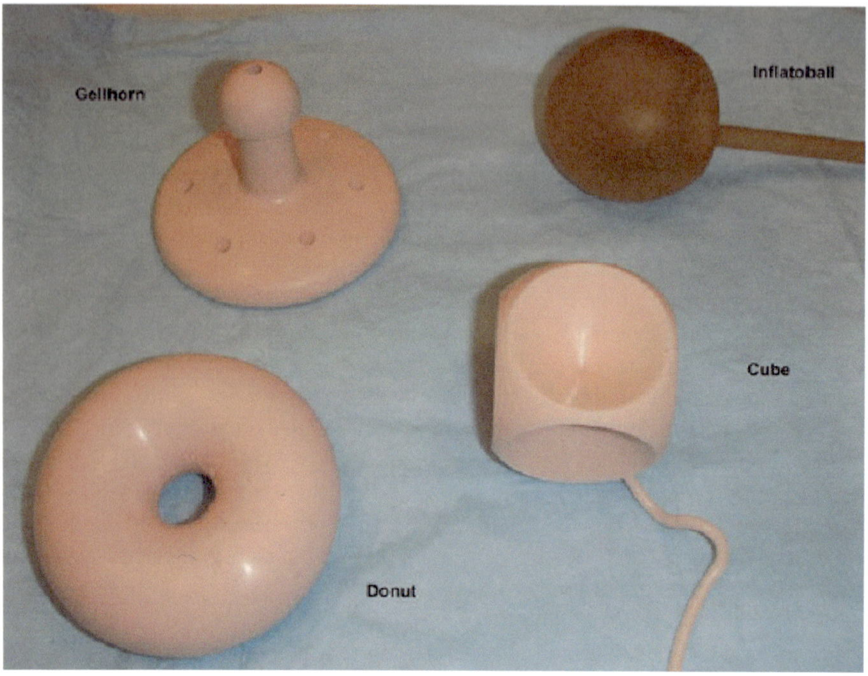

Fig. 18.2 Space-filling pessaries (pelvic organ prolapse)

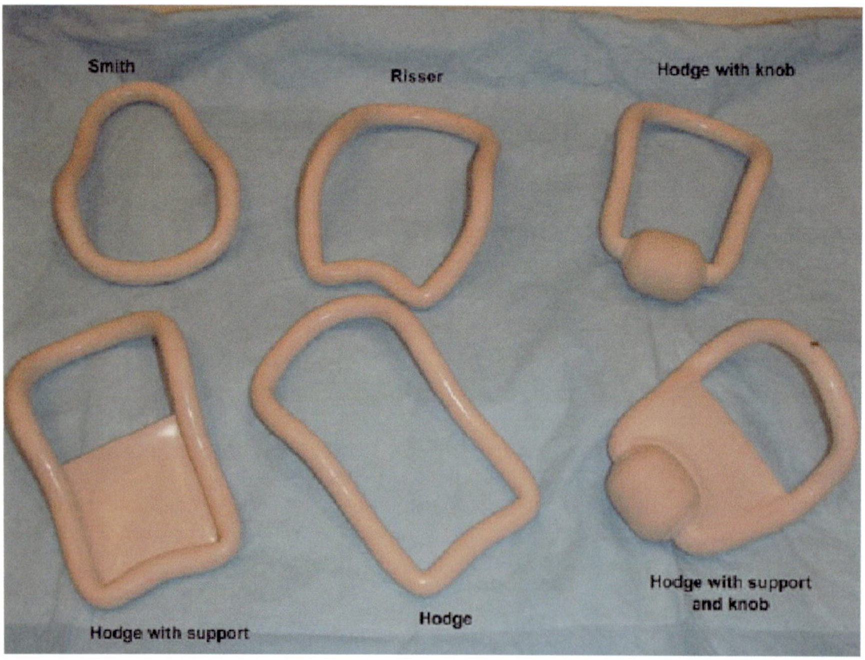

Fig. 18.3 Support pessaries (pelvic organ prolapse)

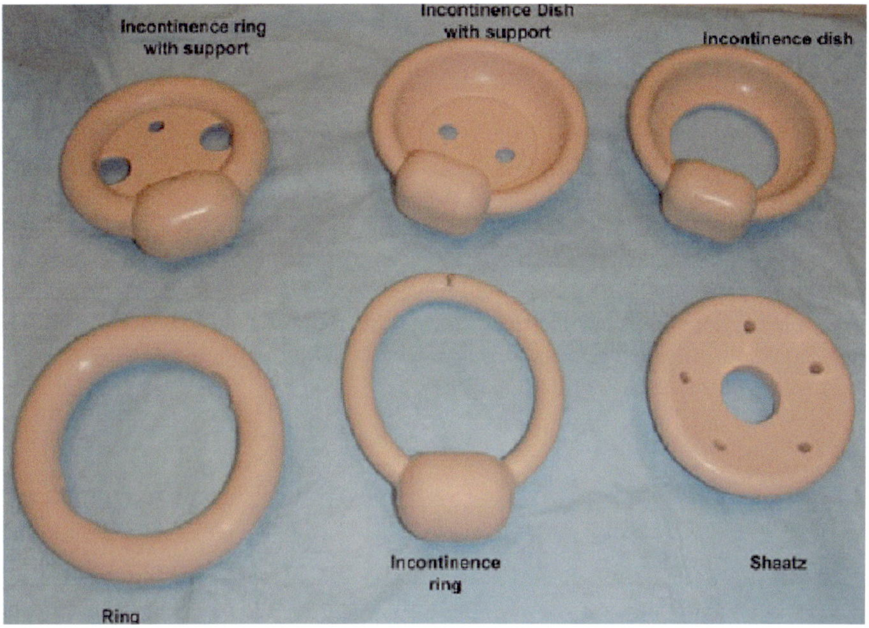

Fig. 18.4 Incontinence pessaries

Fig. 18.5 Saddle pessaries

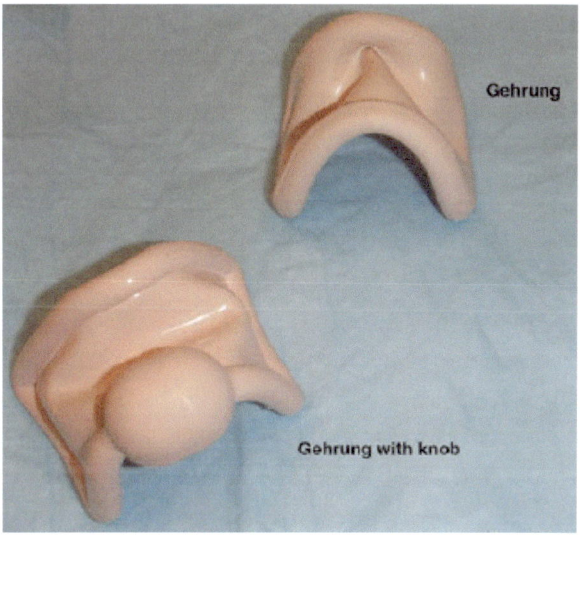

Case Study

Case A

A 36-year-old patient with a past medical history significant for two vaginal deliveries following uncomplicated pregnancies presents to your office for a routine physical examination. After the last pregnancy, she noticed that she occasionally leaked urine when she laughed, coughed, or while she was running. She failed to mention her symptoms at a postpartum checkup because she thought they were normal, but a year later, she is still troubled with the problem and would like to know about treatment options. She performs Kegel exercises only intermittently. Today, the pelvic exam is completely within normal limits.

Case B

A 72-year-old female with a history of a cystocele presents for evaluation. Previously, she has been able to tolerate her symptoms of stress incontinence; however, today, she is interested in available treatment options. On exam, the patient has a grade I cystocele and slight atrophy of vaginal mucosa consistent with chronic estrogen deficiency.

Diagnosis

- Stress incontinence
- Pelvic organ prolapse

Differential Diagnosis

Urge incontinence

Indications (Algorithm 18.1)

- Pelvic organ prolapse
- Vaginal vault prolapse
- Cystocele

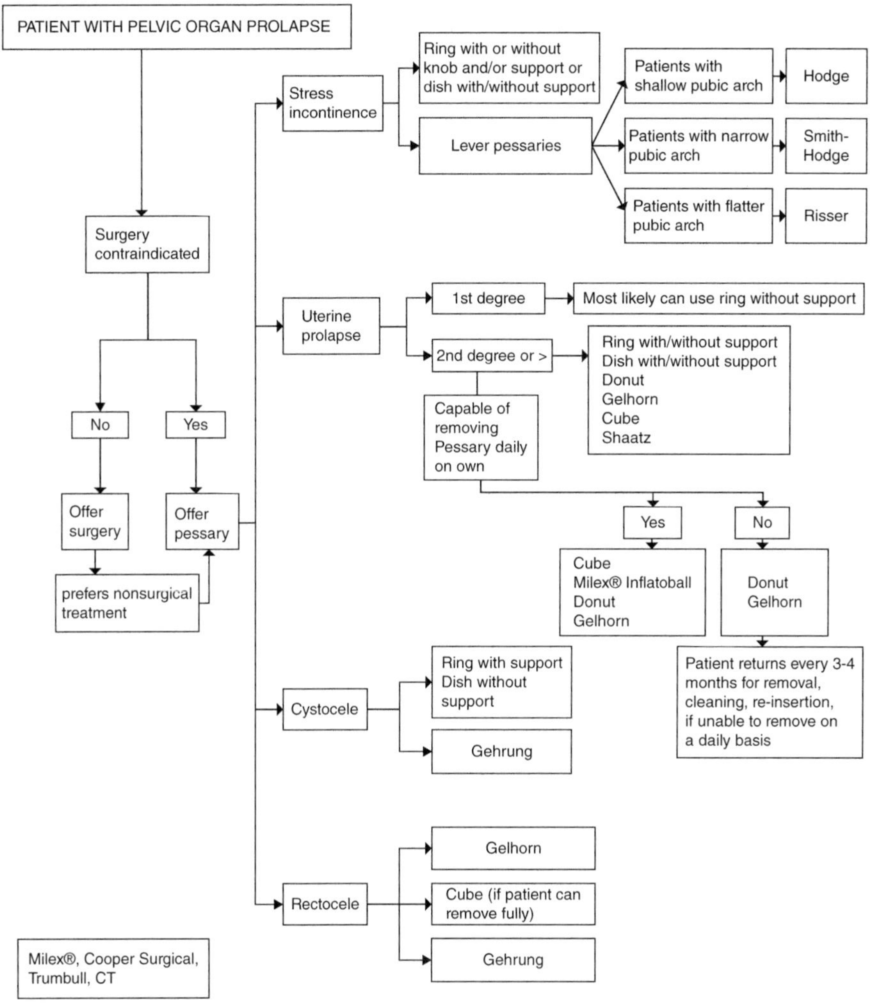

Algorithm 18.1 Decision tree for a patient with pelvic organ prolapse

- Rectocele
- Enterocele
- Uterine prolapse
- Stress urinary incontinence
- Preoperative evaluation for stress incontinence
- Preoperative preparation for eroded prolapsed tissue

Contraindications

- Noncompliance
- Vaginal erosions
- Active vaginal or pelvic infections
- Silicon or latex allergy

Equipment (Figs. 18.6 and 18.7)

- Pessary fitting kit or actual pessaries for fitting (Table 18.1). Note that the pessaries come in a variety of sizes.
- Water-based lubricant

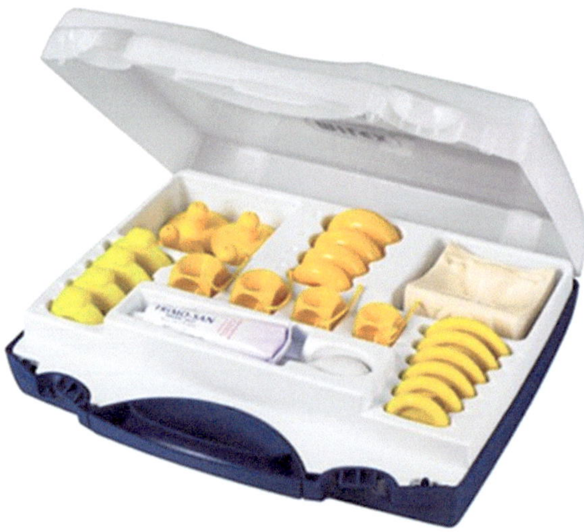

Fig. 18.6 Milex pessary fitting kit with incontinence dish with support, ring with support, Gellhorn, cube and donut pessaries, and Milex Trimo-San Vaginal Jelly (CooperSurgical, Trumball, CT)

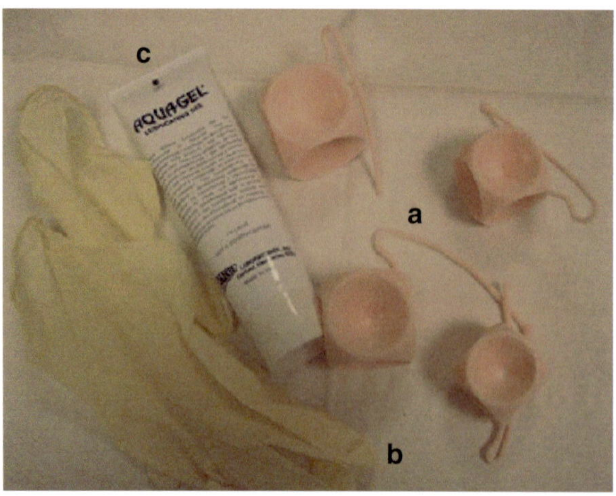

Fig. 18.7 Cube (**a**) pessary set up with gloves (**b**) and Aqua-Gel® Lubricating Gel (Parker Laboratories, Fairfield, NJ) (**c**)

Procedure

1. Patient preparation
   (a) For pelvic organ prolapse, have the patient empty her bladder.
   (b) For incontinence, fit the patient with a full bladder.
2. Place the patient in the lithotomy position.
3. Replace any prolapsed tissue.
4. Perform a bimanual exam to estimate pessary size (Fig. 18.8).
5. Lubricate the tip of the pessary and introitus with water-based lubricant.
6. Insert the pessary into the vagina in a downward fashion, avoiding the urethra.
7. Position the pessary properly (Figs. 18.9, 18.10, 18.11, 18.12, 18.13, 18.14, 18.15, and 18.16). The examiner's fingers should pass easily between the pessary and vaginal wall.
   (a) Have the patient stand, walk, and Valsalva.
   (b) If painful or uncomfortable, try the next smallest size.
   (c) If it falls out or starts to slip out, try the next largest size. The largest pessary that the patient can comfortably wear is generally the most effective.
8. Patient needs to void effectively before leaving the office to ensure there is no urethral obstruction.
9. Schedule follow-up visit within 1 week.
   (a) Remove pessary and inspect vagina for irritation, erosion, or allergic reaction.
10. For those unable to remove their own pessary, schedule routine removal and cleaning visits from 1 to 6 months depending on doctor and patient preference.

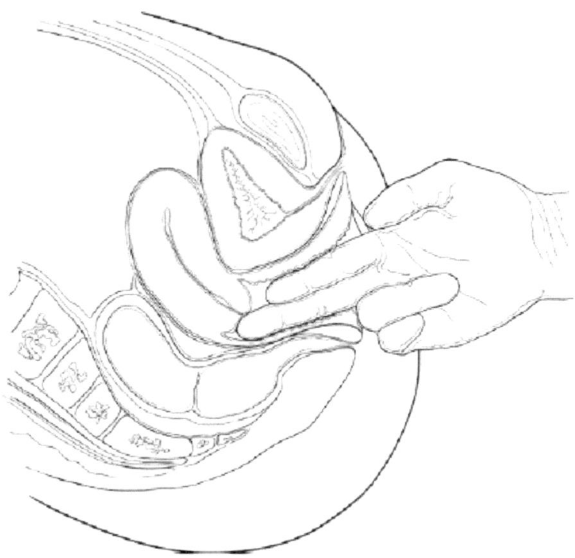

Fig. 18.8 Estimate the pessary size

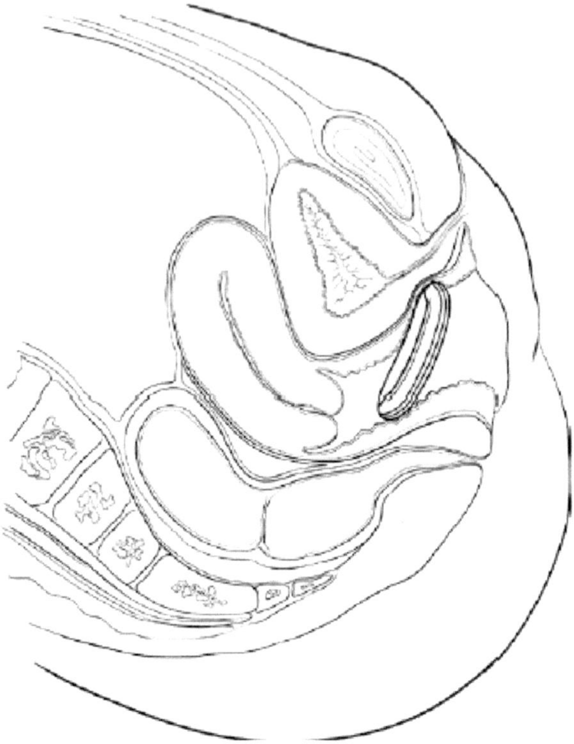

Fig. 18.9 Proper position of the incontinence Ring pessary

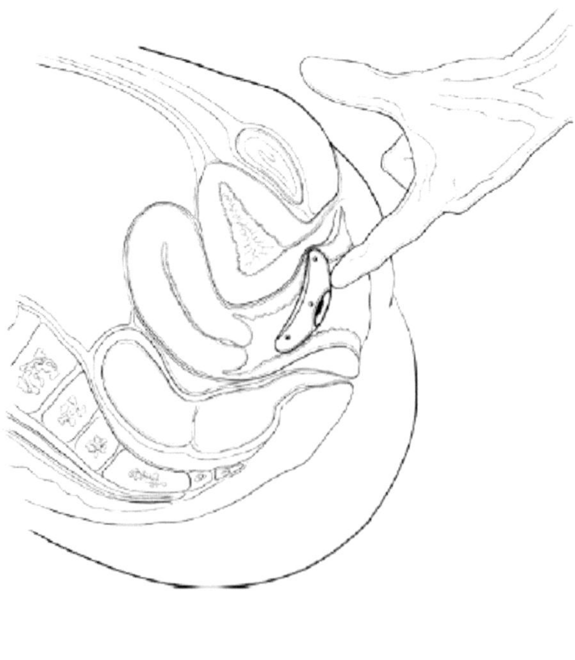

Fig. 18.10 Placement of a Shaatz pessary

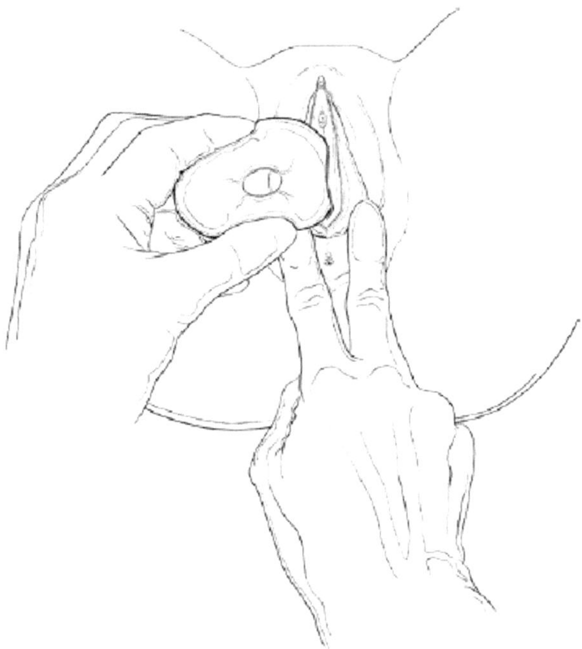

Fig. 18.11 Insertion of a Donut pessary

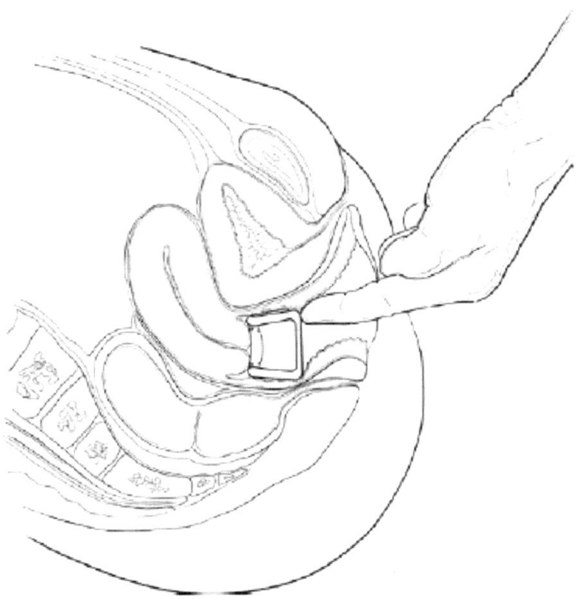

Fig. 18.12 Proper position of the Milex® Regula pessary (CooperSurgical, Trumbull, CT)

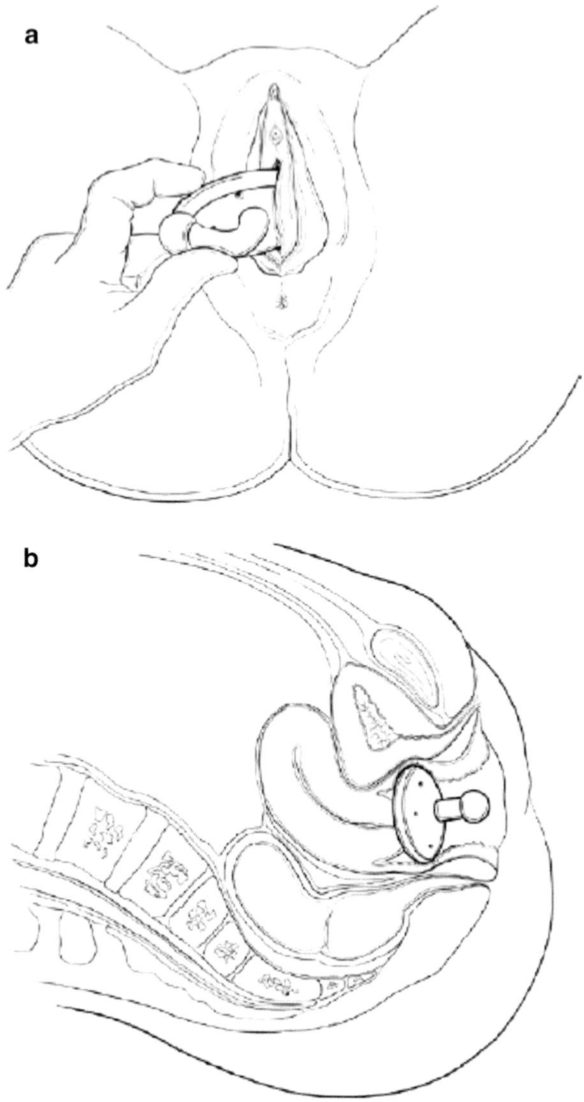

Fig. 18.13 (**a**) Gellhorn knob is folded on its side for easier insertion. (**b**) Proper position of the inserted Gellhorn pessary

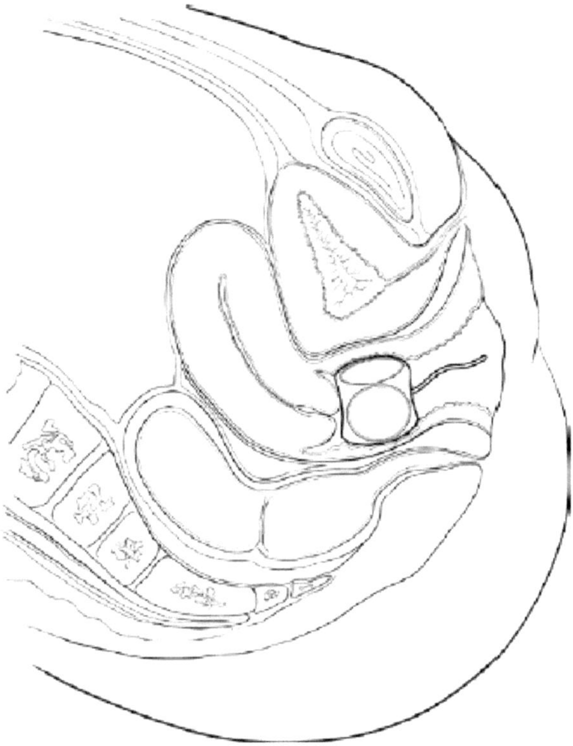

Fig. 18.14 Cube pessary in proper placement

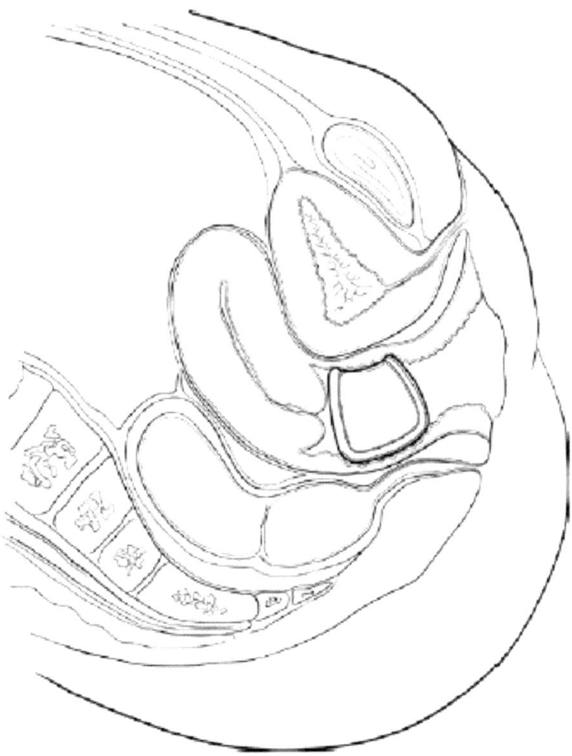

Fig. 18.15 Gehrung pessary placement

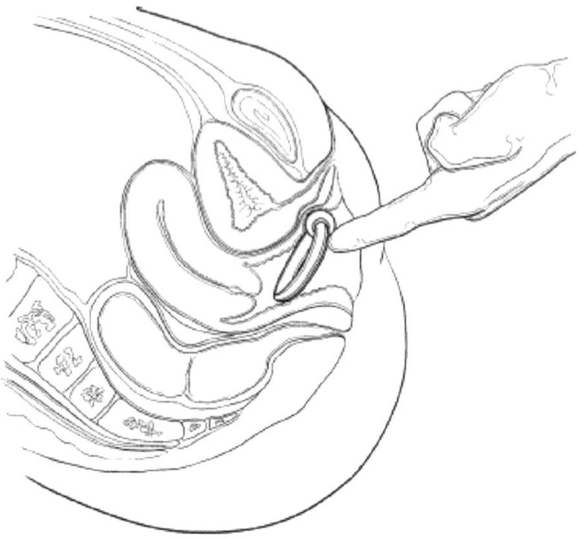

Fig. 18.16 Incontinence Ring with knob in proper position

Complications and Risks

- Vaginal irritation/erosions/bleeding
- Vaginal discharge and odor
- Discomfort
- Infections:
  - Bacterial vaginosis
  - Actinomycosis
  - Urosepsis
- Rectovaginal fistula
- Incarceration
- Dislodgment
- Urinary tract or bowel obstruction
- Hydronephrosis
- Cervical/uterine herniation/entrapment
- Latex allergy

Tricks and Helpful Hints

- For patients with atrophic vaginal tissue, pretreat for 1–2 weeks with estrogen cream (1/2 applicator full at night prior to bedtime) and continue use after successful pessary placement.
- Advise patients that it is not uncommon to need several to get the right size and shape pessary.

- If the patient is not going to be removing the pessary daily, use an acidic vaginal gel, such as Milex® Trimo-San (CooperSurgical, Trumbull, CT), three times a week (may be ordered with the pessary) to prevent odor and discharge.
- For patients who use a diaphragm, their diaphragm size does not correlate with their correct pessary size. (Patients may use a diaphragm to help with incontinence or prolapse.)
- If one size is too large and the next smaller size is too small, try a different style pessary.
- In some patients with long-term pessary use, it may be necessary to switch to a smaller or larger pessary over time.
- The Milex® Regula (CooperSurgical, Trumbull, CT) can be tried when expulsion of the pessary is a problem.
- The Milex® Inflatoball (CooperSurgical, Trumbull, CT) is a good choice for someone who needs a space-filling pessary but has a very narrow introitus and can remove the pessary on a daily basis.
- The Cube can be difficult to remove and needs to be removed daily.

Procedure Note

(Provider to customize as needed.)

Risks and benefits of pessary use were reviewed with the patient. The patient was placed in the lithotomy position. (Prolapsed tissue was inspected and replaced.) A bimanual exam was performed to estimate the pessary size. The chosen pessary was lubricated and gently inserted into the vagina. Fit was ensured as the pessary filled the vagina, and one finger passed easily around it. (If too loose, a larger size was tried. If uncomfortable or too tight, a smaller size was tried.) Patient was asked to stand, ambulate, and Valsalva with the pessary in place to ensure fit. Patient voided without difficulty with a pessary in place. A follow-up appointment was given.

Coding

CPT® Codes (Current Procedural Terminology, AMA, Chicago, IL)	
Pessary fitting	57160
Pessary, rubber	A4561
Pessary, nonrubber	A4562
ICD 10-CM-Diagnostic Codes (International Classification of Diseases, 10th Revision, Clinical Modification, Center for Disease Control and Prevention)	
Incontinence:	
Stress urinary	N39.3
Urge and stress	N39.46

Incompetent cervix	N88.3
Prolapse:	
Cystocele	N81.10
Uterovaginal, incomplete	N81.2
Uterovaginal, complete	N81.3
Uterovaginal, unspecified	N81.4
Uterus prolapse	
First degree	N81.2
Second degree	N81.2
Third degree	N81.3
Unspecified	N81.4
Posterior vaginal wall prolapse	N81.6
Vaginal vault prolapse post hysterectomy	N99.3

Postprocedure Patient Instructions

Have the patient call if the pessary becomes dislodged, falls out, or is uncomfortable or if the patient is having difficulty voiding or having a bowel movement with the pessary in place.

Follow up in 1–2 weeks for confirmation of fitting and vaginal exam to look for irritation, pressure sores, or allergic reaction.

Case Study Outcome

Case A

A size 3 cube pessary was successfully inserted into the vagina and positioned. The patient tolerated the pessary well and was able to walk and Valsalva without it falling out. She voided while at the office and was able to demonstrate removing the pessary. She understands the importance of taking the pessary out daily. She returns in 1 week for follow-up.

Case B

The patient is asked to use estrogen cream nightly for the next week. Upon returning the following week, the vaginal mucosa appears less atrophied. Attempts are made to fit a dish with support, but these prove uncomfortable. Next, the Gehrung is fitted with the patient experiencing no loss of the pessary with walking or a Valsalva maneuver. She also voids without difficulty. She is given a tube of Milex® Trimo-San and returns in 1 week for follow-up.

Postprocedure Patient Handout

(*Provider to fill in blanks/circle applicable choice when given multiple choices and customize as needed.*)

A pessary is a silicone or latex device placed inside your vagina. It can be used to help support your uterus (which can hang down from its original position), vagina (which can lose firm support to its walls), bladder (which can push down into your vagina), or rectum (which can push up into your vagina). A pessary can also be used to help prevent the leakage of urine, which happens during coughing, sneezing, straining, or exercise. This is called stress incontinence.

Today you were fitted with a _____________ pessary. Ideally, your pessary should be removed and cleaned every _____________ day(s). It is important to follow your doctor's directions in caring for your pessary so it will last as long as possible. Remove and clean your pessary as instructed by your doctor today. You can use a mild soap and water to clean it. If you are not going to wear it, make sure to dry it completely and store it in a safe place. Your pessary can be worn even during your period, although it is very important to remove your pessary daily during your menses. Some women will leave their pessaries in for several days; however, if you do this, you may experience more discharge and odor.

Your doctor might have told you today that you do not need to remove your pessary yourself. If this is the case, your doctor will remove and check it for you at your follow-up appointment.

You will need to return for follow-up within 1 week to make sure the pessary fits well and is not causing any irritation in your vagina. Please call your clinician before your appointment if you experience any of the following: vaginal bleeding, vaginal pain, difficulty urinating, or having a bowel movement. Also, call if your pessary is falling out or falls out. After your first follow-up appointment, your clinician will schedule less frequent regular visits.

Many styles of pessaries can be worn during intercourse. Your doctor should have told you today if you can wear your pessary during intercourse.

You may have an increase in vaginal secretions/discharge or odor while using a pessary. Using Milex® Trimo-San cream or gel three times a week may be helpful in decreasing the discharge and odor.

Please call the office if you have any problems or questions.

References

1. Vierhout ME. The use of pessaries in vaginal prolapse. Eur J Obstet Gynecol Reprod Biol. 2004;117:4–9.
2. Barsky M, Kelley R, Bhora FY, Hardart A. Customized pessary fabrication using three-dimensional printing technology. Obstet Gynecol. 2018;131(3):493–7.
3. Long J, Zidan G, Seyfoddin A, Tong S, Brownfoot FC, Chowdary P. An estriol-eluting pessary to treat pelvic organ prolapse. Sci Rep. 2022;12(1):20021. https://doi.org/10.1038/s41598-022-23791-9. PMID: 36414726; PMCID: PMC9681886.

4. Pelvic organ prolapse: ACOG practice bulletin, number 214. Obstet Gynecol. 2019;134(5):e126–42. https://doi.org/10.1097/AOG.0000000000003519.
5. Olsen A, Smith VJ, Bergstrom JO, Colling JC, Clark AL. Epidemiology of surgically managed pelvic organ prolapse and urinary incontinence. Obstet Gynecol. 1997;89:501–6.
6. Wu JM, Matthews CA, Conover MM, Pate V, Jonsson Funk M. Lifetime risk of stress urinary incontinence or pelvic organ prolapse surgery. Obstet Gynecol. 2014;123(6):1201–6. https://doi.org/10.1097/AOG.0000000000000286. PMID: 24807341; PMCID: PMC4174312.
7. Abdool Z, Thakar R, Sultan AH, Oliver RS. Prospective evaluation of outcome of vaginal pessaries versus surgery in women with symptomatic pelvic organ prolapse. Int Urogynecol J. 2011;22:273–8.
8. Ma C, Zhou Y, Kang J, Zhang Y, Ma Y, Wang Y, Tian W, Xu T, Liang S, Fan G, Cui Y, Zhu L. Vaginal pessary treatment in women with symptomatic pelvic organ prolapse: a long-term prospective study. Menopause. 2021;28(5):538–45. https://doi.org/10.1097/GME.0000000000001751. PMID: 33625108.
9. Yurteri-Kaplan LA, Meyn L, Moalli PA, Bradley CS, Foster RT Sr, Andy UU, Guaderrama N, Gutman RE, Anger JT, Hull A, Propst K, Shippey SS, Brown HW. Outcomes of pessary use at 1 year in women treated for pelvic organ prolapse in a large multicenter registry: developed by the pelvic floor disorders registry. Urogynecology (Phila). 2022;28(12):800–10. https://doi.org/10.1097/SPV.0000000000001279. PMID: 36409637.
10. Brown JS, Nyberg LM, Kusek JW, Burgio KL, Dioko AC, et al. Proceedings of the national institute of diabetes and digestive and kidney diseases international symposium on epidemiologic issues in urinary incontinence. Am J Obstet Gynecol. 2003;188:S77–88.
11. Weber AM, Richter HE. Pelvic organ prolapse. Obstet Gynecol. 2005;106(3):615–34.
12. Baden WF, Walker T. Fundamentals, symptoms and classification. In: Baden WF, Walker T, editors. Surgical repair of vaginal defects. Philadelphia: J.B. Lippincott; 1992. p. 14.
13. Farrell SA. Continence pessaries in the management of urinary incontinence in women. J Obstet Gynaecol Can. 2004;26:113–7.
14. Handa VL, Jones M. Do pessaries prevent the progression of pelvic organ prolapse? Int Urogynecol J Pelvic Floor Dysfunct. 2004;13:349–52.
15. Maito JM, Quam ZA, Craig E, Danner KA, Rogers RG. Predictors of successful pessary fitting and continued use in a nurse-midwifery pessary clinic. J Nurse Midwifery. 2006;51:78–84.
16. Mutone MF, Terry C, Hale DS, Benson JT. Factors which influence the short-term success of pessary management of pelvic organ prolapse. Am J Obstet Gynecol. 2005;193:89–94.
17. Clemons JL, Aguilar VC, Tillinghast TA, Jackson ND, Myers DL. Patient satisfaction and changes in prolapse and urinary symptoms in women who were fitted successfully with a pessary for pelvic organ prolapse. Am J Obstet Gynecol. 2004;190:1025–9.
18. Clemons JL, Aguilar VC, Sokol ER, Jackson ND, Myers DL. Patient characteristics that are associated with continued pessary use versus surgery after 1 year. Am J Obstet Gynecol. 2004;190:1025–9.
19. Fernando RJ, Thakar R, Sultan AH, Shah SM, Jones PW. Effect of vaginal pessaries on symptoms associated with pelvic organ prolapse. Obstet Gynecol. 2006;108:93–9.
20. Clemons JL, Aguilar VC, Tillinghast TA, Jackson ND, Myers DL. Risk factors associated with an unsuccessful pessary fitting trial in women with pelvic organ prolapse. Am J Obstet Gynecol. 2004;190:345–50.
21. Manzini C, Morsinkhof LM, van der Vaart CH, Withagen MIJ, Grob ATM. Parameters associated with unsuccessful pessary fitting for pelvic organ prolapse up to three months follow-up: a systematic review and meta-analysis. Int Urogynecol J. 2022;33(7):1719–63. https://doi.org/10.1007/s00192-021-05015-2. Epub 2022 Jan 17. PMID: 35037973; PMCID: PMC9270314.
22. Meriweather KV, Komesu Y, Craig E, Qualls C, Davis H, et al. Sexual function and pessary management among women using a pessary for pelvic floor disorders. J Sex Med. 2015;12(12):2339–49.
23. Dessie SG, Armstrong K, Modest AM, Hacker MR, Hota L. Effect of vaginal estrogen on pessary use. Int Urogynecol J. 2016;27(9):1423–9.

24. Schulz JA, Kwon E. Pelvic organ prolapse: pessary treatment. In: Baessler K, Schussler B, Burgio KI, Moore KH, Norton PA, Stanton SL, editors. Pelvic floor reeducation: principles and practice. London: Springer-Verlag London Limited; 2009. p. 271–7.
25. Viera AJ, Larkins-Pettigrew M. Practical use of the pessary. Am Fam Physician. 2000;61:2719–26, 2729.
26. Nygaard I. Prevention of exercise incontinence with mechanical devices. J Reprod Med. 1195;40:89–94.
27. Bugge C, Adams EJ, Gopinath D, Reid F. Pessaries (mechanical devices) for pelvic organ prolapse in women. Cochrane Database Syst Rev. 2013;(2):CD004010. https://doi.org/10.1002/14651858.
28. Cundiff GN, Amundsen CL, Bent AE, Coates KW, Schaffer JI, Strohbehn K, et al. The PESSRI study: symptom relief outcomes of a randomized crossover trial of the ring and Gellhorn pessaries. Am J Obstet Gynecol. 2007;196(4):405.e1–8.
29. Robert M, Schulz JA, Harvey M. Technical update on pessary use. J Obstet Gynaecol Can. 2013;35(7):664–74.

Additional Resources

Articles

Anders K. Devices for continence and prolapse. BJOG. 2004;111(Suppl 1):61–6.
Farrell SA. Practical advice for ring pessary fitting and management. J Soc Obstet Gynaecol Can. 1997;19:625–32.
Harvey MA, Lemieux MC, Robert M, Schulz JA. Guideline no. 411: vaginal pessary use. J Obstet Gynaecol Can. 2021;43(2):255–266.e1. https://doi.org/10.1016/j.jogc.2020.11.013. Epub 2020 Nov 26. PMID: 33248302.
Miser WF. For want of a pessary, the life was lost. J Am Board Fam Pract. 2002;15(3):249.
Vaginal pessary use and management for pelvic organ prolapse: developed by the joint writing group of the American Urogynecologic Society and the Society of Urologic Nurses and Associates. Individual writing group members are noted in the Acknowledgments section. Urogynecology (Phila). 2023;29(1):5–20. https://doi.org/10.1097/SPV.0000000000001293. PMID: 36548101.
Wheeler LD, Lazarus R, Torkington J, O'Mahoney MS, Woodhouse K. Lesson of the week: perils of pessaries. Age Ageing. 2004;33:510–1.

Miscellaneous

Milex pessary fitting kit (Cooper Surgical, Trumbull, CT) 1-800-243-2974; http://www.coopersurgical.com/ or
Monarch Medical Products 1-866-241-1625, http://www.monarchmedicalproducts.com.
Trimo-San vaginal cream or gel – Milex products, available over the counter.

Chapter 19
Bartholin Gland Cysts and Abscesses

Sandra M. Sulik

Introduction

Bartholin gland cysts are caused when trauma or inflammation obstructs the duct of the Bartholin gland, occurring in approximately 2% of women, most commonly in the reproductive years. The Bartholin gland ducts secrete mucus near the hymenal ring [1]. Cysts are often asymptomatic, and intermittent obstruction of the duct can cause the cyst to fluctuate in size. If secondarily infected, the cyst can become an abscess.

Visual inspection of the vulva will show a soft, compressible mass at approximately 4 o'clock or 8 o'clock on either side of the hymenal ring (Figs. 19.1 and 19.2). If not infected, Bartholin gland cysts are usually nontender. Abscesses are usually tender to palpation and may cause discomfort when walking, sitting, or with sexual intercourse. Abscesses may rupture spontaneously and may have associated cellulitis. When infected, the most common organism is *Escherichia coli*. Other organisms include *Chlamydia trachomatis*, *Brucella melitensis*, *Neisseria gonorrhoeae*, *Neisseria sicca*, *Pseudomonas aeruginosa*, *Staphylococcus aureus*, Bacteroides, *Pasteurella bettii*, or Salmonella enterica serovar Panama. Antibiotics are used when abscesses are present for at-risk patients such as those who are immunosuppressed, are pregnant, or have recurrences or widespread cellulitis. Bartholin's gland carcinoma is rare and tends to occur in women over 40 [2].

In addition to a drainage procedure with re-creation of a gland orifice, local heat to the area can provide relief of discomfort and enhance healing.

S. M. Sulik (✉)
St. Joseph's Health, Professor Emeritus, Upstate Medical Center, Syracuse, NY, USA
e-mail: Sandra.sulik@sjhsyr.org

S. M. Sulik, C. B. Heath (eds.), *Primary Care Procedures in Women's Health*,
https://doi.org/10.1007/978-3-032-07061-6_19

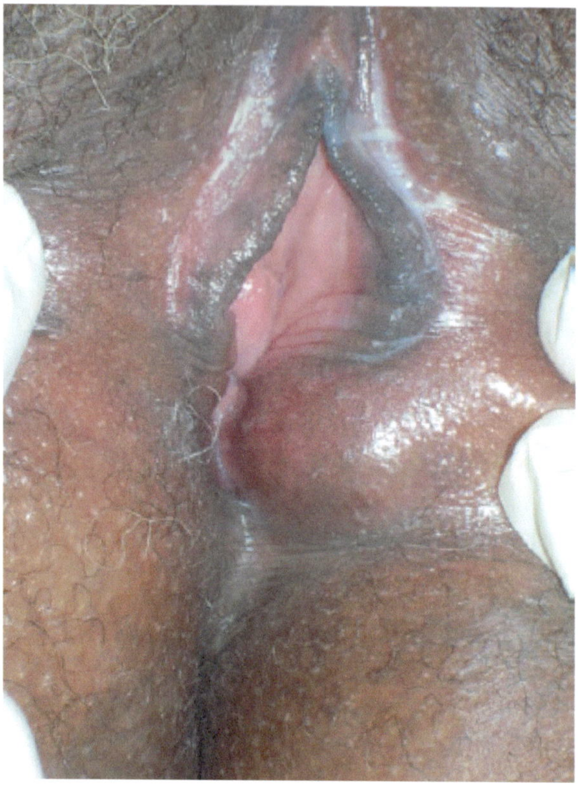

Fig. 19.1 Illustration of Bartholin gland cyst at the 4:00 position

Bartholin gland cysts or abscesses are distinct from other vulvar masses in their location and cystic texture on palpation. Solid or vascular vulvar masses generally do not lie in the same anatomic position as a Bartholin gland cyst or abscess [3]. Bartholin glands are most active during the reproductive years; therefore, masses occurring before puberty or beyond the menopausal period are not likely to be Bartholin cysts.

A number of treatments have been described for Bartholin gland cysts including Word catheter insertion, marsupialization, simple needle drainage, Jacobi ring insertion, silver nitrate gland ablation, or gland excision [4]. The Word catheter, placed inside the Bartholin gland cyst, is a small silicone device with a balloon that allows it to function as a self-retaining drain [5]. It can remain in place within the cyst for several days to up to 4 weeks to allow a new gland opening to epithelialize [4, 6]. A Jacobi ring can be constructed using a piece of rubber tubing (tubing from a butterfly needle can be used) and suture material that is threaded through the tubing, the ring is placed in the cyst, and left to drain and epithelialize similarly to the Word catheter [1]. Alternatively, women may need a marsupialization procedure if the cyst or abscess is recurrent. Studies have shown no significant difference in recurrence rates between Word catheter and marsupialization [7–9] but significantly

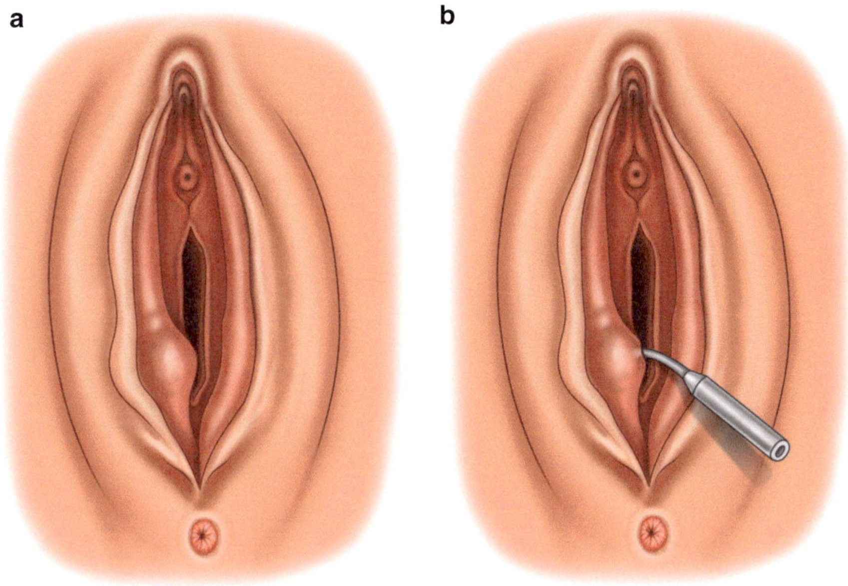

Fig. 19.2 (**a**) Drawing of the Bartholin gland with cyst. (**b**) Word catheter in place within the Bartholin cyst

lower costs with Word catheter or Jacobi ring placement. Quality of life was found to be good during treatment with the Word catheter [8, 9]. A systematic review showed less recurrence with marsupialization, and recurrence rates were reported to be similar with Word's catheters and Jacobi rings; however, patient satisfaction appeared higher in one comparative study with the ring [4, 9].

Case Study

A 35-year-old patient presents for a health maintenance examination and states that she has for 6 months noted a swelling on the right side of her vulva near the vaginal opening. She is concerned because it gets larger at times, and she has had pain when she sits or has intercourse.

Diagnosis (Algorithm 19.1)

Bartholin gland cyst or abscess.

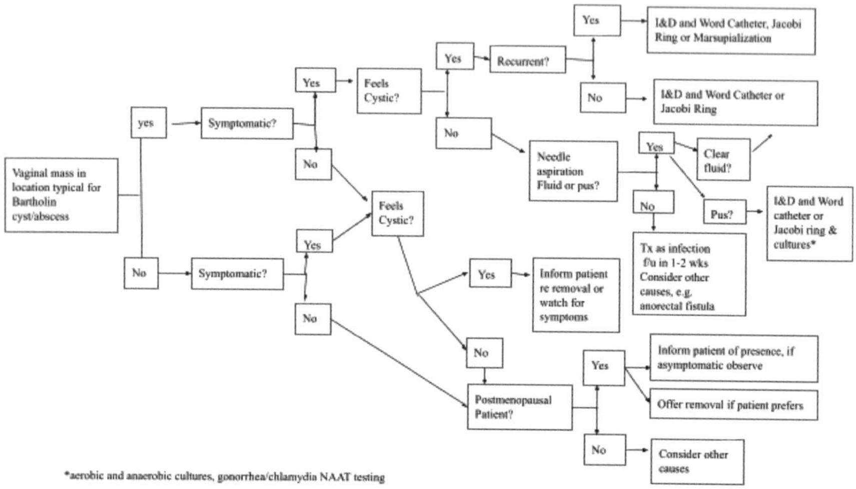

Algorithm 19.1 Decision tree for treatment of a vaginal mass near the hymenal ring

Differential Diagnosis

- Hematoma
- Endometrioma
- Sebaceous cyst
- Hemangioma
- Lipoma
- Malignant neoplasm: primary or metastatic carcinoma
- Sarcoma

Indications (Algorithm 19.1)

Symptomatic cyst or abscess

- The purpose of the procedure is not only to drain the cyst fluid but also to reestablish a gland opening in an optimal anatomical position.
- The procedure of first choice is incision and drainage of cyst/abscess with insertion of Word catheter or Jacobi ring.
- If prior drainage procedures have repeatedly failed, or follow-up is unlikely to occur, marsupialization of the cyst may be the primary management [1, 10].

Contraindications

- Bleeding disorders, systemic anticoagulation.

Equipment (Fig. 19.3)

- Word catheter or Jacobi ring (can be made from 5 cm of tubing from an 18-gauge butterfly needle with 3.0 nylon suture threaded through the tubing and used to tie into a ring)
- Antiseptic solution
- No. 11 or 15 scalpel
- 1% Lidocaine
- 22- or 25-Gauge 1-in. needle for catheter inflation
- 30-Gauge 1-in. needle for infiltration anesthesia
- 3- or 5-cc syringe
- 2 Hemostats: curved mosquito, and straight
- Silver nitrate stick
- 4 × 4 Sterile gauze pads
- Pickups with teeth
- Needle holder: small
- 3-0 or 4-0 Absorbable suture on small cutting needle
- Scissors
- Eye protection
- Mask
- Gloves

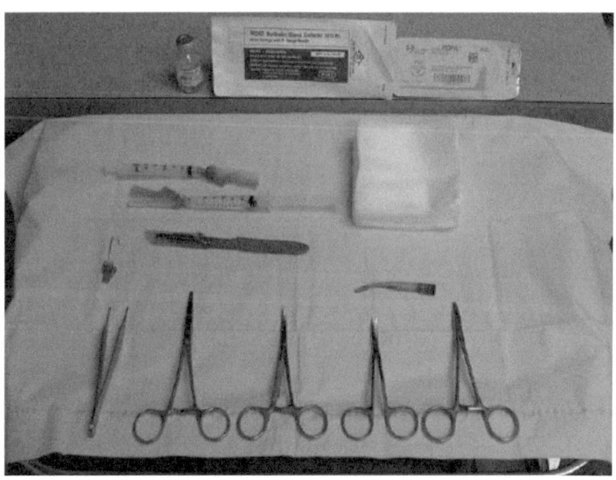

Fig. 19.3 Sterile setup tray for Word catheter insertion: (**a**) 1% lidocaine anesthetic, (**b**) syringe with 3 cc of 1% lidocaine, (**c**) needle driver, (**d**) hemostats, (**e**) scissors, (**f**) pickups, (**g**) scalpel, (**h**) 4 × 4 inch gauze, (**i**) Word catheter, (**j**) 3-cc syringe with water, (**k**) add extra needle 1½″ for a hook

Procedure

Procedure for Incision and Drainage with Word Catheter Placement

1. Remove the Word catheter from the package. Attach a 22- or 25-gauge 1″ needle to a 3-cc syringe filled with tap water.
2. Carefully insert the needle into the center of the wider end of the catheter and test the balloon by filling it with approximately 3 cc of water (Fig. 19.4).
3. Aspirate the water from the catheter and leave the catheter in place on the needle.
   - The syringe will serve as a handle to make the catheter easier to insert into the cyst, and fewer punctures mean less likelihood that the water will leak out.
4. Place the patient in a lithotomy position.
5. Have an assistant place traction on the vulvar skin to provide good exposure to the area.
6. Infiltrate the area over the cyst just inside the hymenal ring with local anesthetic in an area about 1.5 cm across.
7. Cleanse the area with antiseptic solution.
8. Stabilize the cyst with either your fingers or a needle-hook into the cyst (Fig. 19.5).
9. Make a stab incision approximately 1.5 cm deep and 0.5 cm long into the cyst (Fig. 19.6).
10. Insert a hemostat and spread the tips of the hemostat within the cyst or abscess to break up any loculation.
11. Insert the Word catheter into the cyst (Fig. 19.7) and fill the bulb with 2–3 cc of water. Remove the syringe from the catheter (Fig. 19.8).

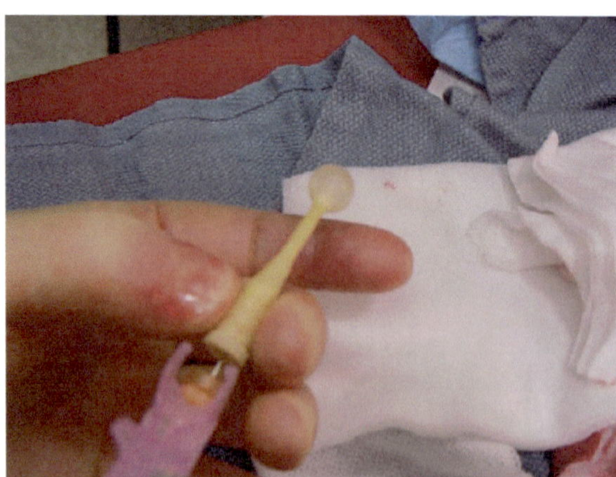

Fig. 19.4 Testing Word catheter balloon system

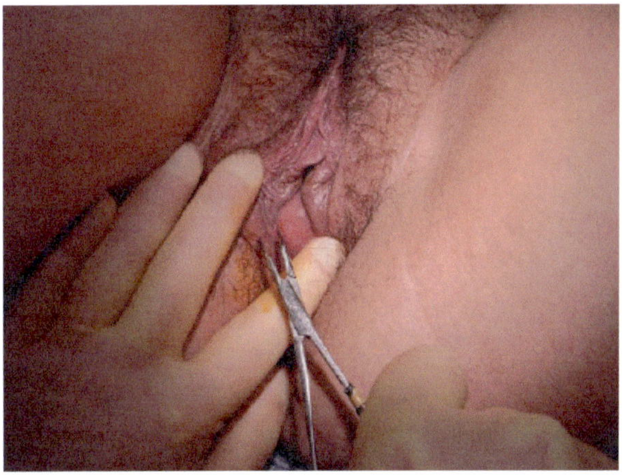

Fig. 19.5 Stabilization of Bartholin cyst prior to incision and drainage

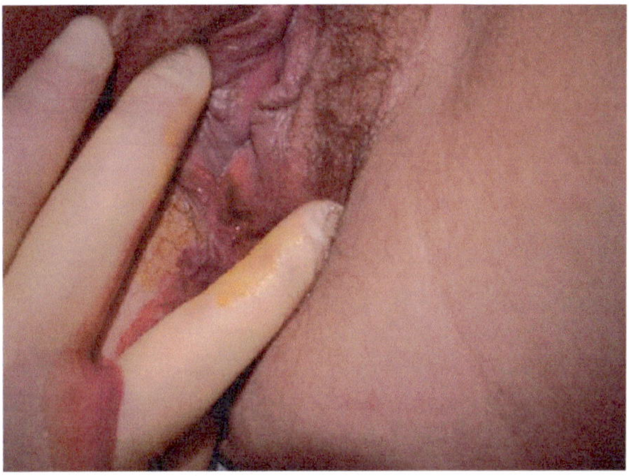

Fig. 19.6 Incision has been made into Bartholin cyst prior to insertion of Word catheter

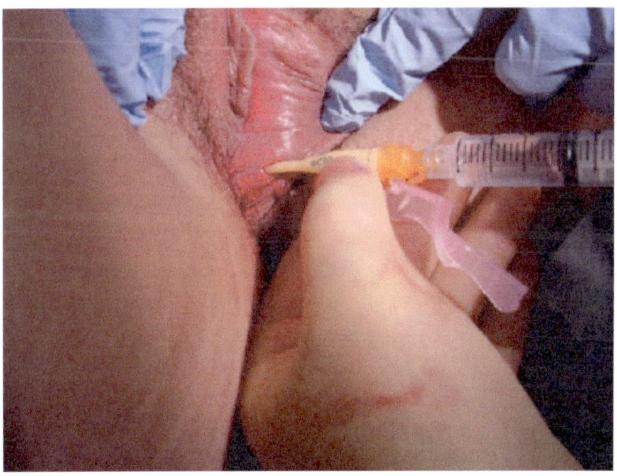

Fig. 19.7 Insertion of Word catheter

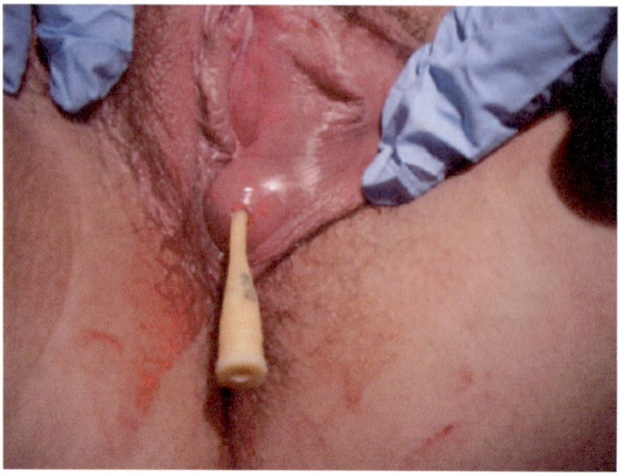

Fig. 19.8 Word catheter in place after insertion

12. If desired, place a small absorbable suture next to the incision, tie a knot, and then tie the suture around the catheter. Do not place a suture through the catheter.
13. Push the external end of the Word catheter up through the hymenal ring into the vagina. Instruct the patient that she can push it back up when it slips out.

Procedure for Jacobi Ring

1. Prepare Jacobi ring: Cut approximately 5 cm of tubing from a 16- or 18-gauge butterfly blood collection set. Thread 3.0 non-absorbable nylon suture through the tubing leaving 2–3 cm of suture on either side of the tubing (Fig. 19.10).
2. Place the patient in a lithotomy position.
3. Have an assistant place traction on the vulvar skin to expose the cyst.
4. Infiltrate the area with 0.5 cc of anesthetic locally.
5. Make a small stab incision in the lower mucosal surface of the abscess (Fig. 19.11).
6. Use the curved hemostat to tunnel to the upper portion of the cyst wall and make a second small incision (Fig. 19.12).
7. Using the tips of the hemostat, grasp the tubing/suture and pull through the cyst (Figs. 19.13 and 19.14).
8. Tie the two ends of the suture, forming a ring (Fig. 19.15).
9. Tuck the ring into the vagina.
10. The ring should stay in place for 4 weeks to allow for epithelization.
11. Have the patient return in 4 weeks, cut the suture, and gently remove the ring [1].

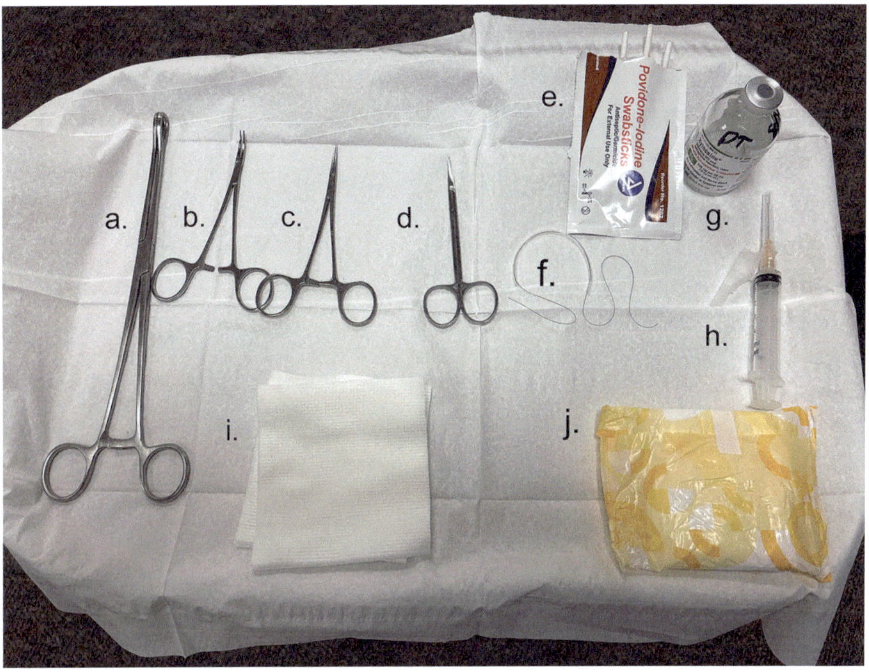

Fig. 19.9 Sterile setup tray for Jacobi ring insertion: (**a**) ring forceps, (**b**) curved hemostat, (**c**) straight hemostat, (**d**) iris scissors, (**e**) antiseptic swabs, (**f**) Jacobi ring, (**g**) lidocaine 1%, (**h**) 3-cc syringe, (**i**) 4 × 4 sterile gauze pads, (**j**) sanitary pad

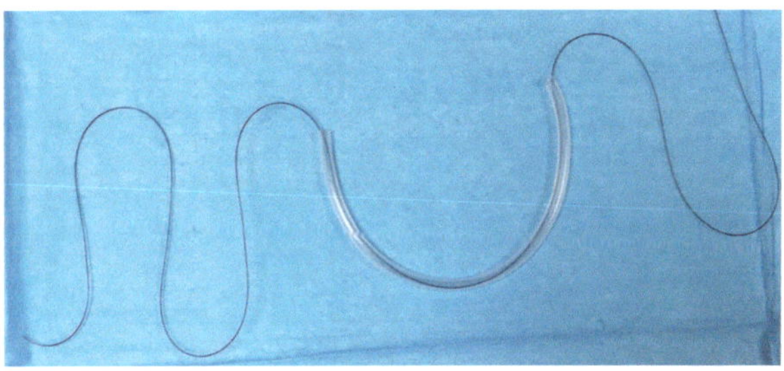

Fig. 19.10 Thread 3.0 nylon suture through the tubing leaving extra suture on each end

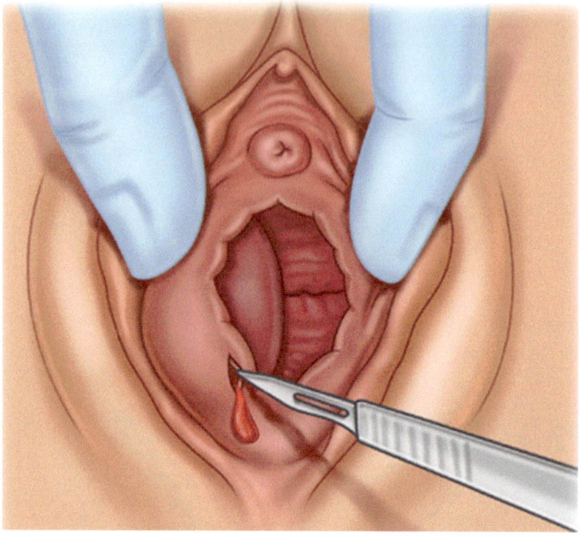

Fig. 19.11 Make a small stab incision into the abscess

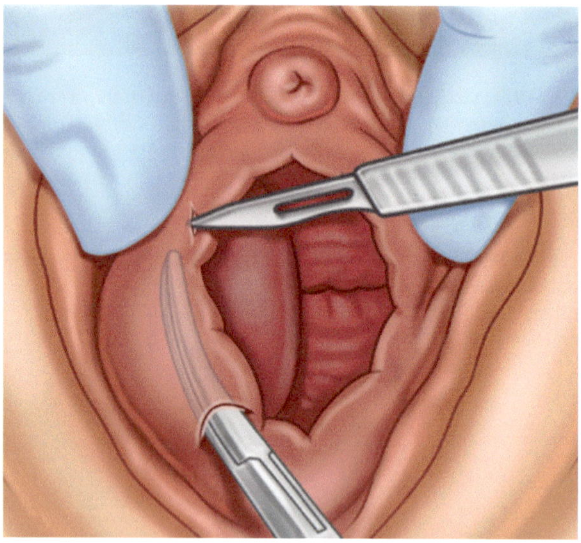

Fig. 19.12 Use the curved hemostat to tunnel to the upper portion of the cyst and make a small incision

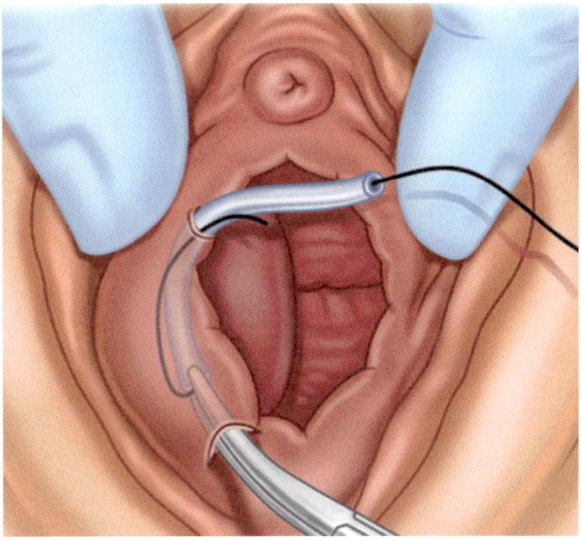

Fig. 19.13 Use the tips of the hemostat to pull the tubing through the cyst

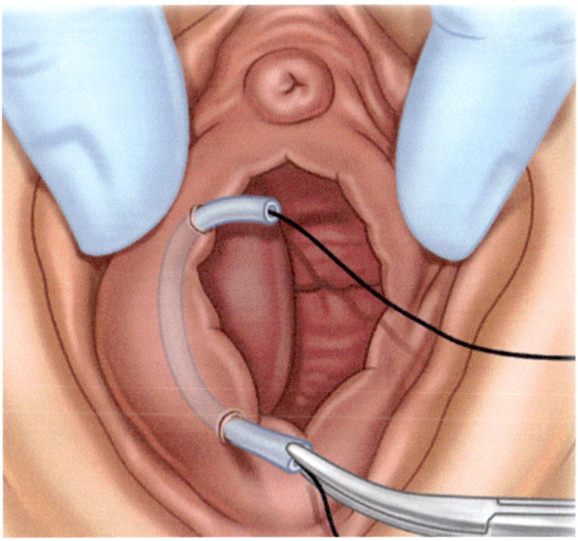

Fig. 19.14 Tubing is through the cyst

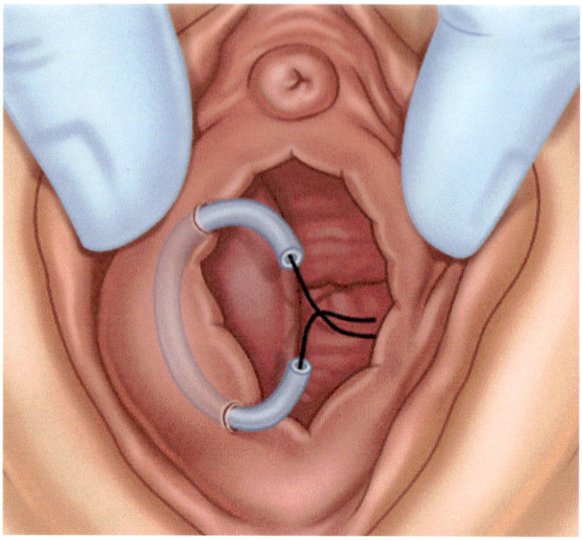

Fig. 19.15 Tie the suture to form a ring

Procedure for Marsupialization

1. Place the patient in a lithotomy position.
2. Have an assistant place traction on the vulvar skin to provide good exposure to the area.
3. Infiltrate the area over the cyst, just inside the hymenal ring, with local anesthetic in an area about 2.5 cm across.
4. Cleanse the area with antiseptic solution.
5. Stabilize the cyst with either your fingers or a needle-hook into the cyst (Fig. 19.16a).
6. Excise an ellipse of mucosa and its underlying cyst wall approximately 1–1.5 cm in diameter (Fig. 19.16b, c).
7. Insert a hemostat and spread the tips within the cyst or abscess to break up any loculation.
8. Suture the vulvar mucosa to the cyst wall around the circumference of the incision, using either running or simple interrupted absorbable sutures (Fig. 19.16d).

Complications and Risks

- Bleeding at the site
- Infection
- Reactions to local anesthetic
- Reactions to latex unless a silicone Word catheter is used

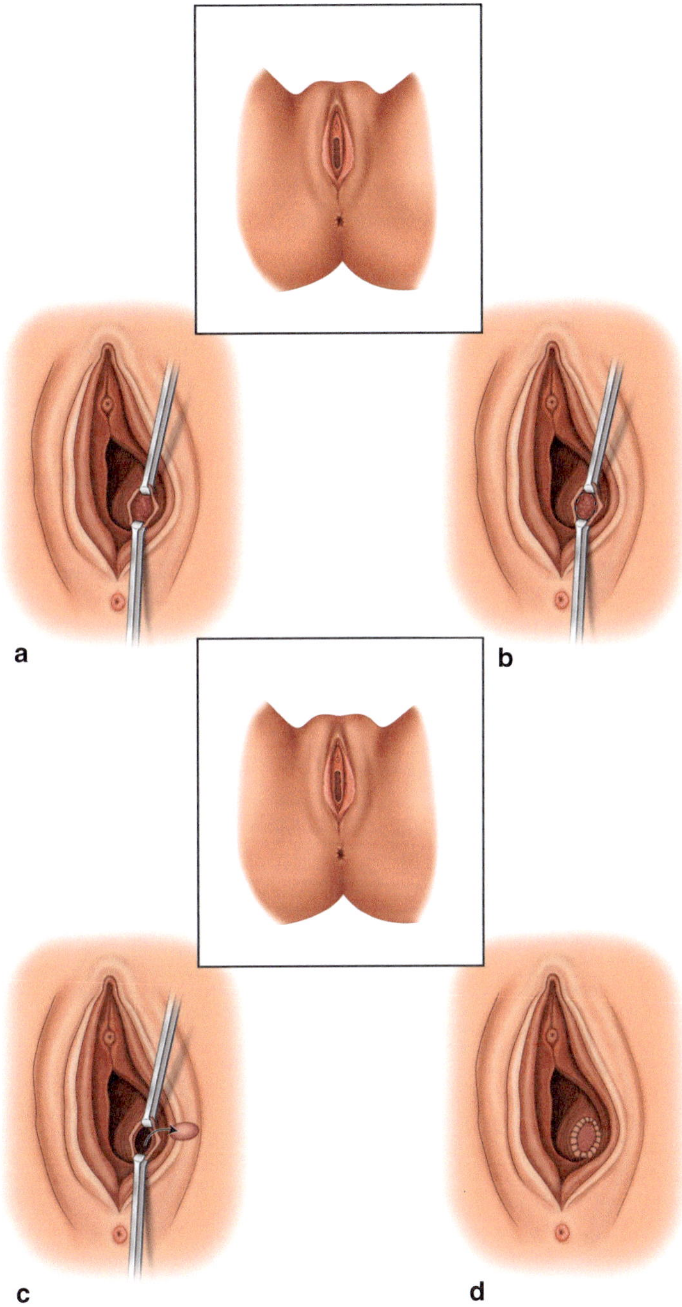

Fig. 19.16 Bartholin cyst Marsupialization steps (**a**–**d**) Bartholin cyst marsupialization. (**a**) Stabilization of the Bartholin cyst. (**b**) An elliptical incision is made on the center of the cyst. (**c**) Excise an ellipse of mucosa and its underlying cyst wall approximately 1–1.5 cm in diameter. (**d**) Suture the vulvar mucosa to the cyst wall around the circumference of the incision, using either running or simple interrupted absorbable sutures

Tricks and Helpful Hints

- Having an assistant to help with maintaining exposure to the area will make the procedure much easier.
- Do not inflate the Word catheter with air: it will leak out too soon. Sterile water is not necessary for filling the catheter, as the vulva is not sterile.
- Take care when inserting the needle into the catheter not to pierce the side or end of the catheter.
- Stabilize the cyst wall by using a curved hemostat or make a needle-hook by using a hemostat to bend a 25-gauge 1½″ needle attached to a small locking syringe. The syringe serves as a handle for the hook, which can be placed into the cyst to stabilize it, facilitate exposure, and make it less likely for the skin and the cyst wall to "eclipse" the incision, which makes proper insertion of the Word catheter difficult (see Fig. 19.17).
- A portable warm soak can be made by folding a washcloth in quarters and then once again to make a rectangle approximately the size of a sanitary pad (Fig. 19.18). Place the washcloth in a sandwich-sized zipper-lock plastic bag, add enough water to soak the cloth, and seal the bag. Heat the bag and cloth in the microwave for a few seconds until it is warm but not hot to the touch. The woman can place this in her underclothing to provide moist heat without wetting her clothing. She can reheat the cloth as necessary without opening the bag.

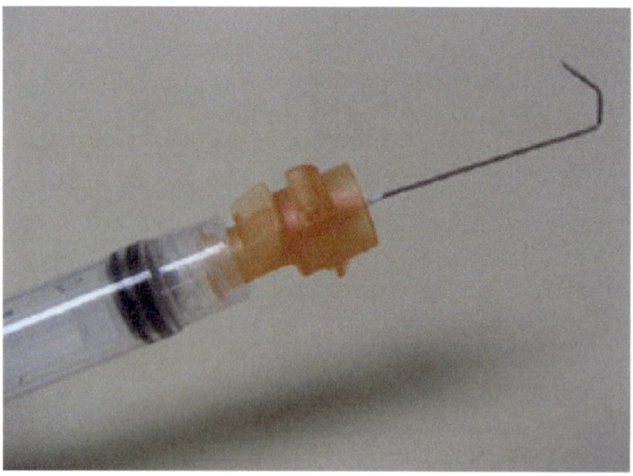

Fig. 19.17 Make a needle-hook by using a hemostat to bend a 25-gauge needle attached to a small Luer-tip syringe. The syringe serves as a handle for the hook, which can be placed into the cyst to stabilize it, facilitate exposure, and make it less likely for the skin and the cyst wall to "eclipse" the incision, making proper insertion of the Word catheter difficult

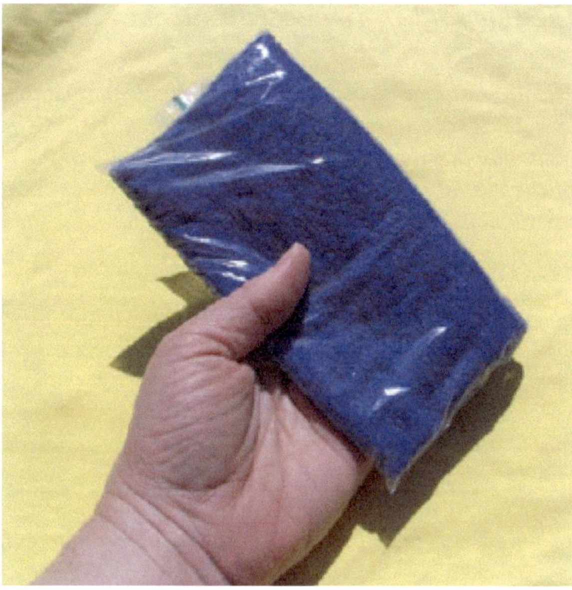

Fig. 19.18 Moist washcloth in a plastic sandwich bag can be microwaved and reused as a heat pack

Procedure Note

(*Provider to customize as needed.*)

Incision and Drainage with Word Catheter Placement

The procedure was discussed with the patient, including the benefits of draining cyst fluid/pus and establishing a new gland opening, as well as the likely relief of discomfort. Risks including bleeding, infection, early dislodging of the catheter, and possible recurrence of the cyst/abscess were discussed, as were alternative treatments for this condition. The patient states no known allergy to iodine or local anesthetics. Aftercare instructions were discussed. The patient signed a consent form for this procedure.

The patient was placed in the lithotomy position. The cyst was identified and palpated near the hymenal ring. Local anesthesia was achieved with 1–2 cc of 1% lidocaine by local infiltration. The area was cleansed with povidone–iodine and manually stabilized, and an incision was made into the cyst. A Word catheter that had been previously tested was placed into the cyst cavity and filled with water to allow retention of the balloon. (A retention suture of 4-0 absorbable suture was placed around the catheter.)

The patient tolerated the procedure well, and aftercare instructions were repeated. She is to return to the office in 2 weeks for follow-up.

Incision and Drainage with Jacobi Ring

The procedure was discussed with the patient, including the benefits of draining the cyst fluid/pus and establishing a new gland opening and relief of discomfort. Risks including bleeding, infection, early dislodging of the ring, and possible recurrence of the cyst/abscess were discussed as well as alternatives to treatment. Aftercare instructions were also reviewed. Consent form for the procedure was signed by the patient.

The patient was placed in the lithotomy position. The cyst was identified and palpated near the hymenal ring. Local anesthesia was infiltrated over the top of the cyst. A small stab incision was made in the lower aspect of the cyst, the cyst drained, and a curved hemostat was threaded through the cyst to the upper aspect, and a second stab incision was made. The Jacobi ring was grasped with the hemostat and pulled through the cyst. The edges were approximated, and the suture was tied. The ring was placed in the vagina.

The patient tolerated the procedure well. Postprocedure instructions were reviewed, and the patient was scheduled for a follow-up visit in 4 weeks.

Marsupialization of Bartholin Gland Cyst

The procedure was discussed with the patient, including the benefits of draining the cyst fluid/pus and establishing a new gland opening, as well as the likely relief of discomfort. Risks including bleeding, infection, and possible recurrence of the cyst/abscess were discussed, as were alternative treatments for this condition. The patient states no known allergy to iodine or local anesthetics. Aftercare instructions were discussed. The patient signed a consent form for this procedure.

The patient was placed in the lithotomy position. The cyst was identified and palpated near the hymenal ring. Local anesthesia was achieved with 1–2 cc of 1% plain lidocaine by local infiltration. The area was cleansed with povidone–iodine and manually stabilized, and an ellipse of mucosa and cyst wall was removed. The edge of the mucosa was sutured to the cyst wall in a circumferential fashion with running absorbable suture.

The patient tolerated the procedure well, and aftercare instructions were repeated. She is to return to the office in 2 weeks for follow-up.

Coding

CPT® Codes (Current Procedural Terminology, AMA, Chicago, IL)

Incision and drainage with Word catheter placement or Jacobi ring placement	
Procedure:	56420
Supplies:	99070
Marsupialization of Bartholin gland cyst	56440
ICD 10-CM-Diagnostic Codes (International Classification of Diseases, 10th Revision, Clinical Modification, Centers for Disease Control and Prevention)	
Bartholin gland cyst	N75.0
Bartholin gland abscess	N75.1

Postprocedure Patient Instructions

Incision and Drainage with Word Catheter or Jacobi ring Placement

- It is best if the catheter can remain in place for 2–4 weeks.
- If using a Word catheter or Jacobi ring, the patient may want to tuck the end of the catheter/ring back into the vagina when it comes out with straining, etc.
- Otherwise, the woman may resume her normal activities immediately after the procedure.
- Antibiotics are not necessary unless there is cellulitis or systemic signs of infection associated with an abscess.
- Instruct the patient to report any heavy bleeding, apply moist heat as much as possible during the first few days after the procedure, and return for follow-up as scheduled.
- Keeping the abscess open is adequate to allow healing in most cases.

Marsupialization of Bartholin Gland Cyst

- Warm moist soaks will help ease the discomfort and speed healing.

Case Study Outcome

At her follow-up visit 4 weeks after the procedure, the patient had good resolution of her symptoms, and the tract around the Word catheter was well-healed. The balloon was deflated with a needle, and the catheter was removed. She will return to the office as needed.

Postprocedure Patient Handout

(*Provider to fill in blanks/circle applicable choice when given multiple choices and to customize as needed.*)

What Is a Bartholin Gland Cyst or Abscess?
The Bartholin glands are small mucus-producing glands on either side of the vaginal opening. If a gland opening becomes blocked due to irritation or infection, the mucus can accumulate and form a cyst. If this fluid becomes infected, it can form an abscess.

How Is a Bartholin Gland Cyst or Abscess Treated?
The purpose of treatment is to drain the fluid and create a new opening for the gland. If the fluid is drained without creating a new opening, the cyst or abscess is more likely to come back. The usual treatment for Bartholin cysts is to drain the fluid and insert a small soft tube, called a Word catheter, which has a balloon that helps keep it in place within the cyst for about 2 weeks. Leaving the tube in place allows the body to heal with a new opening for the gland. The Word catheter procedure can be done in the office with local anesthesia. A Jacobi ring may be inserted in place of the Word catheter.

What Can I Do at Home to Feel Better?
Applying a warm pack to the area can help with the swelling and discomfort. Sometimes an abscess will drain on its own, and moist heat can help it heal more quickly. Getting extra rest will also help your body heal more quickly.

Acetaminophen 650 mg taken every 4–6 hours (h) or ibuprofen 400 mg every 4–6 h will help with your discomfort.

If you have a Word catheter or a Jacobi ring in place, it is OK to have sexual intercourse, and you can bathe normally with the catheter in place.

What if the Cyst or Abscess Comes Back?
If a cyst or abscess has come back more than once after the Word catheter procedure, your healthcare practitioner may recommend a procedure that makes a larger opening in the cyst. This procedure can usually be done in the office.

When Should I Call My Healthcare Practitioner?
If you have:

- Discomfort that is increasing rather than decreasing
- Fever or chills
- Any questions or concerns

Remember to keep your appointment for follow-up in 2–4 weeks.
Your appointment date and time is ____________________.

References

1. Omole F, Kelsey R, Phillips K, Cunningham K. Bartholin duct cyst and gland abscess: office management. Am Fam Physician. 2019;99(12):760–6.
2. Lee M, Dalpia A, Schwamn R, Miao Y, Waltzer W, Khan A. Clinical pathology of Bartholin's glands: a review of the literature. Curr Urol. 2014;8:22–5. https://doi.org/10.1159/000365683.
3. Wilkinson EJ, Stone IK. Atlas of vulvar disease. 5th ed. Baltimore: Williams & Wilkins; 1995. p. 11–5.
4. Wechter ME, Wu JM, Marzano D, Haefner H. Management of Bartholin duct cysts and abscesses: a systematic review. Obstet Gynecol Surv. 2009;64(6):395–404.
5. Word B. Office treatment of cyst and abscess of Bartholin's gland duct. South Med J. 1968;61(5):514–8.
6. Mayeaux EJ Jr, Cooper D. Vulval procedures: biopsy, Bartholin abscess treatment, and condyloma treatment. Obstet Gynecol Clin N Am. 2013;40:759–72.
7. Kroese JA, van der Velde M, Morssink LP, Zafarmand MH, Geomini P, van Kesteren PJM, Radder CM, van der Voet LF, Roovers JPWR, Graziosi GCM, van Baal WM, van Bavel J, Catshoek R, Klinkert ER, Huirne JAF, Clark TJ, Mol BWJ, Reesink-Pteres N. Word catheter and marsupialization in women with a cyst or abscess of the Bartholin gland (Wo-Man-trial): a randomized clinical trial. BJOG. 2017;124:243–9.
8. Reif P, Ulrich D, Bjelic-Radisic V, Hausler M, Schnedl-Lamprecht E, Tamussino K. Management of Bartholin's cyst and abscess using the Word catheter: implementation, recurrence rates and costs. Eur J Obstet Gynecol Reprod Biol. 2015;190:81–4.
9. Gennis P, Li S, Provataris J, Shahabuddin S, Schachtel A, Lee E, Bobby P. Jacobi ring catheter treatment of Bartholin's abscesses. Am J Emerg Med. 2005;23(3):414–5.
10. Reif P, Elsayed H, Ulrich D, Bjelic-Radisic V, Hausler M, Greimel E, Tamussino K. Quality of life and sexual activity during treatment of Bartholin's cyst or abscess with a Word catheter. Eur J Obstet Gynecol Reprod Biol. 2015;190:76–80. Cho JY, Ahn MO, Cha KS. Window operation: an alternative treatment method for Bartholin gland cysts and abscesses. Obstet Gynecol. 1990;76(5 Pt 1):886–8.

Additional Resources

Websites

http://www.operationalmedicine.org/Videos/Bartholin1.mpg: a video of the procedure of Word catheter insertion.

Equipment Companies

Artisan Medical 1-609-654-2613 www.artisanmed.com.
Cook Medical 1-800-457-4500 www.cookmedical.com.
CooperSurgical, 1-800-243-2974, www.coopersurgical.com.

Chapter 20
Endometrial Biopsy

Kristen McNamara

Introduction

The endometrial biopsy is a safe, simple office procedure that can diagnose most abnormal uterine bleeding. The most common indications for the procedure are bleeding after menopause or abnormal uterine bleeding (AUB) in younger patients. Other uses include the workup of an atypical glandular cell (AGC/AGC-US) Pap in patients over 35, evaluation of endometrial cells on a Pap in postmenopausal patients, or evaluation of patients bleeding on tamoxifen therapy. In most cases, office endometrial biopsy has replaced dilatation and curettage (D&C) due to its ease of performance in the outpatient setting. This also allows for the evaluation of patients with abnormal uterine bleeding who are poor candidates for general anesthesia.

Endometrial biopsy has a high overall accuracy when an adequate specimen is obtained. The overall sensitivity for detecting carcinoma is 99.6% in postmenopausal women and 91% in perimenopausal women. Endometrial sampling with a Pipelle® (Unimar, Wilton, CT) also detects atypical hyperplasia with a sensitivity of 81% and a specificity of 98% [1–3]. Some providers also use a uterine ultrasound to assess endometrial lining thickness prior to the endometrial biopsy. While significantly more costly, endometrial sampling with office hysteroscopy provides a higher accuracy for detecting focal lesions and polyps [4].

While no anesthesia is required for most endometrial biopsies, it is recommended that the patient takes a dose of a nonsteroidal anti-inflammatory drug (NSAID) such as ibuprofen prior to the procedure to decrease discomfort and cramping. In

K. McNamara (✉)
Faculty, St. Joseph's Family Medicine Residency, Syracuse, NY, USA
e-mail: kristen.mcnamara@sjhsyr.org

S. M. Sulik, C. B. Heath (eds.), *Primary Care Procedures in Women's Health*,
https://doi.org/10.1007/978-3-032-07061-6_20

addition, the use of local anesthesia with 1% lidocaine via a paracervical block can decrease pain as well. Use of a paracervical block can also decrease the risk of vasovagal events postprocedure [5]. Topical anesthesia can be used locally on the cervix for some reduction of discomfort caused by the placement of the tenaculum [6].

Performing an endometrial biopsy on a patient with a stenotic os is technically difficult for clinicians and uncomfortable for the patient. Nulliparous, breastfeeding, postmenopausal patients, or patients using progestogen-only contraceptives are at greatest risk for cervical stenosis. Treatment for cervical stenosis prior to performing the endometrial biopsy may involve insertion of a laminaria several hours to 1 day prior to the procedure, use of misoprostol intravaginally or orally 1–2 days prior to the procedure, or premedication with estrogen cream vaginally for 2 weeks prior to the procedure.

Case Study

A 56-year-old postmenopausal patient, LMP at age 54, presents to the office complaining of 2 days of vaginal bleeding and abdominal cramping last week that spontaneously resolved. The patient has not had any menses or vaginal bleeding in 2 years and used two pads on the first day of bleeding and one pad on the second day of bleeding. The bleeding spontaneously resolved. The history reveals no medical issues, no medications, and the pelvic exam is unremarkable. The Pap smear is up to date and is normal.

Diagnosis (Algorithm 20.1)

Postmenopausal vaginal bleeding; rule out endometrial malignancy.

Indications (Algorithm 20.1)

- Postmenopausal vaginal bleeding
- Abnormal uterine bleeding over age 45
- AGC-US/AGUS (atypical glandular cells of uncertain significance) Pap in a woman over 35
- Evaluation of endometrial thickness >5 mm in a postmenopausal patient
- Endometrial cells on Pap in a postmenopausal patient
- Evaluation of endometrium prior to the onset of Hormone Replacement Therapy (HRT) use in high-risk patients
- Evaluation of bleeding in patients on tamoxifen
- Abnormal uterine bleeding under age 45 that has not responded to standard treatments

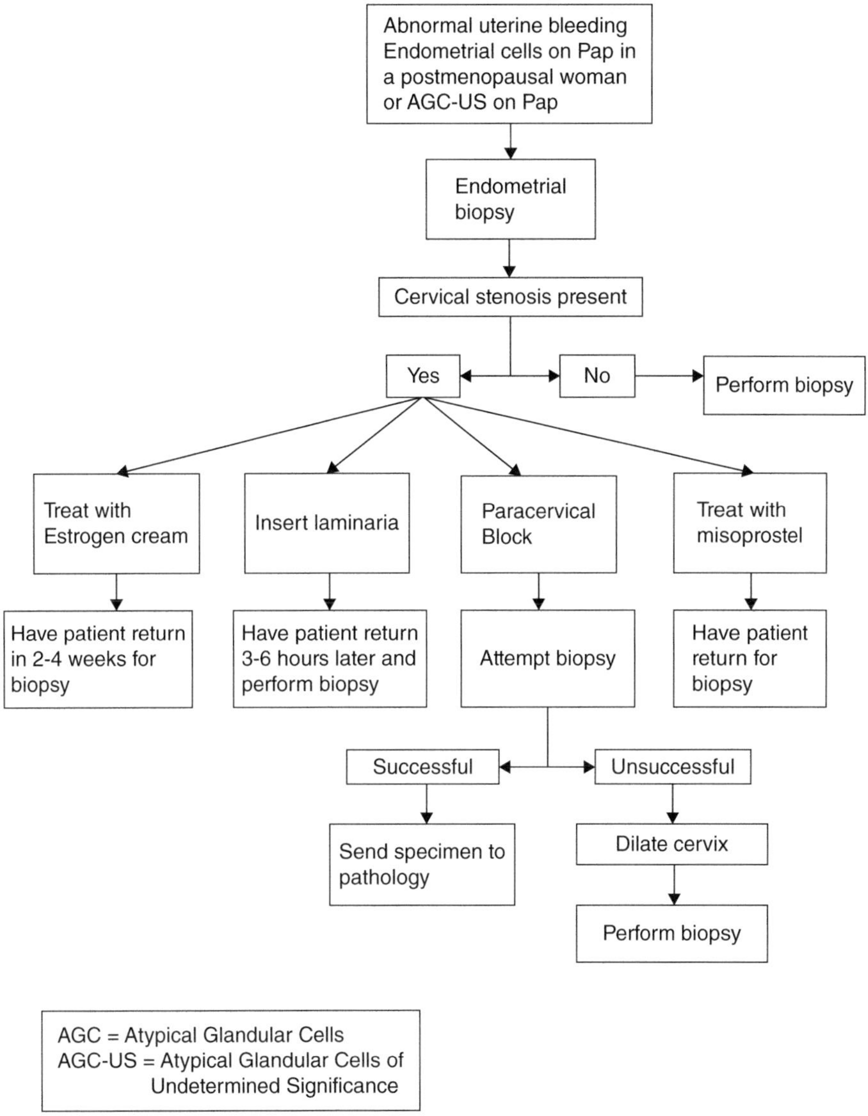

Algorithm 20.1 Decision tree for endometrial biopsy procedure

Contraindications

- Pregnancy
- Known cervical cancer

Relative Contraindications

- Acute cervicitis/pelvic infection
- Active uterine bleeding (may be difficult to obtain a core sample of endometrium adequate for analysis)
- Cervical stenosis
- Difficulty passing a cannula secondary to cervical stenosis, large leiomyomas, marked uterine flexion, and patient discomfort

Equipment (Fig. 20.1)

- Antiseptic solution
- Tenaculum
- Hurricaine® gel (Beutlich LP Pharmaceuticals, Waukegan, IL) (topical anesthetic)
- Vaginal speculum
- Formalin sample bottle with labels
- Endometrial biopsy sampler [Pipelle® (Unimar, Wilton, CT), Endocell™ Endometrial Sampler (Wallach Surgical Devices, Orange, CT), or endometrial aspirator]

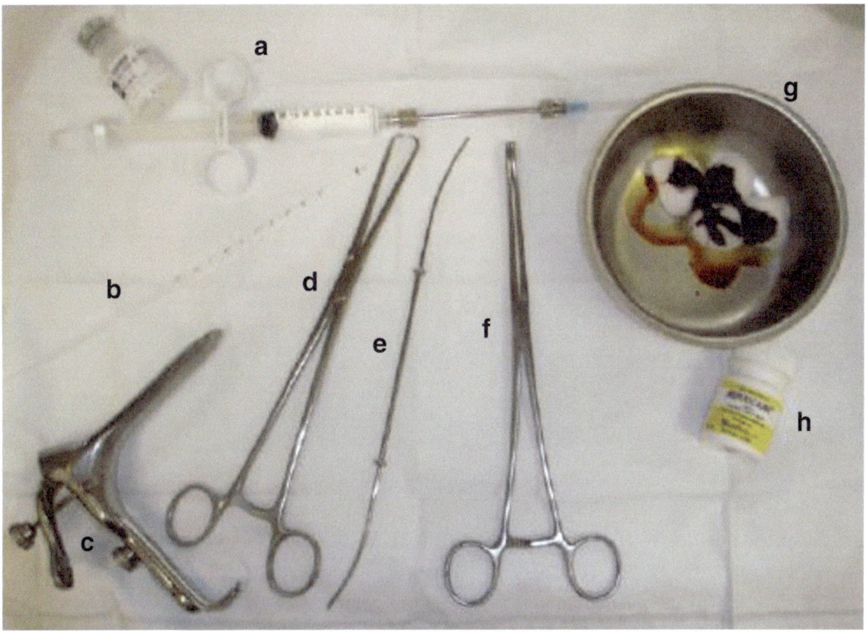

Fig. 20.1 Equipment setup for endometrial biopsy: (**a**) 1% lidocaine with epinephrine anesthetic in 10-cc syringe with needle extender; (**b**) endometrial sampler, sterile; (**c**) sterile speculum; (**d**) sterile cervical tenaculum; (**e**) sterile uterine sound; (**f**) sterile long-looped forceps; (**g**) metal basin with betadine-soaked cotton swabs; (**h**) Hurricaine® gel (Beutlich LP Pharmaceuticals, Waukegan, IL) for topical anesthesia

Optional Equipment

- Uterine sound (endometrial sampler can be used to sound the uterus) or Os-Finder
- 1% lidocaine with epinephrine
- Needle extender
- 10 cc syringe

Procedure

1. Obtain informed consent for the procedure and obtain a urine pregnancy test if the patient is not postmenopausal.
2. Place the patient in a dorsal lithotomy position.
3. Perform a bimanual examination to determine the position and size of the uterus.
4. Insert vaginal speculum and visualize the cervix.
5. Cleanse the cervix with the antiseptic solution.

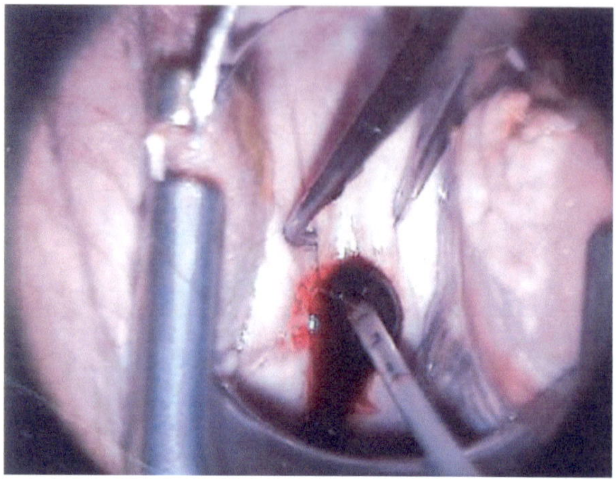

Fig. 20.2 Proper placement of tenaculum and insertion of endometrial sampler

6. Sound the uterus (determine the depth of the uterus to avoid perforation) and document the depth (usually 6–9 cm). Use a uterine sound/os-finder or the biopsy sampler itself inserted through the cervical os.
7. If there is difficulty inserting the sound, straighten and stabilize the cervical canal by using a tenaculum. Apply Hurricaine® anesthetic to the cervix prior to placing the tenaculum. Place the "teeth" of the tenaculum on the cervix horizontally, at 11 o'clock and 1 o'clock positions, approximately 1 cm from the cervical os (Fig. 20.2).
8. Insert the sampler through the cervical os. If resistance is encountered, use gentle pressure. If there is still resistance, terminate the procedure and follow the steps below for stenotic cervical os (Fig. 20.3a).
9. Stabilize the sheath with one hand and draw the piston completely back in one continuous motion. This creates a vacuum, or negative pressure, within the uterus (Fig. 20.3b).
10. Rotate the sheath between the thumb and index finger and move it in and out between the fundus and the internal os three or four times until the sampler is full. These actions pass the sampler opening through a helical arc against the uterine walls. The negative pressure vacuum draws the endometrial tissue into the sampler, do not remove the sampler from the os before obtaining the entire sample. Visualize the tissue in the lumen of the sampler to make sure an adequate specimen is present (Fig. 20.3c).
11. Withdraw the device (with piston still drawn back).
12. Expel the sample into the formalin by advancing the piston back into the sheath. Do not put the tip of the sampler directly into the formalin in the container. Some clinicians use the sampler to repeat the procedure to obtain a second sample (Fig. 20.3d).
13. Some clinicians cut the tip of the sampler and send it with the specimen.

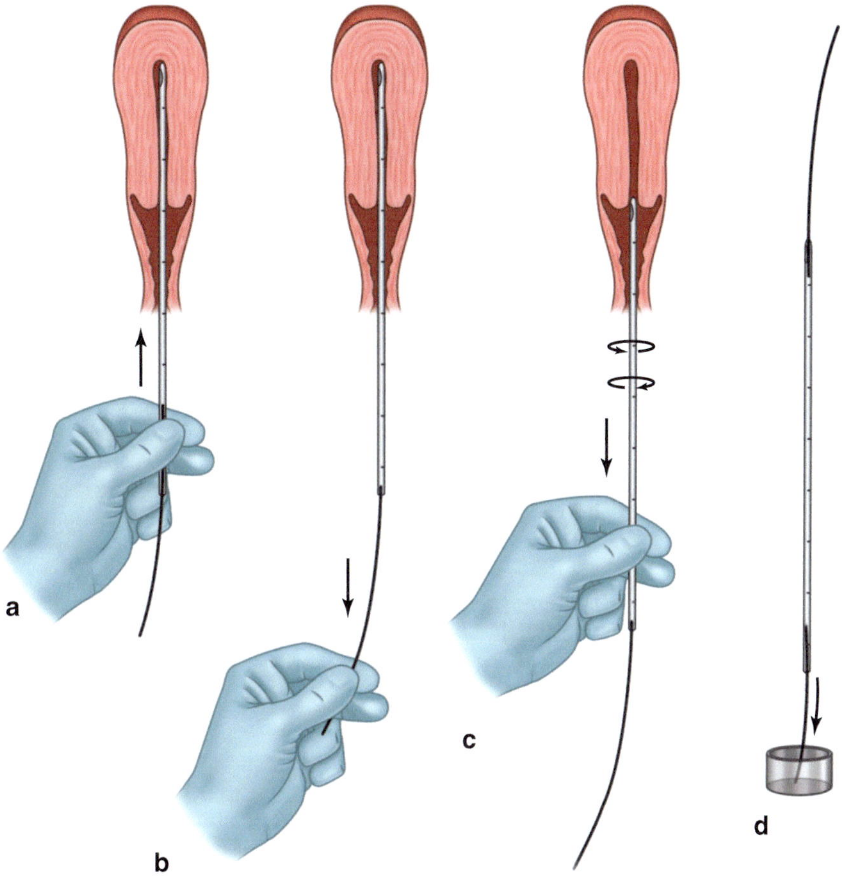

Fig. 20.3 (**a**) Endometrial sampler is inserted to the fundus of the uterus. (**b**) The sampler is stabilized, and the piston is pulled entirely back to the stopper. (**c**) The endometrial sampler is moved in and out and rotated clockwise and counterclockwise to obtain the uterine sample. (**d**) The sample is placed in the formalin container to send to pathology

14. Remove the tenaculum, if applied and apply pressure to achieve hemostasis if needed.
15. Remove the speculum from the vagina and send the specimen to pathology.

For a stenotic cervical os, consider using the Uterine Explora™ Curette in lieu of a traditional endometrial sampling pipelle. A stylus within the sampling curette helps with insertion through a stenotic os.

With this curette, the stylette keeps the unit less flexible. The stylette is removed after the curette is in the appropriate position. Instead of a piston, attach a syringe to

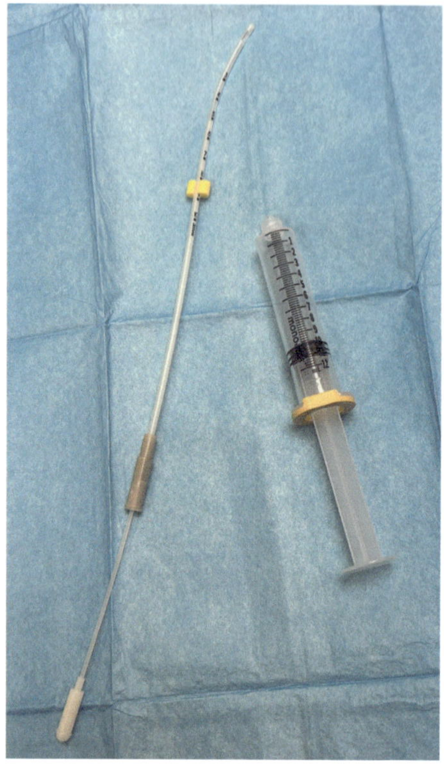

Fig. 20.4 Uterine Explora Curette

the Curette and pull back to 6–8 cc and then lock into position to create a suction within the uterus. The procedure for the biopsy is the same as stated above (Fig. 20.4).

Complications and Risks

- Missed lesion in biopsy sample (5–15% false-negative rate)
- Uterine perforation (0.1–1.0%)
- Infection (0.4%)
- Excessive uterine bleeding
- Cramping (common and brief)
- Vasovagal syncope (10% of patients)

Tricks and Helpful Hints

Storing the sampling device in the freezer stiffens the plastic enough that a tenaculum may be unnecessary.

- Use tenaculum only if necessary to straighten the cervical os, as it increases cramping and may increase postprocedure bleeding.
- Options for patients with cervical stenosis:
  - Pretreat postmenopausal patients or patients who have not had vaginal deliveries with estrogen cream one half-full applicator into the vagina every other night for 2–4 weeks prior to the procedure.
  - Insert a laminaria into the cervical os 1 day prior to the procedure or in the morning and have the patient return later in the day for the procedure.
  - Have the patient insert 200 μg of misoprostol into the vagina or take it orally the day prior to the procedure. (This may cause some mild cramping.)
- For uncomfortable patients:
  - Two to 3 days prior to the procedure, have the patient begin taking ibuprofen or other NSAID to decrease the discomfort felt during the procedure.
  - A paracervical block done just prior to the procedure can decrease the pain during the endometrial biopsy.
  - To perform a paracervical block:
    (a) Use 5–10 cc of 1% or 2% lidocaine with epinephrine.
    (b) Place a needle extender onto the syringe with a 26-gauge needle.
    (c) Stabilize the cervix by placing a tenaculum, as described previously if needed.
    (d) Inject submucosally 1–2 cc of lidocaine into the cervix at the 12, 3, 6, and 9 o'clock positions (can use 2:00, 4:00, 8:00, and 10:00 positions if preferred). Wait for at least 2 minutes for the lidocaine to take effect.
    (e) Proceed with the biopsy as described previously.

Interpretation of Results [7, 8] (Algorithm 20.2)

- *Insufficient tissue*: Follow-up will depend on the reason the biopsy was done. *Further workup for postmenopausal bleeding is necessary to rule out malignancy.*
- *Proliferative or secretory endometrium*: Normal findings, no follow-up required, and confirms ovulation.
- *Atrophic endometrium*: No treatment needed.
- *Hyperplasia*:

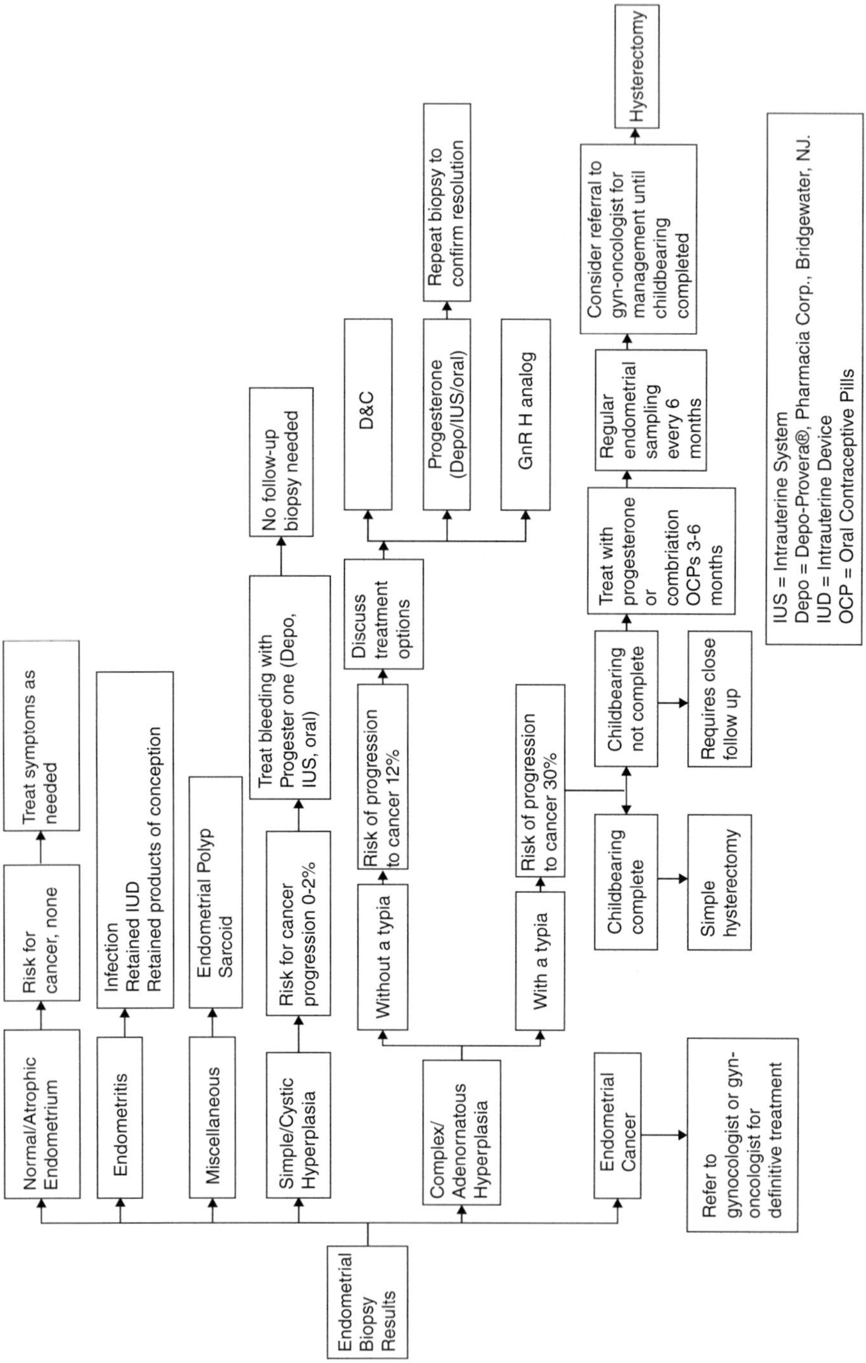

Algorithm 20.2 Decision tree for endometrial biopsy results

- Simple (cystic)
  - (a) 0–2% progress to cancer
  - (b) If bleeding persists, treat with progesterone.
  - (c) No follow-up biopsy is needed.
- Complex (adenomatous) *without* atypia
  - (a) 12% progress to cancer—close follow-up is required.
  - (b) Treatment with progesterone and follow-up biopsy to confirm resolution is necessary.
- Complex (adenomatous) *with* atypia
  - (a) 30% progress to cancer
  - (b) If childbearing is *not* completed:
    - Progesterone treatment for 3–6 months
    - Regular endometrial sampling every 6 months
  - (c) If childbearing is completed, a simple hysterectomy is recommended.

- *Carcinoma*: Refer to gynecology oncology for staging and hysterectomy.
- *Endometritis*: Multiple causes
  - Acute: infection, necrosing endometrial polyp
  - Chronic: infection, sarcoidosis, radiation effects, carcinoma, retained IUD, retained products of conception (post miscarriage or termination)

Procedure Note

(*Provider to customize as needed.*)

Preoperative diagnosis:
Postoperative diagnosis:
Indications:
Procedure details: Urine pregnancy test was done and is negative. The risks (including infection, bleeding, pain, and uterine perforation) and benefits of the procedure were explained to the patient, and written consent was obtained.

The patient was placed in the dorsal lithotomy position. Bimanual exam showed the uterus to be in the anteverted position. A speculum was inserted, and the cervix prepped with iodine solution. Endocervical curettage was not performed.

A tenaculum was applied to the anterior lip of the cervix for stabilization. A sterile uterine sound was used to sound the uterus to a depth of 7 cm. A pipelle was used to sample the endometrium. The sample was sent for pathological examination.

Condition: *Stable*
Complications: *None*
Plan: The patient was advised to call for any fever or for prolonged or severe pain or bleeding. She was advised to use over the counter analgesics for pain. We will call her with the pathology results.

Coding

CPT® Codes (Current Procedural Terminology, AMA, Chicago, IL)	
58100	Endometrial sampling (with or without endocervical sampling, without cervical dilatation, any method)
57800	Dilation of cervical canal, instrumental
59200	Insertion of cervical dilator, laminaria
ICD 10-CM-Diagnostic Codes	
C54.1	Cancer uterus
D28.2	Benign neoplasm, uterus
D07.0	Cancer in situ, uterus
N85.00	Endometrial hyperplasia
R10.2	Pelvic pain
N93.8	Dysfunctional uterine bleeding
N93.9	Abnormal uterine bleeding
N92.4	Premenopausal menorrhagia
N95.0	Postmenopausal bleeding
R87.628	Atypical glandular cells
Z79.890	Postmenopausal HRT
Z85.42	Personal cancer uterus

Postprocedure Patient Instructions

- The patient may experience dizziness/syncope after the procedure: Have the patient sit up slowly on the exam table postprocedure.
- Mild cramping is expected: The patient may take ibuprofen.
- Vaginal bleeding/spotting is a common postprocedure. The patient can resume sexual activity after her bleeding has stopped.
- Postprocedure infection is uncommon. Instruct the patient to call the office if a fever, foul-smelling vaginal discharge, or abdominal pain develops.
- Have the patient return in 1 week to discuss the results of the biopsy.

Case Study Outcome

The patient's biopsy showed secretory endometrium. The patient was reassured that the biopsy did not have cancer or precancerous cells. The patient will follow up with the clinician as directed.

Patient Handout

(*Provider to customize as needed.*)

An endometrial biopsy evaluates the tissue inside the uterus and is used to check for cancerous or precancerous cells. This procedure involves passing a small tube into your uterus and removing part of the endometrium (lining) of your uterus. Your clinician may be doing this test to evaluate any abnormal vaginal bleeding, check on the lining of the uterus if you are on hormones, or check for endometrial cancer.

The endometrial biopsy can be uncomfortable, and we recommend you start taking ibuprofen, three 200 mg tablets three times daily, with food for 2 days prior to the procedure. This will help alleviate the discomfort during the procedure.

The procedure takes less than 10 min, and after the procedure, the sample from your uterus will be sent for microscopic evaluation by a pathologist. Please return to the office in 1 week to discuss those results.

After the procedure, you may have some mild cramping. If this happens, you may take ibuprofen, three 200-mg tablets three times a day with food. Some vaginal bleeding or spotting is common after your procedure. If you have heavy vaginal bleeding, more than one pad every 2 hours, please call your clinician. Infection following this procedure is also uncommon. If you develop fever, foul-smelling vaginal discharge, or lower abdominal pain, please contact the office.

References

1. Clark TJ, Mann CH, Shah N, et al. Accuracy of outpatient endometrial biopsy in the diagnosis of endometrial cancer: a systematic quantitative review. Br J Obstet Gynaecol. 2002;109:313–21.
2. Rezak M, Sayyed T, Dawood R. The effectiveness and acceptability of Pipelle endometrial sampling versus classical dilatation and curettage: a three-year observational study. Gynecol Obstet Investig. 2016;81:537–42.
3. vanHanegem N, Prins MM, Bongers MY, et al. The accuracy of endometrial sampling in women with postmenopausal bleeding: a systematic review and meta-analysis. Eur J Obstet Gynecol Reprod Biol. 2016;107:147–55.

4. Vitale SG, Buzzaccarini G, Riemma G, et al. Endometrial biopsy: indications, techniques and recommendations. An evidence-based guideline for clinical practice. J Gynecol Obstet Hum Reprod. 2023;52(6):102588. https://doi.org/10.1016/j.jogoh.2023.102588. Epub 2023 Apr 13. PMID: 37061093.
5. Cincelli E, Didonna T, Schonauer LM, Stragapede S, Falco N, Pansini N. Paracervical anesthesia for hysteroscopy and endometrial biopsy in postmenopausal women: a randomized, double-blind, placebo-controlled study. J Reprod Med. 1998;43:1014–8.
6. Leclair C. Anesthesia for office endometrial procedures: a review of the literature. Curr Womens Health Rep. 2002;2(6):429–33.
7. Trimmble CL, et al. Society of gynecologic oncology clinical practice committee. Management of endometrial precancers. Obstet Gynecol. 2012;120(5):1160–75.
8. Armstrong AJ, Hurd WW, Elguerro S, et al. Diagnosis and management of endometrial hyperplasia. J Minim Invasive Gynecol. 2012;19:562–71.

Chapter 21
Vulvar Skin Punch Biopsy

Matthew L. Picone

Introduction

Vulvar lesions consist of a wide array of benign, premalignant, and malignant lesions that involve the vulva (Fig. 21.1). The decision to biopsy is determined by many factors including the time course of the lesion, uncertainty of diagnosis, symmetry of the lesion, irregularity of the borders, bleeding tendencies of the lesion, family history of vulvar malignancy, and patient concerns. All these factors independently play a role in the decision to biopsy.

Cancer of the vulva is statistically the fourth most common gynecologic malignancy (following cancer of the endometrium, ovary, and cervix) and comprises 5% of malignancies of the female genital tract. In the United States in 2021, 2.7/100,000 women were diagnosed with vulvar carcinoma [1, 2]. The most common subtype is squamous cell linked with the human papilloma virus (HPV). Vulvar carcinoma presents most commonly in the postmenopausal female. Risk factors include cigarette smoking, history of lichen sclerosis or any vulvar dystrophy, cervical cancer, immunodeficiency syndromes, and human papillomavirus (HPV).

Often asymptomatic, vulvar lesions present in a variety of ways to the clinician. Pruritus is usually the most common symptom complaint. Pain, ulcerations, or a lump found by the patient are other presenting factors. Clinicians are often the first to see these lesions and bring them to the patient's attention [3]. Non healing lesions, suspicious looking lesions, treatment resistant areas, and indurated areas of the vulva should all be considered for biopsy.

A thorough history (before patient undresses) and complete gynecologic exam are necessary to make the diagnosis and to determine the appropriate treatment plan. Hygiene habits and personal care products used (including detergents, fabric

M. L. Picone (✉)
Faculty, St. Joseph's Hospital Family Medicine Residency, Syracuse, NY, USA
e-mail: matt.picone@sjhsyr.org

S. M. Sulik, C. B. Heath (eds.), *Primary Care Procedures in Women's Health*,
https://doi.org/10.1007/978-3-032-07061-6_21

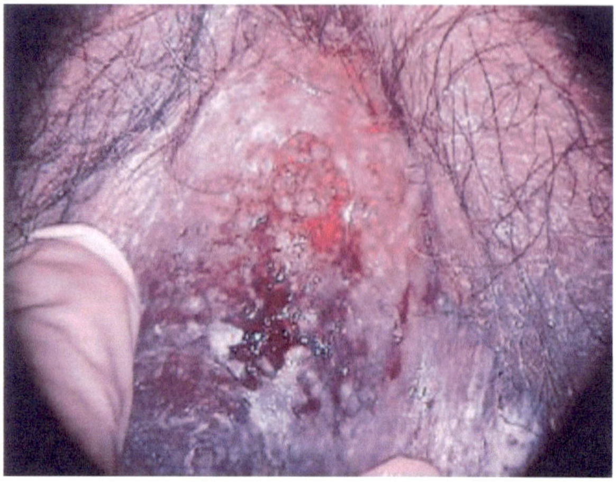

Fig. 21.1 Paget's skin lesion of the vulva

softeners, soaps, feminine hygiene sprays, sanitary napkins, and habits of douching) should be evaluated. Soaps, shaving products, hair removal techniques, and spermicides are all irritants that cause several different dermatoses in the vulvar area. Hormonal status can be determined based on the physical exam of the vulva to assess for hypoestrogenism. A discussion of the potential "home cures" that the patient has tried should be explored, as these remedies can often make visual diagnosis difficult. Finally, patient concerns for cancer should be elicited.

Performing a vulvar biopsy is a simple procedure easily done in the office setting. A recent study done in dermatology residents showed 50% had never performed a vulvar skin biopsy during their training leading to many who are uncomfortable with the procedure. Easily taught and learned, the comfort and skill of the primary care provider in performing this simple procedure allows the patient to receive care without referral to a specialist [4].

There are a variety of videos showing punch biopsy techniques that can be used for teaching or reviewing the procedure prior to performing it [5].

A vulvar biopsy should be performed in the area that is most suspicious. It is important to avoid the midline structures such as the clitoris, urethra or anus when choosing the site to biopsy. It is important to biopsy each morphologically distinct area if the lesion is not uniform. When doing a biopsy on an ulcerated lesion, it is best to biopsy at the periphery. Hyperpigmented lesions should be biopsied in the thickest area. The recommended technique is a punch biopsy, although studies have looked at cervical forceps biopsy with equal effectiveness [6]. Use of lidocaine for local anesthesia is common practice; however, application of 5% lidocaine-prilocaine cream placed 10 min prior to the biopsy may provide better pain relief [7].

Case Study

A 65-year-old presents to your office for her annual physical exam and cervical cancer screening. Review of systems reveals that the patient has been postmenopausal for the past 13 years with no history of hormone replacement therapy. During the physical exam, an irregularly shaped, nonulcerated, raised, and flesh-toned plaque measuring approximately 1.5 × 1.5 cm in diameter is noted. The patient was unaware that the lesion was present. A biopsy was suggested based on the uncertainty of the diagnosis.

Diagnosis

Vulvar lesion, Not otherwise specified (NOS)

Differential Diagnosis [4, 5] (Algorithm 20.1)

- Vulvar intraepithelial neoplasia
- Cancer: the most common is squamous cell carcinoma
- *Condyloma Acuminata*: genital warts
- Lichen sclerosis
- Vestibular papillae
- Acrochordon: skin tags
- Cysts: Bartholin, pilonidal, dermoid, and mucus cysts
- Molluscum contagiosum: immunosuppressed disorders
- Hyperkeratosis or lichen simplex: white patches
- Paget's Disease
- *Acanthosis nigricans*: pigmented macules/plaques
- Junctional nevi: common
- Seborrheic keratosis
- Dermatofibroma
- Extramammary breast found along the nipple line
- Fox-Fordyce disease
- Kaposi's sarcoma: immunodeficiency syndromes
- Dysplastic nevi
- Melanoma: family history sometimes present
- Dermatitis: chemical or allergic
- Psoriasis
- Infection

Indications

Diagnostic

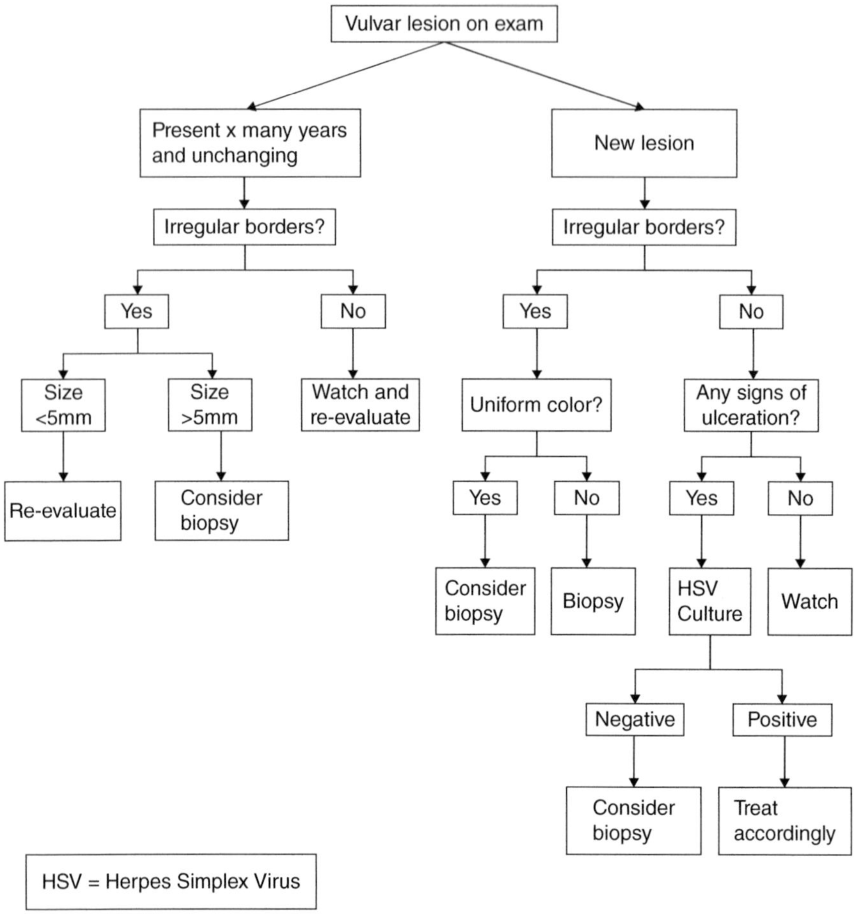

Algorithm 20.1 Decision tree for vulvar skin lesion

Contraindications

- Bleeding or coagulation disorders
- Patient uncomfortable with having procedure done

Equipment (Fig. 21.2)

Nonsterile tray for anesthesia:

- Nonsterile gloves
- 4 × 4-inch gauze pads

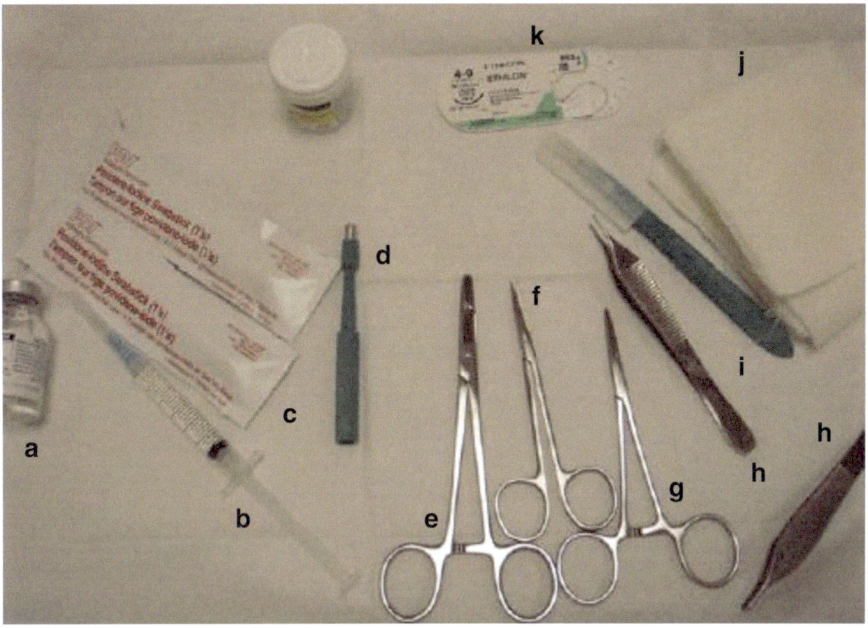

Fig. 21.2 Equipment tray for vulvar skin biopsy. (**a**) Lidocaine; (**b**) 1% lidocaine in 5-cc syringe; (**c**) PDI® povidone-iodine swab sticks (Orangeburg, NY); (**d**) punch biopsy; (**e**) needle driver/holder; (**f**) fine scissors; (**g**) hemostat; (**h**) needle nose pick-ups; (**i**) scalpel; (**j**) gauze; (**k**) Ethilon™ 4–0 Nylon Absorbable Suture. (Ethicon Inc., West Somerville, NJ); (**l**) formalin specimen container

- 3-cc syringe filled with 1% lidocaine with epinephrine and 25–27-gauge needle
- Labelled formalin container(s) for the number of biopsies

Sterile tray for the procedure:

- Sterile gloves
- Desired punch biopsy instrument (2–6 mm)
- Scalpel with blade if preferred
- Needle holder for suturing if needed
- Desired size of suture usually 4-0 or 5-0 nylon absorbable
- Iris scissors
- Small-gauge needle

Procedure

1. Explain the procedure and have the patient sign consent for the procedure.
2. Clean the skin with povidone iodine solution after determining the selection of the site.

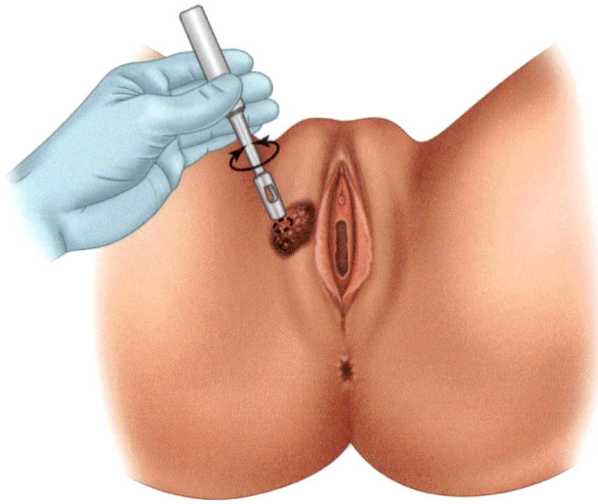

Fig. 21.3 Identify the vulvar lesion and perform a biopsy in the center of the lesion

3. Pick the site for biopsy at the center of the lesion and not at the periphery—be sure to include 1–2 mm of normal skin for analysis [5] (Fig. 21.3).

4. Use generous local anesthesia to surround the lesion. Allow 3–5 min for anesthesia to be fully absorbed. Or place the lidocaine-pilocarpine cream on the area at least 10 min prior to the procedure.
5. Identify the lines of least skin tension (the lines vertical to the vulva).
6. Stretch the skin around the site perpendicular to the skin lines with the opposite hand (Fig. 21.4a).
7. Hold the punch biopsy vertically to the skin and rotate downward between the first and second fingers in a clockwise and counterclockwise fashion, penetrating the dermis and subcutaneous tissues.
8. Lift the lesion with a small-gauge needle and cut the base with iris scissors, and place in formalin. Properly label the specimen and send to pathology with identification of biopsy, any pertinent history, and presumed diagnosis (Fig. 21.4b).
9. Place sutures perpendicular to the tension lines for the vulva that were identified earlier using 4–5.0 nylon suture.
10. Apply antibiotic ointment and a bandage. Patients may find using Vaseline or antibiotic ointment with a pad more comfortable then applying a bandage to the vulvar area.
11. If preferred, the entire lesion can be removed. Follow the steps previously delineated. Once the area is anesthetized, make a fusiform incision with the scalpel that encompasses the entire lesion. The blade should be pressed firmly to penetrate the entire thickness of the dermis.
12. Grasp the corner of the incision with a pair of forceps and cut the lesion free with the scalpel or iris scissors.
13. Close the incision as above.

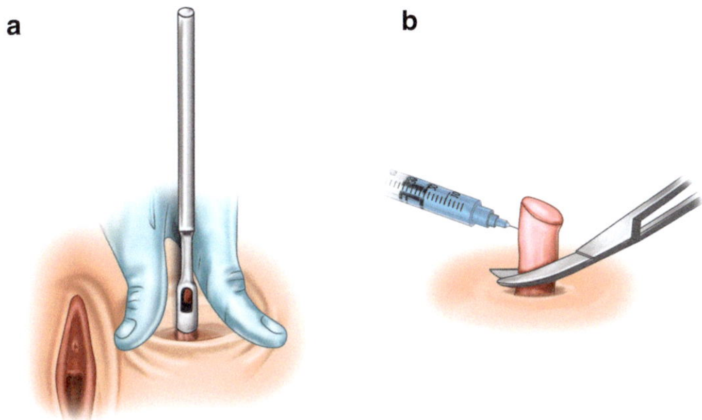

Fig. 21.4 (**a**) Stretch the skin at the biopsy site perpendicular to the skin lines with the non-dominant hand. (**b**) Lift the punch biopsy with a needle and cut the base to avoid crushing the tissue

Complications and Risks

- Bleeding—a suture placed after the biopsy will achieve hemostasis
- Recurrence
- Scarring/keloids
- Infection: rare
- Pain

Tricks and Helpful Hints

- Use a small gauge needle instead of forceps to avoid crushing the lesion and interfering with pathology interpretation.
- If a 6-mm punch is needed to remove the entire lesion, it may be better to perform a fusiform incisional removal.
- Consider delaying submission for payment until pathology returns, as payment is based on pathology results.
- Consider applying lidocaine-prilocaine cream 10–60 min prior to procedure to decrease pain as an alternative or an adjunct to intradermal local anesthesia.

Interpretation of Results

Treatment is determined by the final pathology. If cancerous, then referral to a specialist is indicated. See Algorithm 20.1.

Procedure Note (Provider to Customize as Needed)

Surgical consent was discussed and signed by the patient. The patient was placed in the lithotomy position. The area was cleansed, and sterile technique was utilized. After local anesthesia was administered, a 4-mm punch biopsy to the region of concern was performed. The lesion was placed in formalin and sent to pathology. Hemostasis and closure of the wound were obtained by placing two 5-0 interrupted sutures. The patient tolerated the procedure well and will return in 10 days for the pathology report and suture removal.

Coding

CPT® Codes (Current Procedural Terminology, AMA, Chicago, IL)	
56605	Biopsy of vulva or perineum [one lesion]
56606	Biopsy of each additional vulvar or perineal lesion
ICD-10 CM 10th Revision (International Classification of Diseases, 10th Revision, Clinical Modification, Center for Disease Control and Prevention)	
N90.89	Vulvar lesion
N 90.0	Mild vulvar dysplasia
N 90.1	Moderate vulvar dysplasia
N 90.3	Vulvar dysplasia
N 90.4	Leukoplakia of the vulva
N 90.5	Atrophy of the vulva
N90.9	Noninflammatory lesion of the vulva
N90.3	Vulvar dysplasia moderate
D 07.1	Vulvar intraepithelial neoplasia (VIN) III
L98.9	Skin tag
D28.0	Benign vulvar neoplasm
A63.0	*Condyloma acuminata*

Postprocedure Patient Instructions

- Instruct the patient to keep the bandage in place for the next 24–36 h followed by air drying the area and keeping it clean and dry until the follow-up appointment.
- Have the patient call the office for signs of infection, pain, redness, fever, discharge, or wound opening.
- Tell the patient to return to the office in 10 days for suture removal and pathology report.

Case Study Outcome

The biopsy was successfully obtained, and sutures were removed 10 days post biopsy with excellent approximation of the site. Pathology report revealed a vulvar intraepithelial neoplasm (VIN) 3. The patient was referred to a specialist for complete excision. She will follow up 2 months after the surgery has been performed.

Patient Handout (Provider to Customize as Needed)

A vulvar biopsy is a procedure done to take a small piece of an abnormal area that is found on the vulva. The procedure is done in the office to help determine or clarify what type of growth is present.

You may want to take Tylenol (650 mg) or Ibuprofen (600 mg) 1 h prior to the visit for some mild discomfort that may occur. There will be a local anesthesia given to the area before a biopsy is performed; this may cause mild pain and possibly burning. After the area is numb, you may experience nothing at all or a pressure sensation.

After the procedure is performed, the lesion will be sent out to a pathology lab that will help us determine the cause of the abnormal growth. At the follow-up visit, we will have the report and will discuss any future treatment plans.

There is a small risk for bleeding, infection, and possibly excessive scar formation or discoloration that persists at the biopsy site. You should call the office if signs of infection should occur, such as redness, swelling, increased pain, or discharges from the biopsy site.

References

1. U.S. Cancer Statistics Working Group. U.S. Cancer Statistics Data Visualizations Tool. U.S. Department of Health and Human Services, Centers for Disease Control and Prevention and National Cancer Institute; https://www.cdc.gov/cancer/dataviz, released in June 2024.

2. Siegel RL, Miller KD, Jemal A. Cancer statistics, 2017. CA Cancer J Clin. 2017;67(1):7–30. https://doi.org/10.3322/caac.21387. Epub 2017 Jan 5
3. Olawaiye AB, Cuello MA, Rogers LJ. Cancer of the vulva: 2021 update. Int J Gynaecol Obstet. 2021;155 Suppl 1(Suppl 1):7–18. https://doi.org/10.1002/ijgo.13881. PMID: 34669204; PMCID: PMC9298362
4. Panez S, Sattler S, Dobry AS, Kraus CN. A survey of practices and perceptions of vulvar biopsies in academic dermatology. Int J Womens Dermatol. 2021;7(5 Part B):763–5. https://doi.org/10.1016/j.ijwd.2021.10.011. PMID: 35028378; PMCID: PMC8714558
5. Levitt J, Bernardo S, Whang T. Videos in clinical medicine. How to perform a punch biopsy of the skin. N Engl J Med. 2013;369(11):e13. https://doi.org/10.1056/NEJMvcm1105849.
6. Tuil A, Bergeron C, Lucet JV, Dabi Y, Favier A, Da Maia E, Uzan C, Mergui JL, Canlorbe G. Vulvar biopsy: Punch biopsy or cervical forceps biopsy? J Gynecol Obstet. Hum Reprod. 2023;52(10):102667. https://doi.org/10.1016/j.jogoh.2023.102667. Epub 2023 Sep 12
7. Williams LK, Weber JM, Pieper C, Lorenzo A, Moss H, Havrilesky LJ. Lidocaine-Prilocaine Cream Compared With Injected Lidocaine for Vulvar Biopsy: A Randomized Controlled Trial. Obstet Gynecol. 2020;135(2):311–8. https://doi.org/10.1097/AOG.0000000000003660.
8. Mayeaux EJ Jr, Cooper D. Vulvar procedures: biopsy, bartholin abscess treatment, and condyloma treatment. Obstet Gynecol Clin N Am. 2013;40(4):759–72. https://doi.org/10.1016/j.ogc.2013.08.009.

Chapter 22
Treatment of Genital Warts

Cathryn B. Heath

Introduction

Infections of Human papillomavirus (HPV) are the most common sexually transmitted disease in the United States. Prior to the HPV vaccination, the rate of HPV among the US population was 14 million new infections occurring yearly, with half of those infections being in the 15–24-year-old age group [1]. There is an estimate of 291 million women worldwide who have contracted HPV [2]. There are currently 150 known types of HPV. An increased number of sexual partners, a new partner within the previous 12 months, smoking history, and immunosuppression are risk factors associated with HPV infection. External genital warts are most commonly types 6 and 11 and are rarely associated with cancer causing high-risk types of HPV. With the advent of the quadrivalent HPV vaccine, there has been a significant decline in the rates of HPV in countries with high vaccination coverage. Consistent condom usage also confers a reduction in the HPV rate. A number of studies have shown a consistent decline in HPV in all sexes with vaccination. A lower risk was seen with even one dose of the vaccine. Recurrence rates of HPV have has reduced in those vaccinated [3].

Genital warts are soft, moist, fleshy colored lesions on the genital area. Warts can also be flat, cauliflower-like, papular, or rounded, keratotic with a thick horny surface, multiple or single lesions on the labia, vulva, vagina, cervix, penis, scrotum, glans, urethra, perianal area, oropharynx, or rectum. There is a broad spectrum of disease presentation ranging from asymptomatic external lesions to invasive

C. B. Heath (✉)
Rutgers University Student Health, New Brunswick, NJ, USA
e-mail: heathcb@scarletmail.rutgers.edu

S. M. Sulik, C. B. Heath (eds.), *Primary Care Procedures in Women's Health*,
https://doi.org/10.1007/978-3-032-07061-6_22

carcinoma. Lesions may appear within weeks or months of initial contact. Two-thirds of individuals who have had sexual contact with a partner with genital warts will develop lesions within 3 months. In the anogenital area, warts, dysplasia, and carcinoma are all indistinguishable. There should be a higher index of suspicion for advanced lesions in patients older than 40, immunocompromised patients, patients with lesions refractory to treatment, and patients with any large atypical appearing lesions. A biopsy should be performed whenever the clinician is unsure of the diagnosis or when lesions do not respond to treatment.

The expression of anogenital warts varies considerably, although most individuals have a subclinical infection that is cleared spontaneously by the host immune response. Anogenital HPV types are divided based on their oncogenic response into low- and high-risk types. Almost all cervical cancers and 50–80% of vulvar, vaginal, and anal carcinomas are due to high-risk types of HPV. Over 90% of genital warts, however, are due to the low-risk oncogenic types 6 and 11 and do not become cancerous. However, individuals who have one type of HPV may harbor other types of HPV and other types of sexually transmitted infections (STIs); therefore, it is important to perform STI screening on all patients with genital warts.

Genital warts develop anywhere in the anogenital tract or oropharynx. Many warts are asymptomatic and are found only on physical examination; however, symptoms may include burning, anogenital pruritus, vaginal discharge, bleeding, and, rarely, dyspareunia. Most warts are visible with the naked eye, but a magnifying glass or colposcope can aid in identifying additional or smaller lesions.

Prevention

In 2006, the quadrivalent HPV vaccine Gardasil® (Merck & Co., Inc., Whitehouse Station, NJ) became available to immunize patients against HPV types 6, 11, 16, and 18. Types 6 and 11 are responsible for most anogenital warts, and types 16 and 18 account for over 80% of cervical cancer types worldwide. In the phase III trial of this medication, the rate of vulvar, vaginal, and anogenital lesions of the vaccinated population decreased by a rate of 34%, while the rate of cervical lesions decreased by 20% [4]. Vaccination has been approved in patients aged 9–45 years and is considered most effective prior to exposure to the HPV virus. The vaccine requires a series of two immunizations if given from 9 to 14 years of age, with an interval of 6–12 months between the immunizations. Immunizations initiated at 15 years of age or older require three immunizations and are given at an interval of 2 months after the initial vaccine and then 6 months after the first vaccination [5]. Cervarix 2 (manufactured by GlaxoSmithKline Biologicals) is a bivalent vaccine that targets HPV types 16 and 18 and is given at the same intervals as Gardasil. Gardasil-9 (Merck) covers 9 subtypes of HPV, including 6, 11, 16, 18, 31, 45, 52, and 58. Within 6 years of vaccine introduction, there was a 64% decrease in HPV type (6,11,16,18) prevalence among females aged 14–19 years and a 34% decrease among those aged 20–24 years [6]. In the United States, the rate of HPV types 6, 11,

16, and 18 currently have decreased 85% in females between ages 14 and 19 in the 10 years following the introduction of the vaccination and 71% decrease in females aged 20–24 [1]. Gardasil-9 covers HPV subtypes 6 and 11, which are two subtypes that commonly cause genital warts. A more recent study published in New England Journal of Medicine showed vaccinated Swedish women between the ages of 10 and 30 had a substantial decrease in cervical cancer with an incidence ratio of 0.37 (95% CI 0.21-0.57) [15].

Treatments

For some patients, warts may spontaneously resolve without any treatment. However, most patients prefer to have them treated to hasten the process. A variety of treatments exist for anogenital warts, both patient-administered (podofilox solution or gel, 5% imiquimod cream, and 15% sinecatechins) and provider-administered (podophyllin resin, trichloroacetic acid (TCA), cryotherapy, laser vaporization, or intralesional interferon [7]). Many clinicians use a combination of provider-administered and patient-administered treatments. Patient preference and affordability are important in choosing a regimen for each patient. There are no treatments that are 100% effective, recurrence is common, and up to 70% of patients have been treated more than once for their warts. Several therapies are contraindicated in pregnancy, and therefore, the patient's pregnancy status and method of contraception must also be considered.

Patient-Administered Treatments

The patient-administered therapies allow for privacy of treatment, which helps reduce the psychological discomfort and stress associated with this condition. Available treatments have been 0.5% podofilox (Condolox® Gel, Corona, CA), 5% imiquimod cream (Aldara™, 3 M Company, St. Paul, MN), and sinecatechin (Veregen®, MediGene, Germany). Treatment with podophyllin, interferon α, or 5-fluorouracil is no longer recommended for use [8].

Podofilox is an antimitotic agent that works by arresting the formation of the mitotic spindle in metaphase, preventing cell division. Podofilox can be applied by patients at home. They should wash their hands prior to applying the podofilox gel as well as afterwards. Podofilox solution should be applied using a cotton-tipped applicator. Both Podofilox gel and solution should be applied twice daily for 3 days and then remain without using it for 4 days. With podofilox the surface area treated must not exceed 10 cm^2 and no more than 0.5 cc should be used at any one application [9]. Clearance rates vary from 45 to 88%, with recurrences common. Podofilox should not be used during pregnancy and cannot be used in the vagina or rectum.

Five percent topical imiquimod (Aldara®) cream is a local immune modulator that induces interferon and cytokine release, stimulating both innate and cell-mediated immune responses. The cream is applied to the individual lesions three times per week for up to 12–16 weeks. Patients should apply the cream to the affected area with clean hands and keep it on for 6–10 hours and then wash the cream off. A small amount of cream is used at each treatment, and a single sachet packet can cover most areas effectively. Local erythema and some swelling are the most common side effects and are reported in over 50% of patients. Clearance rates range from 72 to 84% in women with higher clearance rates reported in women compared to men. Up to 81% of patients report at least a reduction in the wart area if not completely resolved. Recurrence rates are reported from 5 to 19%, which is less than the rates reported by cytodestructive methods. Imiquimod is category B and is safe for use in pregnancy, although its safety has not been firmly established.

Veregen®, an ointment derived from a water extract of green tea, was approved by the US Federal Drug Administration (FDA) in late 2007 for use on external and perianal warts. Sinecatechins ointment (Veregen®) is composed of eight catechins, which may act to inhibit proinflammatory enzymes and proteases found in HPV. It is approved for immunocompetent patients above the age of 18. In the phase III trials of the medication, 56.8% of women cleared the virus versus 34.1% of the placebo patients. Men had a clearance rate of 60.1% versus 40.5% who cleared with placebo [10]. The most common side effects of the ointment were redness (70%), itching (69%), burning (67%), pain (56%), and erosions/ulcerations (49%) [11]. Sexual contact needs to be avoided while undergoing treatment. In addition, sinecatechin ointment was found to weaken condoms and diaphragms; use of these contraceptives with Veregen® is not recommended. Sinecatechin ointment is pregnancy category C.

Clinician-Administered Treatment

The clinician-administered treatment modalities depend on the expertise and equipment availability of the provider. Chemical agents that can be applied in the provider's office include podofilox, podophyllin resin, and trichloroacetic acid (TCA). Bichloroacetic acid is no longer available.

TCA is used in concentrations of 80–90% and can be used on both skin and mucosal surfaces. They are not systemically absorbed and can be used during pregnancy. Application causes burning, and this is reduced by applying petroleum jelly to the surrounding skin before application of the acid. Multiple applications are usually necessary, and clearance rates approach 80%. Recurrence rates are similar to other treatment modalities.

Cryotherapy can be used to treat genital warts. Both nitrous oxide and liquid nitrogen may be used. The freeze-thaw cycle with cryotherapy causes cell lysis and is cytodestructive. The ice ball should extend 2–3 mm past external lesions. Both nitrous oxide and liquid nitrogen can be used for anogenital and vulvar warts; however, cryotherapy of the cervix should be done only with nitrous oxide as liquid nitrogen is not cold enough to produce adequate freezing of the area. With weekly treatments until clear, approximately 90% resolve with recurrence rates up to 40%. Cryotherapy may be used safely during pregnancy. Cryotherapy does not leave permanent scarring but can cause hypopigmentation in darker skin colors.

Surgical removal of condyloma can be accomplished with scissors, scalpel, electrocautery, or loop excision [12]. These methods are appropriate as first-line therapy for large or obstructing lesions. Excision with scissors or a scalpel is best for smaller lesions or when a biopsy is needed to rule out cancer or dysplasia. Clearance rates approach 70% with recurrence often at the surgical margins. Large condyloma are very vascular and may require a surgical setting where bleeding can be easily controlled, and better anesthesia can be used.

Laser vaporization can also be used for treatment, although this requires extensive expertise of the provider and costly equipment. Clearance rates approach 87% with recurrence rates also at the margins of approximately 50%. Laser is especially effective in the vagina and for extensive external genital and perianal warts. Clinicians using laser vaporization should wear a well-fitted N95 respiratory protection as HPV particles can aerosolize [13]. Intralesional interferon has also been used with success rates up to 60%; however, it is costly, is painful, and has multiple systemic side effects.

Due to the extensive recurrence rates with individual treatment modalities, combination therapies have been proposed, but there are no established guidelines for their use. A recent systematic review compared the success of a combination of self-administered treatment with ablative therapy vs ablative therapy alone and found that combination therapy resulted in higher complete clearance rates than ablative therapy alone [13, 14].

Case Study

A 25-year-old G0P0 presents with bumps on the labia. During her history, the patient relates that she has been sexually active with one male partner having just started a relationship within the last 3 months. On physical examination, five lesions are found scattered on the patient's introitus. The patient was never immunized for HPV.

Differential Diagnosis (Algorithm 21.1)

- Microglandular papillomatosis (normal papillary tissue in the vestibule of the female single base for each projection versus multiple projections with papilloma)
- Hymenal remnants
- Condyloma lata
- Bowenoid papulosis
- Buschke-Lowenstein tumors

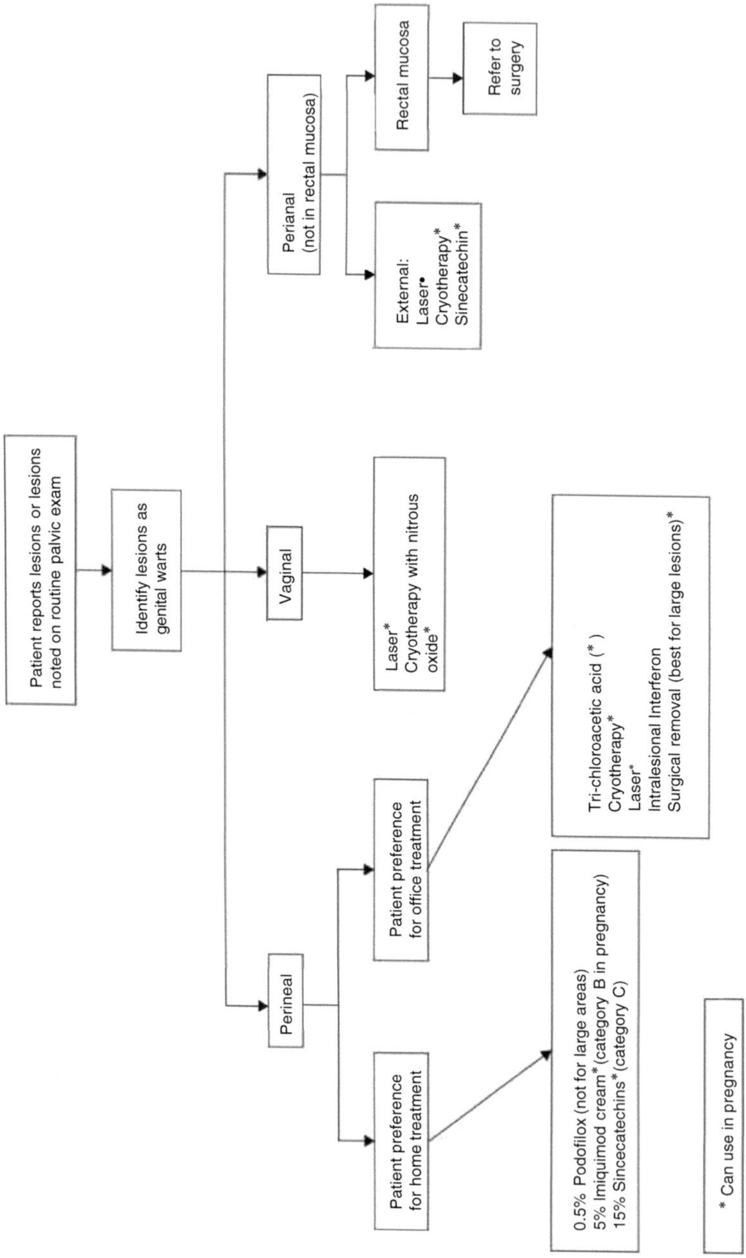

Algorithm 21.1 Decision tree for treatment of genital warts based on location

- Nevi
- Seborrheic keratosis
- Molluscum contagiosum
- Squamous cell Cancer

Indications (Algorithm 21.1)

- Noted lesions present on examination
- Symptomatic lesions
- Patient desire for treatment
- Lesions that obstruct the vaginal opening

Contraindications (Algorithm 21.1)

- Some methods should not be used during pregnancy (podophyllotoxin, podophyllum resin, or imiquimod).
- Some methods are not for use with vaginal lesions (podofilox, podophyllin).
- Lesions in the rectal mucosa or in the urethra should be referred to a specialist.

Equipment

Equipment is variable depending on the method chosen:

- Cryotherapy: liquid nitrogen or nitrous oxide, water-based gel, cryoprobe, cotton-tipped applicator, or handheld cryogen
- Podophyllin: 10–25% podophyllin resin, pregnancy test, cotton-tipped applicator, and petroleum jelly
- TCA: TCA, cotton-tipped applicator, talc or baking soda, petroleum jelly
- Surgical excision: EMLA® (AstraZeneca, London, UK) or 1% xylocaine, iris scissors, scalpel, electrocautery, or aluminum chloride solution

Procedure

Patient-Directed Methods (Suggest First Time Use in Office)

Podophyllotoxin 0.5 mg Solution or Gel

1. Gently wash and dry the application area.
2. Apply with a cotton swab or on a finger directly on the lesion.
3. Apply twice daily for 3 days to each lesion; then do not apply for 4 days. Repeat this cycle up to four times.
4. Patient should wash hands after application.

Imiquimod 3.75% or 5% Cream

1. Gently wash and dry the application area.
2. Rub cream on each lesion until the cream is no longer visible.
3. Wash hands before and after application.
4. Remove all cream by washing the area 6–10 h posttreatment.
5. When applying 5% cream, apply a thin layer over each lesion on alternate days, either according to a Monday, Wednesday, Friday regimen or a Tuesday, Thursday, Saturday regimen.
6. May be repeated for a total of four cycles.
7. When using imiquimod 3.75% cream, may apply daily for up to 8 weeks.

Sinecatechins 15% Ointment

1. Is approved for external genital and perianal warts in immunocompetent women and men 18 years or older.
2. Ointment should be applied after bathing or showering.
3. Hands should be washed prior to and after application.
4. Up to 250 mg per application applied topically three times a day.
5. Itching and burning frequently occur; continuation of application until side effects are intolerable or until warts disappear is recommended.
6. Applied up to 16 weeks or until complete clearance of warts.
7. Medication to be refrigerated or kept up to 77 °F.

Clinician-Directed Methods

Cryotherapy

1. Place the patient in the dorsal lithotomy position.
2. Cotton-tipped application or Cryoprobe method or Cryogun (Fig. 22.1).

   Cotton-tipped application:

- Apply liquid nitrogen on the lesion with a large cotton-tipped applicator until the ice ball extends 3 mm beyond the perimeter of the lesion.
- May need to exchange applicators, as liquid nitrogen will evaporate in less than 15 seconds.

   Cryoprobe method or Cryogun (Fig. 22.1):

- Apply water-based gel solution to the tip of the cryoprobe.
- Put cryoprobe on wart and apply freezant until ice ball covers wart and 2–3 mm beyond wart, approximately 20 s.
- Consider "freeze–thaw–freeze" method on recalcitrant lesions.
- Patients may return every 1–2 weeks for repeat treatment.

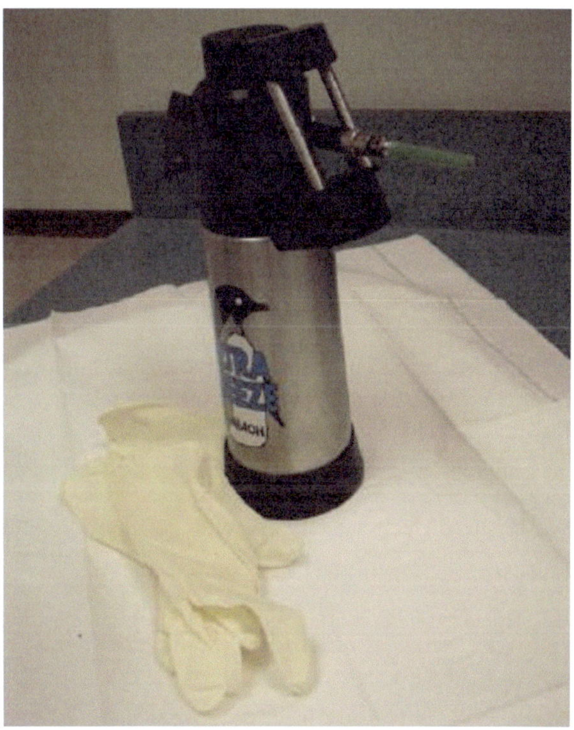

Fig. 22.1 Setup for cryotherapy (e.g., Ultrafreeze™ Liquid Nitrogen Cryosurgical System, Wallach Surgical Devices, Orange, CT)

Podophyllum Resin: 10–25% Podophyllin

- Pregnancy test should be done prior to the start of treatment.
- Apply petroleum jelly around each lesion to protect the skin.
- Apply podophyllin with a small cotton-tipped applicator.
- Air dry.
- Use no more than 0.5 ml of podophyllin in a 10 cm^2 area.
- Instruct patient to wash off in 1–4 h.
- May be reapplied weekly until the lesion is gone.

TCA (Trichloroacetic Acid) (Fig. 22.2)

- Apply petroleum jelly or surgical lubricant around each lesion to protect the skin.
- Transfer a small amount of the TCA into a small test tube. Apply TCA to the lesions with a small cotton-tipped applicator; need to apply with care as TCA is runny and can easily destroy surrounding tissue.
- Allow to air-dry. A whitish frost should appear on the lesion after application.
- Apply talc or baking soda to absorb any remaining acid.
- May be reapplied weekly up to 6 weeks.

Laser Treatment

- Carbon dioxide laser can be used.
- Suggest local anesthetic, such as xylocaine 1% (injected) or topical EMLA® cream, be used prior to procedure.
- Surgeons should use a fitted N-95 mask during application as the HPV is present in smoke flumes created by the laser.

Surgical Removal

- Anesthetize patient with xylocaine 1% subcutaneously, or EMLA® cream to be applied topically 45 min prior to procedure.
- May use electrocautery or a scalpel.
- Alternatively, may use the tangential scissors technique by cutting off exophytic lesion.
- May need electrocautery or aluminum chloride solution to create hemostasis.

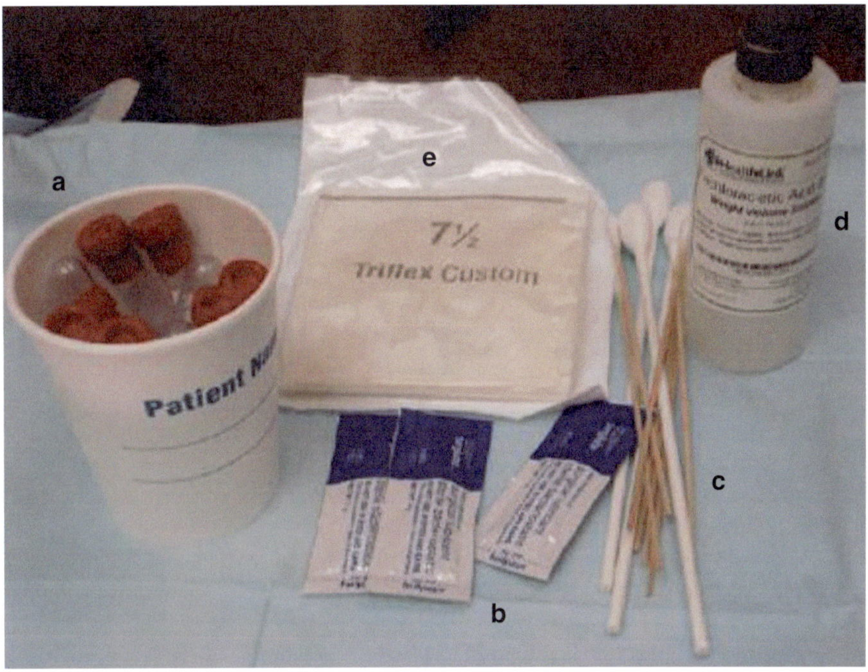

Fig. 22.2 Setup for trichloroacetic acid. (**a**) Small test tubes for acid solution; (**b**) Surgilube® (Fougera, Melville, NY) lubricant for protecting surrounding skin; (**c**) cotton-tipped applicators; (**d**) trichloroacetic acid (e.g., HealthLink®, Jacksonville, FL); (**e**) surgical nonlatex gloves

Complications and Risks

- Erythema and pain at the treatment site
- Blistering (uncommon)
- Severe side effects from absorption of podophyllin include the following:
  - Nausea
  - Vomiting
  - Renal failure
  - Fetal death

Tricks and Helpful Hints (Algorithm 21.1)

- Recommend the patient take a nonsteroidal anti-inflammatory drug (NSAID) 1 hour (h)prior to appointment time.
- Vaginal lesions: use laser, cryotherapy with a cotton applicator only, or TCA.

- Pregnancy: use cryotherapy, TCA, or surgical removal.
  - Important to minimize exposure of neonate to HPV lesions that may cause laryngopapillomatosis (risk 0.04%).
- Anal warts: use cryotherapy, TCA, or surgical removal.
  - If there are anal warts, check the patient by anoscopy for rectal mucosal warts.
  - Do *not* treat warts in the rectal mucosa; these are best treated by a surgeon.
- Genital or anal lesions in prepubescent girls may be associated with sexual abuse.
- Persons with immunodeficiency may have particularly difficult warts to treat; imiquimod may be most effective.
- Patients should be warned to be vigilant for the next 3 months and check for recurrence of warts.
- While most subtypes of external warts are low risk, patients should have HPV testing or it should be obtained at the time of treatment.
- For imiquimod: treatment can be stopped for several days and then restarted if a significant erythematous reaction occurs.
- For any self-applied creams or ointments: If the patient wishes to use tampons, it is recommended that they do so prior to application of antiviral topical medications.
- Cryoprobes should be avoided in the vagina and rectum as there is a higher risk of fistula formation in these areas secondary to the greater depth of freezing.
- For podofilox: Redness and itching may occur after use.
- Patients who have performed oral sex on a male partner are at risk for oropharyngeal warts and need a thorough examination of the oropharynx. Consider referral to an otolaryngologist for a complete laryngeal evaluation.
- Offer HPV vaccination to those who are not fully immunized as it offers protection against multiple subtypes of HPV.
- Have the patient set the alarm on their cellphone to remind them when to remove the chemical treatment in a timely manner.

Procedure Note (Depends on Treatment Used)

(Provider to fill in blanks/circle applicable choice when given multiple choices and customize as needed.)

Patient placed in dorsal lithotomy position. Petroleum jelly applied/Local anesthetic applied. ____method was used to treat ______number of condylomata. Patient instructed to wash off podophyllin within 1–4 h/TCA within 6 h of treatment. Patient tolerated the procedure well. A follow-up appointment for retreatment was made.

Coding

CPT® Codes (Current Procedural Terminology, AMA, Chicago, IL)	
Per lesion: the same coding is used for all treatments	
17110 56501	Destruction of genital warts up to 14 vulvar areas
11420	Excision diameter of 0.5 cm or less
ICD 10-CM-Diagnostic Codes(International Classification of Diseases, 9th Revision, Clinical Modification, Center for Disease Control and Prevention)	
A63.0 O98.319	Genital warts due to HPV Genital warts complicating pregnancy

Postprocedure Patient Instructions

Patients should be instructed to wash off the podophyllin 1–4 h or TCA within 6 h of treatment. Some burning or swelling may be experienced and can be relieved with additional NSAIDs and a warm bath. They should be encouraged to have male partners use condoms while being treated for their genital warts. Partners should also be seen in a physician's office.

Case Study Outcome

Patient treated in the office with cryotherapy. Subsequent follow-up revealed no lesions.

Postprocedure Patient Handout (Provider to Customize as Needed)

You have just been treated for genital warts. Warts are caused by a highly infectious virus. It is important that you refrain from having sex or even contact with skin which has warts until these lesions are gone as they commonly spread to sexual partners. Even skin-to-skin contact with the wart without actually having sex will spread external genital warts. It is especially important to avoid pregnancy while undergoing treatment for genital warts. Your partner should see a physician and be checked for genital warts as well.

A nonsteroidal anti-inflammatory (ibuprofen or naproxen) can help with the pain of treatment 1 h prior to the treatment and the evening after the treatment. If you have been treated with a liquid, cream, or gel, be sure to follow the instructions regarding the timing for removal of the compound. Set the alarm on your cellphone to remove the treatment at the appropriate time. If you have severe pain or swelling, be sure to wash the medication off immediately. Most lesions need to be rechecked by a physician. If your doctor treated you with cryotherapy or trichloroacetic acid (TCA), please make a follow-up appointment within 1–2 weeks for a recheck.

References

1. Gargano J, Meites E, Watson M, Unger, E, Markowitz L. Human Papillomavirus. In Manual for the Surveillance of vaccine preventable disease. HPV - Vaccine Preventable Diseases Surveillance Manual | CDC. Updated March 9, 2022. Accessed 3.10.2024.
2. World Health Organization. Global Health Sector Strategy on Sexually Transmitted Infections 2016-2021. Global health sector strategy on Sexually Transmitted Infections, 2016-2021 (who.int). Accessed 3.10.2024.
3. Tyros G, Mastraftsi S, Gregoriou S, Nicolaidou E. Incidence of anogenital warts: epidemiological risk factors and real-life impact of human papillomavirus vaccination. Int J STD AIDS. 2021;32(1):4–13. https://doi.org/10.1177/0956462420958577. Epub 2020 Nov 9
4. Meites E, Kempe A, Markowitz LE. Use of a 2-dose schedule for human papillomavirus vaccination – updated recommendations of the advisory committee on immunization practices. MMWR Morb Mortal Wkly Rep. 2016;65:1405–8.
5. Garland SM, Hernandez-Avila M, Wheeler CM, Perez G, Harper DM, Leodolter S, Tang GWK, Ferris DG, Steben M, Bryan J, Taddeo FJ, Railkar R, Esser MT, Sings HL, Nelson M, Boslego J, Sattler C, Barr E, Koutsky LA. Quadrivalent vaccine against human papillomavirus to prevent anogenital diseases. N Engl J Med. 2007;356(19):1928–43.
6. Markowitz LE, Liu G, Hariri S, Steinau M, Dunne EF, Unger ER. Prevalence of HPV after introduction of the vaccination program in the United States. Pediatrics. 2016;137(3):1–9.
7. Eschenbach D. Pelvic and sexually transmitted diseases. In: Gibbs RS, Karlan BY, Haney AR, Nygaard IE, editors. Danforth's obstetrics and gynecology. Lippincott Williams & Wilkins; 2008.
8. Delmonte S, Benardon S, Cariti C, Ribero S, Ramoni S, Cusini M. Anogenital warts treatment options: a practical approach. G Ital Dermatol Venereol. 2020;155(3):261–8. https://doi.org/10.23736/S0392-0488.18.06125-4. Epub 2018 Sep 24
9. Podophloxin description; RxList: available at https://www.rxlist.com/podofilox-topical-solution-drug.htm. Accessed 10 Mar 2024.
10. Gross G, Meyer K-G, Pres H, Thielert C, Tawfik H, Mescheder A. A randomized, double-blind, four-arm parallel-group, placebo-controlled Phase II/III study to investigate the clinical efficacy of two galenic formulations of Polyphenon® E in the treatment of external genital warts. J Eur Acad Dermatol Venereol. 2007;21(10):1404–12.
11. Veregen description; Rxlist: the internet drug Index. 2007. Available at: http://www.rxlist.com/cgi/generic/veregen.htm. Accessed 24 June 2018.
12. Workowski KA, Bachmann LH, Chan PA, Johnson CM, Muzny CA, Park I, Reno H, Zenilman JM, Bolan GA. Sexually transmitted infections treatment guidelines. 70(4) 7/23/2021. Accessed 3/10/2024
13. Fox-Lewis A, Allum C, Vokes D, et al. Human papillomavirus and surgical smoke: a systematic review. Occup Environ Med. 2020;77:809–17.
14. Feng C, Li W, Wang X, Zhang H, Si L, Chen Z, Bai M. A systematic review evaluating the efficacy and safety of a combination of ablative treatment and self administered treatment versus ablative treatment alone for external anogenital warts. Int J Dermatol. 2020;59(10):1210–6. https://doi.org/10.1111/ijd.14863. Epub 2020 Apr 16
15. Lei J, Ploner A, Elfström KM, Wang J, Roth A, Fang F, Sundström K, Dillner J, Sparén P. HPV Vaccination and the Risk of Invasive Cervical Cancer. N Engl J Med. 2020 Oct 1;383(14):1340–1348. https://doi.org/10.1056/NEJMoa1917338. PMID: 32997908.

Chapter 23
Cervical Polyp Removal

Ryan Planer

Introduction

Cervical polyps are pedunculated red masses which vary in size from several millimeters to centimeters (Fig. 23.1). They are usually found in the endocervical canal and protrude from the cervical os. Occasionally, polyps protruding from the cervical os are endometrial in origin. Cervical polyps are often single but can be multiple; they are the most common cervical lesion and occur in 2–5% of women [1]. They are usually bright red, spongy in nature, and friable. Management of cervical polyps in the primary care setting may be accomplished through either expectant management or polypectomy, with close considerations of the patient's risk factors. The clinician must review factors such as the patient's symptoms, pregnancy, or menopausal status.

Most often asymptomatic, polyps are commonly found on a routine gynecological exam. They can also be detected on colposcopy, seen as filling defects on hysterosalpingograms, and seen on abdominal and transvaginal ultrasound. Patients with polyps can also present with intermenstrual spotting, post-coital bleeding, persistent leukorrhea, postmenopausal bleeding, or heavy menses (i.e., symptomatic polyp). The cause of polyps is unknown, although they may be a secondary reaction to cervical inflammation or hormonal stimulation and are thus seen more often with increasing age, inflammation, trauma, and pregnancy. Cervical polyps are most frequently seen in parous, perimenopausal, and postmenopausal women in the second through fifth decades of life [1, 2]. Symptomatic polyps tend to be more common in premenopausal women. More pathological conditions are associated with symptomatic polyps and tend to occur more commonly in the postmenopausal age group. While malignant potential is rare, if symptomatic in the postmenopausal woman,

R. Planer (✉)
Faculty, St. Joseph's Family Medicine Residency, Syracuse, NY, USA
e-mail: Ryan.Planer@sjhsyr.org

S. M. Sulik, C. B. Heath (eds.), *Primary Care Procedures in Women's Health*,
https://doi.org/10.1007/978-3-032-07061-6_23

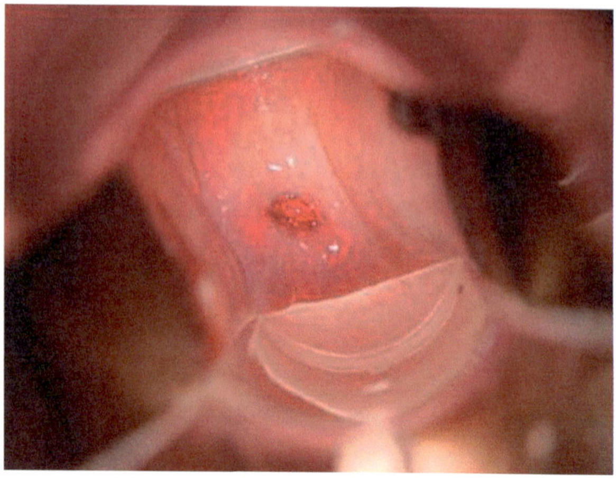

Fig. 23.1 Endocervical polyp

hysteroscopy or uterine dilatation and curettage (D&C) should be considered as part of the evaluation [2].

Asymptomatic Cervical Polyp

In the asymptomatic premenopausal female, a cervical polyp may be treated as a normal variant, and expectant management may be utilized to minimize procedure risk, return visits, and overall healthcare expenditure. A shift in the management of asymptomatic cervical polyps over the last three decades is well supported in the literature, although currently there are no practice guidelines from professional societies. Large research studies (*n* of 898–5488) demonstrate that asymptomatic cervical polyps in a premenopausal patient with normal cytology reported no cases of malignancy or significant pathology [3]. When found, polyps are generally removed as they can become symptomatic over time. Important discussion with the patient about individualized risks, prior Pap smear results, and proper consent with documentation are prudent in either expectant management or polypectomy.

Symptomatic Cervical Polyp

Symptomatic polyps most often present with complaints of intermenstrual spotting, postcoital bleeding, persistent leukorrhea, postmenopausal bleeding, or heavy menses. Several studies have noted an association of endocervical polyps and endometrial polyps, with one study showing that 25% of women with cervical polyps had endometrial polyps as well [4–6]. Combination oral contraceptives reduce the incidence of cervical polyps in this population from 25 to 8.3%. Postmenopausal women with polyps had a 56.8% incidence of cervix-related endometrial polyps [4]. Because of this association between endometrial and cervical polyps, some advocate that removal of cervical polyps should be done with hysteroscopy which would allow for evaluation of the endometrial cavity. This would help clarify the initial diagnosis as well as allow for precise visualization of the polyp peduncle and treat concurrent asymptomatic intrauterine pathology [4].

Histologically, cervical polyps are composed of endocervical epithelium with a fibrovascular stalk. Most are benign, some will show squamous metaplasia or squamous dysplasia, and malignancy is very rare [7]. All polyps should be sent to pathology for evaluation.

Pregnancy

The removal of cervical polyps during pregnancy has been shown to increase the risks of chorioamnionitis, spontaneous abortion, and preterm delivery [8, 9]. Polypectomy during pregnancy is reserved for clinical situations in which there is a high suspicion of possible malignancy. The provider may also consider removal at the time of delivery, and if a concern for malignancy, provide for close coordination with obstetrical and oncological colleagues [9] (Algorithm 23.1). Expectant management during pregnancy is also associated with a higher risk of preterm birth before 34 weeks of gestation [10].

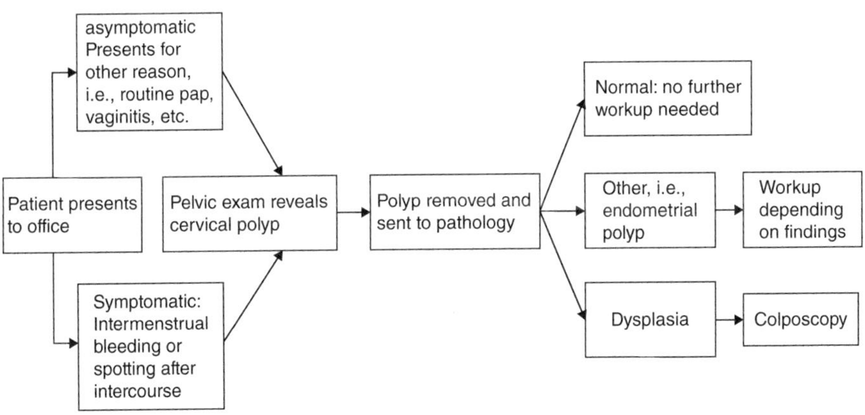

Algorithm 23.1 Decision tree for endometrial polyp removal

Case Study

A 45-year-old G2P2presents to your office for an annual exam and a Pap smear. Review of systems reveals regular menses, with occasional spotting after intercourse. No other spotting noted. On pelvic exam, a pedunculated red mass at the endocervical os is found.

Diagnosis

Cervical polyp

Differential Diagnosis

- Cervical polyp
- Condyloma
- Nabothian cyst
- Prolapsed myoma
- Cervical malignancy
- Squamous papilloma
- Sarcoma
- Retained products of conception

Indications for Polyp Removal

- Intermenstrual spotting or bleeding
- Spotting after intercourse
- Removal to prevent future irritation, bleeding, or discharge

Contraindications

- Pregnancy—delay removal until postpartum, unless significant bleeding exists
- Inability to visualize the base of the polyp
- Bleeding or coagulation disorder

Complications

- Bleeding/spotting
- Recurrence (11%)
- Infection (rare)

Equipment (Fig. 23.2)

- Vaginal speculum
- Nonsterile gloves
- Long Kelly or ring forceps
- Monsel's solution or silver nitrate sticks
- Topical anesthetic
- Formalin container
- Optional equipment (Fig. 23.3):
  - Endocervical curette (ECC)
  - Tischler biopsy forceps
  - Colposcope

Procedure

1. Obtain consent for polyp removal.

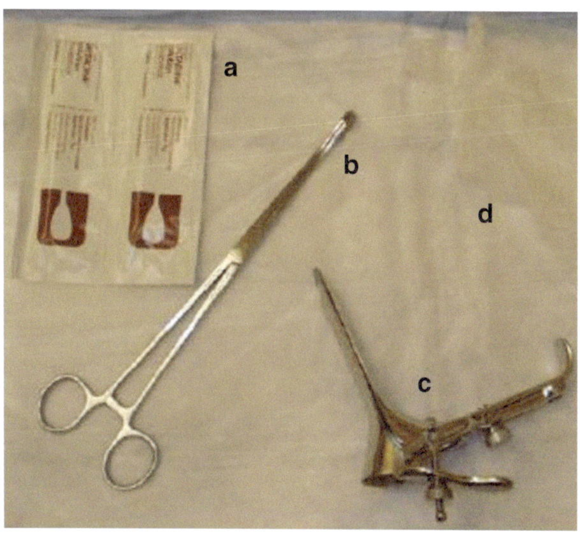

Fig. 23.2 Nonsterile equipment for endocervical polyp removal: (**a**) Betadine® Solution Swabsticks (Purdue Pharma, Stamford, CT); (**b**) ring forceps; (**c**) Pederson speculum; (**d**) gloves

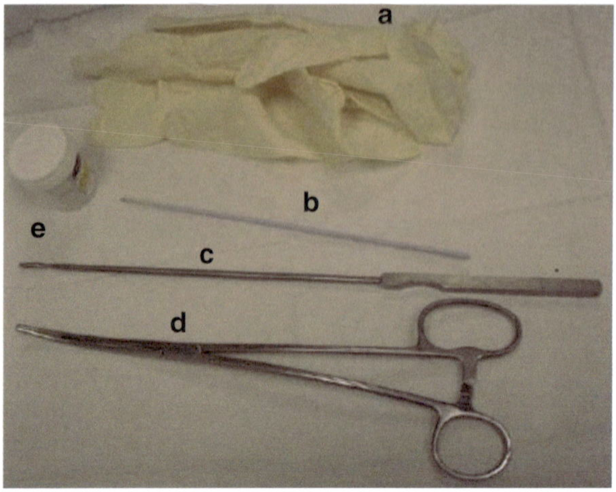

Fig. 23.3 Optional Equipment for endocervical polyp removal: (**a**) nonlatex, nonsterile gloves; (**b**) endocervical brush; (**c**) endocervical curette; (**d**) long Kelly forceps; (**e**) cytology fixative jar

2. Insert the speculum into the vagina and identify the polyp.
3. Place long Kelly or ring forceps as close to the base of the polyp as possible and clamp.
4. Twist the polyp in one direction until it easily breaks off.
5. An ECC curette can be used to curette the base of the endocervical canal in order to remove any polyp remnants. An endocervical brush can also be used.
6. Send specimen to pathology for review.
7. Silver nitrate or Monsel's solution can be used to treat any bleeding.

Helpful Hints

Use the colposcope to identify the base of the polyp, and then remove the polyp using a Tischler biopsy forceps.

Interpretation of Results

- Report usually indicates benign tissue.
- If dysplasia is noted on a polyp, consider colposcopy.
- Any abnormal finding (i.e., sarcoma) requires additional therapy.

Procedure Note

The patient was placed in the lithotomy position, a speculum was inserted into the vagina, and the cervix was identified. The polyp was identified. A long Kelly was placed at the base of the polyp, and the polyp was removed in its entirety by gentle twisting. An ECC curette was used to remove any polyp fragments in the endocervical canal. The specimen was sent to pathology. The patient tolerated the procedure without difficulty.

Coding

There is no separate CPT code for cervical polyp removal.

57500 Cervix uteri biopsy
57505 Endocervical curettage
58100 Endometrial sampling with or without endocervical sampling, without cervical dilation, any method

ICD 10-CM Diagnostic Codes
N84.1 Polyp of cervix uteri
N85.0 Endometrial hyperplasia
D26.0 Benign neoplasm of the cervix uteri
A63.0 Condyloma acuminatum

Postprocedure Patient Instruction

The patient should be told to avoid douching or intercourse until all bleeding/spotting has resolved. Any excessive bleeding should be reported immediately, and the patient re-evaluated. Pathology is usually benign, and no further treatment is usually necessary. Routine follow-up with an annual exam is recommended.

Case Study Outcome

The polyp was easily removed with minimal bleeding. Pathology revealed normal benign epithelium.

Patient Handout

Cervical Polyp Removal

Cervical polyps are small pieces of tissue that are found within the canal of your cervix. While these are usually benign tissue pieces, the sample is always sent to the pathologist for review to ensure that no cancer or other abnormality is present.

Today, your clinician removed a cervical polyp from your cervix. You should expect to have some minimal spotting/bleeding. This should not be heavier than a normal period. If you experience heavier bleeding, please call your clinician right away.

Cramping is usually transient, but if it persists, please take 3 ibuprofen 200 mg tablets every 6 hours (h) as needed or acetaminophen 650 mg every 4–6 h as needed.

You should avoid intercourse, douching, or tampon use for several days.

Your clinician will inform you of the results of the polyp when they receive the information from the pathologist.

Please call the office if you have any problems or questions.

References

1. Ozaran AA, Itil IM, Sagol S. Endometrial hyperplasia coexisting with cervical polyps. Int J Gynecol Obstet. 1999;66(2):185–6.
2. Neri A, Kaplan B, Rabinerson D, Ovadia J, Braslavsky D. Cervical polyp in the menopause and the need for fractional dilatation and curettage. Eur J Obstet Gynecol Reprod Biol. 1995;62(1):53–5.
3. Nelson AL, Papa RR, Ritchie JJ. Asymptomatic cervical polyps: can we just let them be? Womens Health. 2015;11(2):121–6.
4. Stamatellos I, Stamatopoulos P, Bontis J. The role of hysteroscopy in the current management of the cervical polyps. Arch Gynecol Obstet. 2007;276(4):299–303. https://doi.org/10.1007/s00404-007-0417-2. Epub 2007 July 25
5. Spiewankiewicz B, Stelmachow J, Sawicki W, Cendrowski K, Kuzlik R. Hysteroscopy in cases of cervical polyps. Eur J Gynaecol Oncol. 2003;24(1):67–9.
6. Vilodre LC, Bertat R, Petters R, Reis FM. Cervical polyp as risk factor for hysteroscopically diagnosed endometrial polyps. Gynecol Obstet Investig. 1997;44(3):191.
7. Schnatz PF, Ricci S, O'Sullivan DM. Cervical polyps in postmenopausal women. Menopause. 2009;16(3):524–8.
8. Tokunaka M, Hasegawa J, Oba T, Nakamura M, Matsuoka R, Ichizuka K, et al. Decidual polyps are associated with preterm delivery in cases of attempted uterine cervical polypectomy during the first and second trimester. J Matern Fetal Neonatal Med. 2014;28(9):1061–3.
9. Panayotidis LC. Cervical polypectomy during pregnancy: the gynaecological perspective. J Genit Syst Disord. 2013;02(02)
10. Wakimoto T, Hayashi S, Koh I, Yamamoto R, Ishii K. Relationship between unremoved cervical polyp in pregnancy and spontaneous preterm birth. Am J Obstet Gynecol. 2022;227(6):899.e1–6. https://doi.org/10.1016/j.ajog.2022.06.064. Epub 2022 July 13

Chapter 24
Colposcopy

Roshan Ghimire and Laurie Turenne-Kolpan

Introduction

Colposcopy is a procedure used to evaluate the abnormal Pap smear as well as to visualize abnormalities noted anywhere along the lower female reproductive tract. The colposcope is an illuminating instrument that enables the provider to examine the vulva, vagina, cervix, and anus under magnified view. The goal of colposcopy is to identify areas of abnormal epithelium and perform directed biopsies, which will allow for a histological evaluation of abnormal cytological results. This chapter will focus on colposcopy of the cervix and its guidelines.

The procedure is simple and can be performed in the outpatient office; however, recognition of the normal versus abnormal cervix requires a certain level of expertise. Practitioners performing colposcopy should be adequately trained. Such training courses are offered by the American Society for Colposcopy and Cervical Pathology (ASCCP).

R. Ghimire (✉)
Faculty, St. Joseph's Family Medicine Residency, Syracuse, NY, USA
e-mail: turenne-kolpan.laurie@hunterdonhealthcare.org

L. Turenne-Kolpan
Faculty, Department of Family Practice, Hunterdon Medical Center, Flemington, NJ, USA
e-mail: lturenne-kolpan@hhsnj.org

S. M. Sulik, C. B. Heath (eds.), *Primary Care Procedures in Women's Health*,
https://doi.org/10.1007/978-3-032-07061-6_24

Case Study

A 26-year-old female presents to your office for a gynecology exam and Papanicolaou (Pap) smear. The patient is sexually active with male partners, uses oral contraceptives, has never had a Pap smear, has no history of any sexually transmitted diseases, and never had Human Papillomavirus (HPV) vaccination. The exam is normal. Pap smear results return as low-grade squamous intraepithelial lesion (LSIL).

Diagnosis

Abnormal Pap Smear with LSIL

Indications: (Algorithm 24.1)

Colposcopy is indicated when the immediate risk of cervical intraepithelial neoplasia (CIN) 3+ is 4% or greater, as determined by their current HPV and cytology results as well as past screening and clinical history. The American Society for Colposcopy and Cervical Pathology provides excellent tools to help determine this risk including a free web page https://app.asccp.org/; or a smartphone app available at nominal cost https://www.asccp.org/mobile-app.

Other indications for colposcopy include the following:

- Leukoplakia
- Suspicious lesion seen or palpated on exam
- History of intrauterine Diethylstilbesterol (DES) exposure (last used in the US in 1971 and in Europe in 1978) [1]

Contraindications

- Pregnancy is only a contraindication for endocervical curettage (ECC); biopsies are performed for suspicion of cancer only.
- Heavy menses at the time of procedure.
- Active cervicitis.

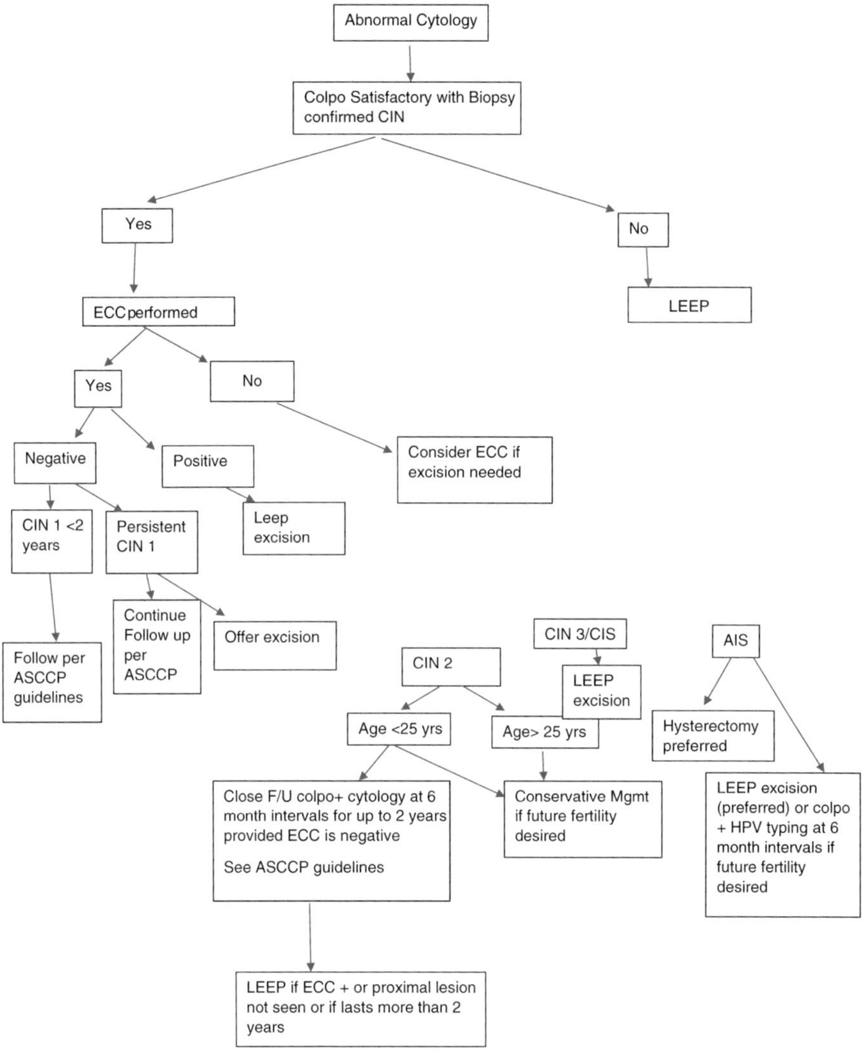

Algorithm 24.1 Management after colposcopy biopsy report

Equipment (Fig. 24.1)

- Vaginal speculum (metal or plastic)
- Small and large cotton-tipped applicators
- 3–5% acetic acid (vinegar)
- Lugol's solution
- Specimen containers

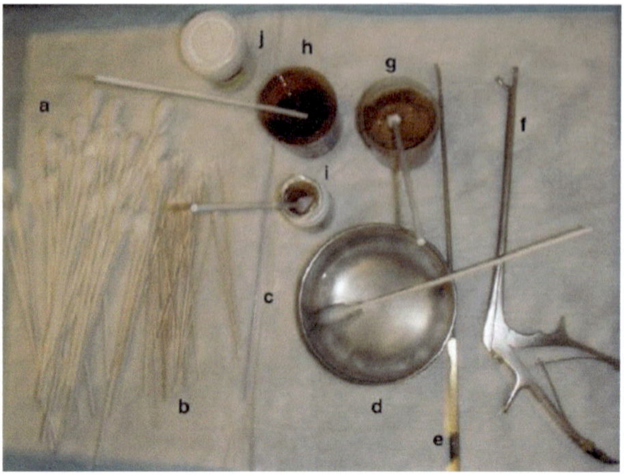

Fig. 24.1 Setup tray for colposcopy: (**a**) large cotton swab applicators; (**b**) small cotton swab applicators; (**c**) endocervical brush; (**d**) basin with acetic acid; (**e**) sterile endocervical curette; (**f**) sterile Kevorkian punch biopsy; (**g**) Monsel's solution; (**h**) Lugol's solution; (**i**) topical anesthetic; (**j**) formalin specimen container

- Kogan endocervical speculum
- Endocervical curette with or without basket
- Tischler or Kevorkian biopsy forceps
- Cervical hook
- Monsel's solution
- Silver nitrate sticks
- Toothpicks
- Papanicolaou smear supplies

Optional Equipment

Cytobrush with a straw (sleeve), ring forceps, or long Kelly, non-stick gauze pads cut into small squares to collect the specimen.

Procedure

1. Check a urine pregnancy test prior to the procedure and obtain surgical consent.
2. Place the patient in the dorsal lithotomy position.
3. Insert the speculum into the vagina and visualize the cervix under medium magnification (12–15×). Ensure the entire cervix can be visualized.
4. Wipe off excess mucus with a large cotton swab and identify landmarks. The squamocolumnar junction is the area of delineation between squamous and columnar epithelium (Fig. 24.2). The active transformation zone is the area where prior columnar epithelium has been changed or is in the process of changing into squamous epithelium, and thus is the area where dysplasia is most likely

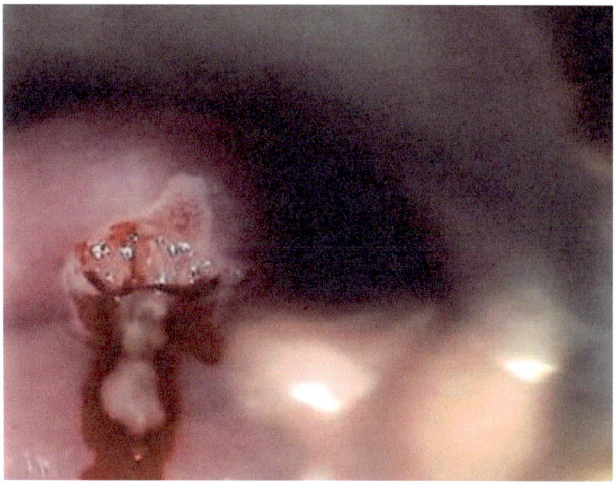

Fig. 24.2 Colposcopic view of squamocolumnar junction

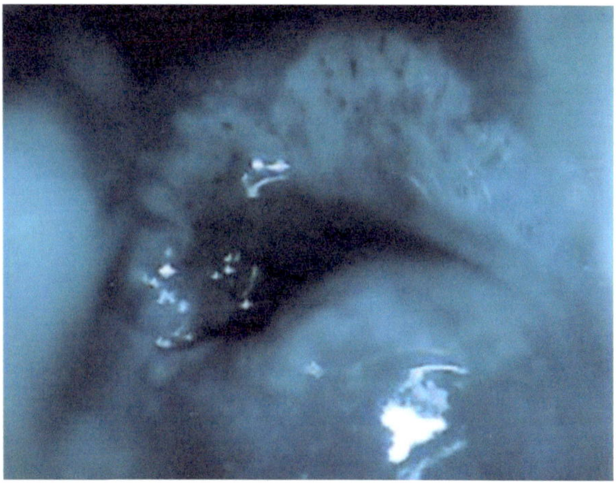

Fig. 24.3 Higher magnification view of cervix with green filter

to occur. Gland openings, crypts, or Nabothian cysts are usually seen in this area. An adequate colposcopy requires that the entire transformation zone and squamocolumnar junction be seen.

5. Perform a Pap smear if desired. Recent evidence shows this practice is rarely useful even if the first cytology was obtained by a conventional smear [2, 3]. One practice could be to repeat cytology if the interval between colposcopy and the original Pap smear is greater than 6 months as abnormal cervical cytology findings may resolve or progress over time.
6. Use the green filter and higher magnification (25–40×) to identify any abnormal vessels (Fig. 24.3).

   - Normal saline can be used with the green filter if preferred.
   - Abnormal vascular patterns include the presence of mosaicism, which is caused by vessels lying along the superficial area of the cervix forming a

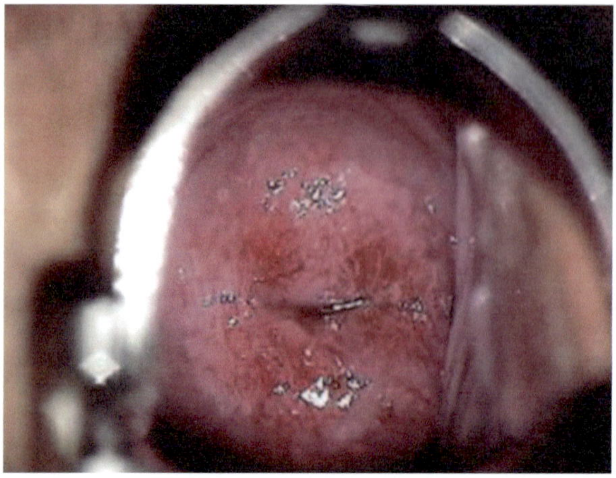

Fig. 24.4 Cervix with mosaic tile pattern pattern seen at 8:00 position on the cervix

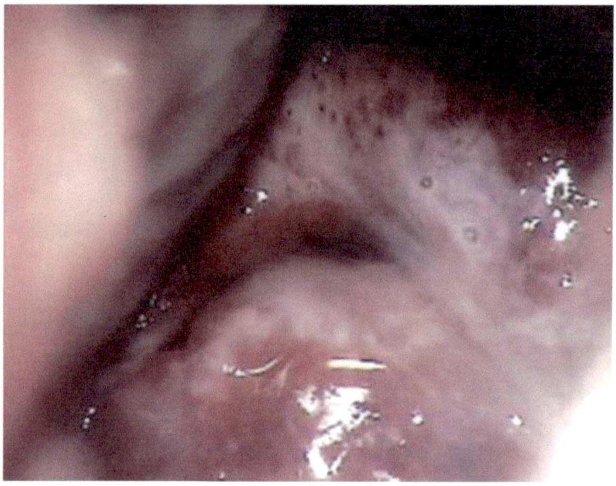

Fig. 24.5 Cervix with coarse punctation seen at 12:00

pattern similar to mosaic tiles (Fig. 24.4), punctation which is caused by vessels lying perpendicular to the cervical surface and creates an appearance of the cervix being dotted with a red marker (Fig. 24.5), and atypical vessels, which are evidence of the presence of a blood vessel lying on top of the cervical surface (Fig. 24.6). The presence of larger or more coarse vessels in any of these vascular patterns is associated with higher-grade dysplasia.

7. Return to white light, medium magnification, and apply 3–5% acetic acid with large cotton swabs or cotton balls (Fig. 24.7)
   - These need to be held against the cervix for at least 1 min. Acetic acid may cause minor stinging, which will quickly abate.
   - Identify any areas of whitened epithelium (acetowhite). Look for all borders of the lesion.

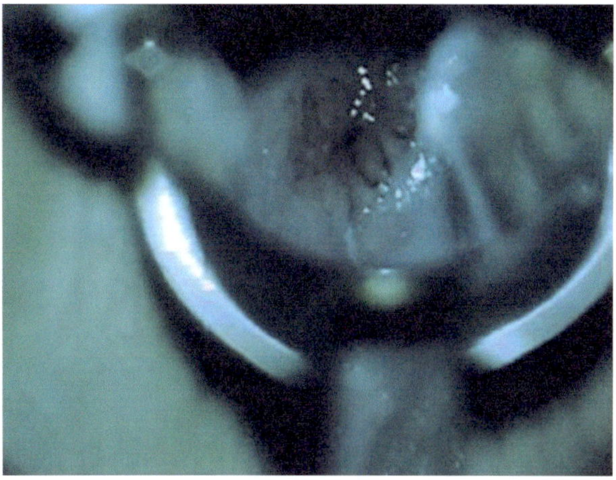

Fig. 24.6 Cervix with green filter showing superficial horizontal abnormal blood vessels.

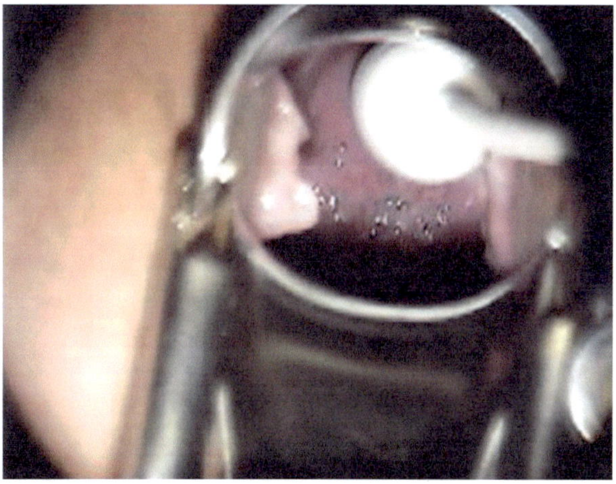

Fig. 24.7 Application of acetic acid under medium magnification

- Identify which areas are the most densely white. High-grade dysplasia is typically associated with thick, well-demarcated areas of acetowhite. The acetowhite reaction will fade quickly (especially in low-grade disease), and more acetic acid may need to be applied (Fig. 24.8).

8. If the entire squamocolumnar junction is not seen or if an acetowhite area enters the cervical canal, place the Kogan speculum into the cervical os and open slowly and gently.
   - If you are still unable to see the entire squamocolumnar junction or acetowhite area, or if you cannot get the Kogan speculum through the os, the colposcopy is considered unsatisfactory.
   - Remove the endocervical speculum.

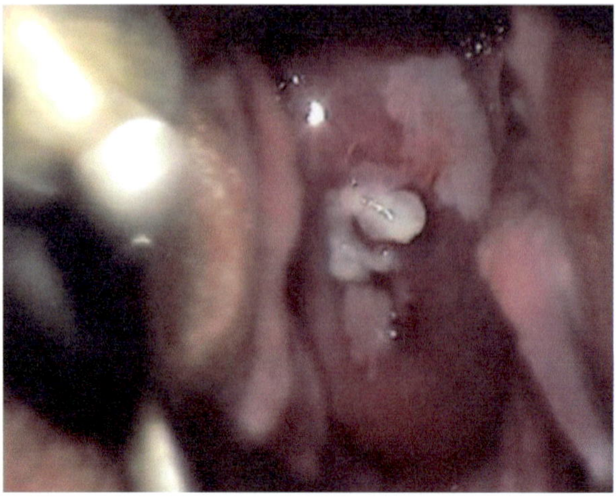

Fig. 24.8 Thick, well-demarcated lesions with acetowhite reaction indicating potential high-grade lesion.

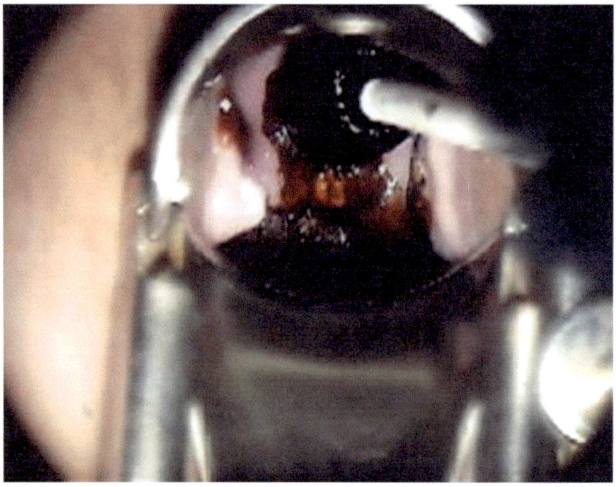

Fig. 24.9 Application of Lugol's solution to the cervix with a large cotton-tipped applicator

9. Apply Lugol's solution if desired (Fig. 24.9).
    - Abnormal epithelium has low levels of glycogen and does not take up iodine well; therefore, abnormal areas will remain light (mustard yellow in color) or "Lugol's Negative." Normal epithelium remains a deep dark brown stain.
    - Be aware that glandular and columnar epithelium will also not take up Lugol's solution.
10. Perform the Endocervical Curettage (ECC) by inserting the curette through the external os, and, with firm pressure, scrape the sides of the canal using downward strokes around the entire canal (360° × two rotations) (Fig. 24.10).
11. Place the specimen from the curette into a formalin container. This can be facilitated by using a small square of nonstick gauze to wipe the curette and then

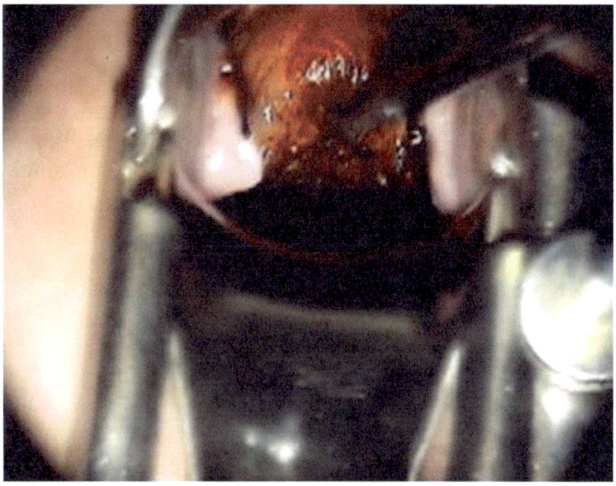
Fig. 24.10 Endocervical curettage performed after application of Lugol's solution.

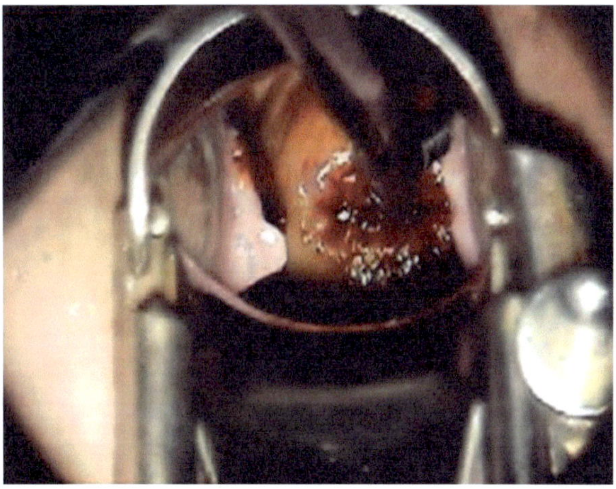
Fig. 24.11 Cervical biopsy with Tischler forceps

placing the gauze in the container. If an additional sample is seen at the os, it can be grasped with a ring forceps or a long Kelly forceps.

- Alternatively, a cytobrush can be used to obtain any residual sample from the os, and the tip of the brush can be cut off into the container.

12. Use the Tischler forceps to biopsy the most abnormal areas of the cervix. Start with the abnormal area most posterior on the cervix so as to avoid bleeding into the next area for biopsy (Fig. 24.11).
    - Recent evidence has shown that even in the hands of the most expert colposcopists, taking more than one biopsy increases the sensitivity of detecting CIN 3 [4]. Therefore, it is recommended that liberal biopsies be taken of the abnormal cervix. It is *not currently recommended*, however, that random biopsies be taken of the normal cervix.

13. Place biopsies in a formalin container. A toothpick or broken stem of a wooden cotton-tipped applicator can be used to remove the biopsy from the forceps. Do not place the forceps directly into the formalin.
    - Although all biopsies can be sent in the same specimen container, the more common approach is to use a separate container for each specimen, allowing the provider to compare the histology results obtained with the visual abnormality seen.
14. Remove excess blood/clot from the vagina.
    - Apply pressure to all bleeding sites with large cotton-tipped applicators.
    - Apply Monsel's solution to all bleeding areas by using firm pressure over the bleeding site. Silver nitrate sticks may also be used (occasionally will stain the cervix).
    - Visualize the cervix under medium magnification to ensure hemostasis.
15. Remove the speculum and have the patient return to a sitting position slowly. Rapid sitting can cause a vasovagal response.

Complications and Risks

1. Discomfort
2. Bleeding
3. Infection
4. Missed disease

Tricks and Helpful Hints

- An alternate way of performing the ECC is to use intensive cytobrushing. A cytobrush is inserted through a straw and into the os. It is rotated 360° five times and then removed through the straw. The purpose of the straw is to prevent contamination of the endocervical sample with ectocervical disease. A recent study has shown this method to be more sensitive and less painful than the traditional ECC [5].
- There is no standard recommendation for obtaining ECC before or after cervical biopsy. Some colposcopists prefer to perform the ECC after the biopsies as this is the most uncomfortable part of the procedure. The concern with this method is contamination of the endocervical specimen with ectocervical disease and interference with visualization of the endocervical canal, so care must be taken to avoid this.
- If a colposcopy is unsatisfactory because the os is stenotic, the patient may be given intravaginal estrogen 2 g inserted nightly for 2 weeks, or 200–400 μg of

misoprostol inserted intravaginally 6 hours (h) before the procedure. The colposcopy is repeated. Either of these techniques has been shown to open the os, often enough to allow for an adequate exam.

Interpretation of Results

There are multiple different pathways for diagnosis and treatment that ultimately depend on the patient's age, dysplasia history, and childbearing goals. Refer to the ASCCP Consensus Guidelines (https://www.asccp.org/managment-guidelines) for detailed algorithms [6]. It is also important to relate the histological results to the colposcopic and cytological results. If significant discrepancies are present, further evaluation needs to be done. This can initially be accomplished by having the pathologist review the slides from both the Pap smear and histological samples obtained at colposcopy. If the discrepancy is not resolved, the patient warrants referral to a provider who can perform a diagnostic excisional procedure (Loop Electrode Excisional Procedure or cold knife cone biopsy).

Unsatisfactory Colposcopy

The colposcopy is considered unsatisfactory if the cervix cannot be fully visualized, the entire squamocolumnar junction cannot be fully visualized, or the limits of the lesion cannot be seen. If the initial cytology was high-grade squamous intraepithelial lesion (HSIL), or histology is shown to be CIN-2 or CIN-3, the patient should undergo a diagnostic excisional procedure. If the cytology was less severe than HSIL and the colposcopy and histology were normal, the patient may be followed up either by HPV-based testing or HPV-based testing and colposcopy at 1 year [6, 7].

Normal Colposcopy

See ASCCP guidelines.

CIN 1
See ASCCP guidelines.
Observation is preferred to treatment for CIN 1.

CIN 2/3
See ASCCP Updated Consensus Guidelines.

Treatment is required for most cases of CIN 2 and 3, although this may depend on age, dysplasia history and pregnancy history, and future fertility plans. This can be performed by either ablative (cryotherapy, laser ablation, cold coagulation, or electrofulguration) or excisional (LEEP, cold knife cone, or laser excision) methods and should include treatment of the entire transformation zone. Excisional treatment is preferred for the management of CIN 2/3; however, treatment with ablation is acceptable. Exceptions to this are when the lesion extends into the canal, when the lesion covers 75% or more of the ectocervix, or the ECC shows CIN 2 or higher [6].

Most current guidelines do allow for an option to observe CIN 2 and 3 in patients younger than age 25 with a combination of cytology (or HPV-based testing) and colposcopy performed at 6-month intervals. If both consecutive evaluations are less than CIN 2, subsequent surveillance should occur at 1 year using HPV-based testing. If there are 3 negative annual HPV-based tests, then the patient may return to normal screening. If CIN 2 persists for more than 2 years, then treatment is recommended [6, 8].

Procedure Note

(Provider to fill in blanks/circle applicable choice when given multiple choices and to customize as needed.)

Name:_________________________________ Date:_________________

Chart #: ___________________________

Dae of Birth:________________ Contraception:

_________________________________ HCG__________________________

G____ P____ A—— Pap Smear History:

____

Reason for Colposcopy:

–

____

____

____

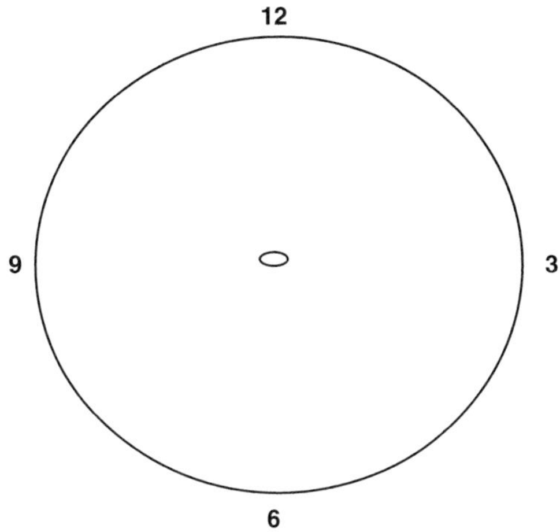

_Smoking: ___________
Colposcopic Exam () Satisfactory () Unsatisfactory
TZ = Transformation zone
Go = Gland openings
NC = Nabothian cysts
CO = Condyloma
WE = White epithelium
MO = Mosaic punctation
LK = Leukoplakia
AV = Atypical vessels
X = Biopsy site
X = Biopsy site
SCJ SEEN: (X)Y N
ECC DONE: (X)Y N
Impression:

____

Disposition:

____

Suggest subsequent examination and/or follow-up: ______________________

____

Physician's Signature

Coding

CPT® Codes (Current Procedural Terminology, AMA, Chicago, IL)
57452 Colposcopy of the upper vagina and cervix
57454 Colposcopy with biopsy(ies) and ECC
57455 Colposcopy with biopsy(ies)
57456 Colposcopy with ECC
57450 Colposcopy of the entire vagina and cervix

ICD 10-CM-Diagnostic Codes (International Classification of Diseases, 9th Revision, Clinical Modification, Center for Disease Control and Prevention)
R87.89 Abnormal Pap Smear of cervix and cervical HPV
R87.619 Abnormal Pap Smear, glandular
N87.9 Dysplasia, cervix, unspecified
N87.0 Dysplasia, cervix, mild (CIN 1)
N87.1 Dysplasia, cervix, moderate (CIN 2)
D06.9 Dysplasia, cervix, severe (CIN 3)

Postprocedure Patient Instructions

Explain to the patient that menstrual-like cramps are common and can be treated with ibuprofen 600 mg every 6 hours as needed. Spotting will occur, but bleeding should not persist beyond a week and should not be heavier than a menstrual period. If Monsel's solution or iodine was used, inform the patient that her vaginal discharge may be brown or black over the next several days. The patient should be instructed not to put anything in the vagina until all bleeding has resolved for 24 hours to reduce the likelihood of infection. She should be advised to avoid vaginal intercourse for 24–48 hours after cervical biopsies are taken to minimize trauma to the cervix to decrease bleeding risk. She should be counselled on the signs of infection and should be told to call for any abdominal pain beyond cramping and for fevers, shaking chills, and foul-smelling vaginal discharge. A follow-up visit should be scheduled with the patient to review her results and make a definitive treatment plan.

Case Study Outcome

The biopsy showed CIN 2, and the patient was referred for a LEEP procedure.

Patient Handout (Provider to Customize as Needed)

A colposcopy is a procedure by which your provider can examine your vulva, vagina, and cervix more closely to evaluate for any possible abnormalities. Most patients are requested to have a colposcopy for further evaluation of an abnormal Pap smear. The procedure is done similarly to a Pap smear in that a speculum is placed into the vagina while you lie on the exam table. The provider will then use a colposcope, which is an instrument that shines light on the cervix and magnifies the view. A vinegar solution, and perhaps an iodine solution, will be applied to your cervix to better identify any areas of potential concern. If such areas are noted, your doctor will take a biopsy, which is the removal of a small amount of tissue, and this will be examined in a lab. If you are not pregnant at the time of your colposcopy, a scraping of the inside of your cervix will also be performed and sent to the lab.

The cervix does not have the same kind of nerve endings as your skin, so while you may feel some pinching with a biopsy, it will not be severe. More likely, you will feel menstrual-like cramps. These can be reduced by taking three tablets (600 mg) of over-the-counter ibuprofen 1 hour prior to the procedure. DO NOT take this if you are pregnant or allergic to aspirin, ibuprofen, or naproxen.

We ask that you do not douche, do not use tampons or vaginal medications, and do not have sexual intercourse for 24 hours prior to your procedure.

After the procedure, you may have some brownish/black vaginal discharge from the medicines used to stop any bleeding. You may also have some spotting for 1–3 days and some menstrual-like cramps. These should improve with additional doses of ibuprofen. Do not put anything in the vagina (douches, tampons, etc.) and do not have intercourse until all spotting has stopped for 24 hours.

References

1. Diethylstilbestrol (DES) exposure and cancer. National Cancer Institute. 2021. https://www.cancer.gov/about-cancer/causes-prevention/risk/hormones/des-fact-sheet
2. Mao C, Balasubramanian A, Koutsky L. Should liquid-based cytology be repeated at the time of colposcopy? J Low Genit Tract Dis. 2005;9(2):82–8.
3. Rieck G, Bhaumik J, Beer H, Leeson S. Repeating cytology at initial colposcopy does not improve detection of high-grade abnormalities: a retrospective cohort study of 6595 women. Gynecol Oncol. 2006;101(20):228–33.
4. Burness JV, Schroeder JM, Warren JB. Cervical Colposcopy: Indications an Risk Assessment. Am Fam Physician.2020;102(1): p39–48.
5. Maksem J. Endocervical curetting vs. endocervical brushing as case finding methods. Diagn Cytopathol. 2006;54(5):313–6.
6. Perkins R, Guido R, Castle P. ASCCP risk-based management consensus guidelines for abnormal cervical cancer screening tests and cancer precursors. Journal of Lower Genital Tract Disease 2020;24(2): p102–131. https://doi.org/10.1097/LGT.0000000000000525
7. Dresang L. Colposcopy: an evidence-based update. J Am Board Fam Pract. 2005;18(5):383–92.

8. Massad S, Einstein M, Huh W, Katki H, Kinney W, Schiffman M, Solomon D, Wentzensen N, Lawson H. 2012 updated consensus guidelines for the management of abnormal cervical cancer screening tests and cancer precursors. J Low Genit Tract Dis. 2013;17(5):s1–27.

Additional Resources

Articles

Aggarwal R, Suneja A, Agarwal N, Mirshra K. Role of misoprostol in overcoming an unsatisfactory colposcopy: a randomized double-blind placebo-controlled clinical trial. Gynecol Obstet Investig. 2006;62(2):115–20.

Massad S, Perkins R, Naresh A. Colposcopy standards: guidelines for endocervical curettage at colposcopy. J Lower Genit Tract Dis. 2023;27(1):97–101.

Wright T, Cox T, Massad L, Twiggs L, Wilkinson E. 2001 consensus guidelines for the management of women with cervical cytological abnormalities. JAMA. 2002;287:2120–9.

Wright T, Cox T, Massad L, Carlson J, Twiggs L, Wilkinson E. 2001 consensus guidelines on the management of women with cervical intraepithelial neoplasia. Am J Obstet Gynecol. 2003;189(1):295–304.

Wright T, Massad S, Dunton C, Spitzer M, Wilkinson E, Solomon D. 2006 consensus guidelines for the management of women with abnormal cervical cancer screening tests. Am J Obstet Gynecol. 2007;197(4):346–55.

Books

Apgar B, Brotzman G, Spitzer M. Colposcopy principles and practice: an integrated textbook and atlas. Philadelphia: W.B. Saunders; 2002.

Website

https://app.asccp.org

Chapter 25
Cervical Cryotherapy

Laurie Turenne-Kolpan

Introduction

Cryotherapy is an ablative technique that has been used to treat all grades of cervical dysplasia for more than 50 years. In low-resource settings, it is a preferred method of many primary care providers because of its cost-effectiveness, safety, and ease in performance. A 2017 Cochrane review concluded that excisional procedures are associated with a small increase in the risk of preterm birth, and these risks increase with the depth of excision. Ablative procedures like cryotherapy have not been associated with adverse pregnancy outcomes, making this a potentially attractive procedure for reproductive-aged women [1]. Cryotherapy causes destruction of cells by producing a rapid freezing of tissue followed by a slow thaw. This causes intracellular ice crystals to form, followed by expansion of intracellular material, leading to rupture of the cells. The depth of freezing is directly proportional to the length of ice ball formation around the side of the probe, so that an ice ball 7 mm thick around the probe will yield a depth of freezing equal to 7 mm. It is important to note that the temperature of the tissue in the distal 2 mm of the ice ball is insufficient to cause cell death, so the level of actual tissue destruction is generally 2 mm less than the thickness of the ice ball [2].

Treatment in properly selected patients with cryotherapy for cervical intraepithelial neoplasia 1 (CIN) and CIN 2 can be as high as 95% effective; however, for larger CIN 2 (>2 cm) and CIN 3 lesions, the effectiveness may be significantly reduced. This is not due to the severity of the lesion but to the depth of dysplasia that occurs with more severe lesions. Cervical crypts have a depth up to 7 mm. Most mild and moderate dysplasia will be confined to an area above 5 mm, making cryotherapy a good choice for treatment. Crypt involvement, however, is a characteristic

L. Turenne-Kolpan (✉)
Faculty, Department of Family Practice, Hunterdon Medical Center, Flemington, NJ, USA
e-mail: turenne-kolpan.laurie@hunterdonhealthcare.org

S. M. Sulik, C. B. Heath (eds.), *Primary Care Procedures in Women's Health*,
https://doi.org/10.1007/978-3-032-07061-6_25

of high-grade lesions such as CIN 3; therefore, treatment of these lesions using cryotherapy should be limited to small lesions 1 cm or less in size [2].

As cryotherapy does not allow for tissue exam, it is essential that the colposcopy performed is adequate and that the histology does not differ more than one degree of severity from the cytology on the Pap smear. Other criteria for use of cryotherapy of the cervix include that the probe tip must cover the entire lesion and transformation zone, the lesion does not comprise more than 75% of the ectocervix, that endocervical sampling was performed and was negative for dysplasia, and that the patient is reliable for follow-up [2, 3]. If these conditions are not met, a diagnostic excisional procedure must be performed [2, 4]. Because the majority of cases of CIN 1 will spontaneously regress, the consensus guidelines set forth by the American Society of Colposcopy and Cervical Pathology (ASCCP) recommend observation without treatment. If the patient continues to have CIN 1 after 2 years, treatment versus further observation can be offered [4]. Treatment failures do occur; however, in properly selected patients, similar success rates have been shown with cryotherapy, laser ablation, fulguration, cold coagulation, Loop electrical excision procedure (LEEP), laser conization, and cold knife conization [5].

Studies comparing the flat and shallow conical probe tips show no difference in effectiveness for eradicating CIN, but they do show a slight increase in posttreatment migration of the squamocolumnar junction into the canal with the conical tip [6]. Nipple-tipped probes should be avoided, however, as they can cause cervical stenosis postprocedure [2].

Cryotherapy may also be used to treat chronic cervicitis that is culture negative. It is also effective in the treatment of external genital warts keeping in mind that the provider must use a different freezing regimen (see Chap. 22) [2].

Case Study

A 27-year-old G2P2 had a colposcopy performed in your office for a Pap smear result of low-grade intraepithelial lesion (LSIL). The histology report returns as CIN 1, and an endocervical curettage (ECC) shows benign endocervical cells. You review her chart and see that the colposcopy was adequate and showed an acetowhite lesion approximately 1 cm in length at the 12 o'clock position. This is the patient's third colposcopy, and prior histology reports have also revealed CIN 1. The patient does not smoke and is on oral contraceptives. At this point, after discussing the options of treatment including further observation, the patient opts for definitive treatment.

Diagnosis

Persistent low-grade dysplasia

Indications (Algorithm 25.1)

- Persistent low-grade squamous intraepithelial lesions that cover 75% of the cervix or less
- CIN 2 with a lesion sized as 2 cm or less confirmed by adequate colposcopy

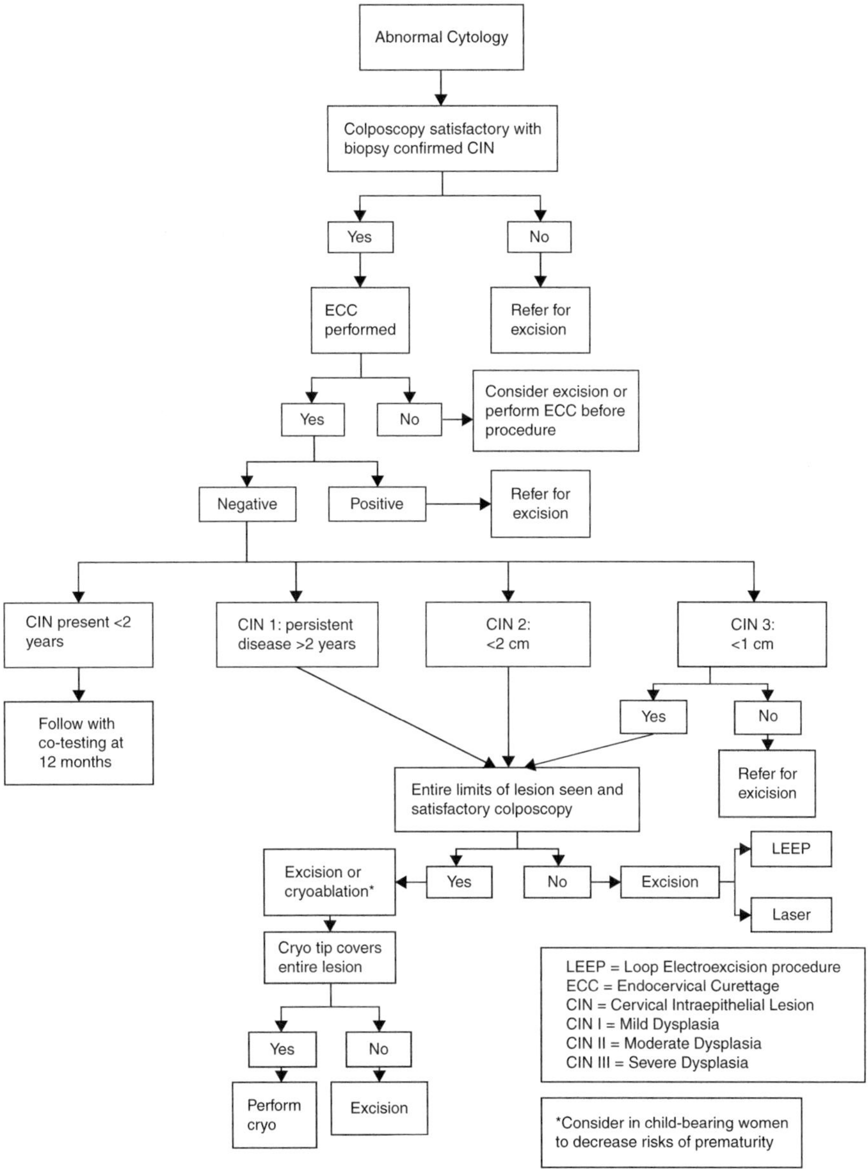

Algorithm 25.1 Decision tree for treatment of an abnormal pap smear with cryotherapy

- CIN 3 confirmed by adequate colposcopy 1 cm or less where LEEP is not available or accessible to the patient
- Chronic cervicitis that is culture negative
- External genital warts (see Chap. 22 on genital warts)

Contraindications (Algorithm 25.1)

- Large lesions that are not covered completely by the probe tip or comprise >75% of the ectocervix
- Inadequate colposcopy
- Positive endocervical curettage for CIN 2+
- Histology that differs more than 1° from the cytology of the Pap smear
- Lesions that extend more than 5 mm into the canal
- Current heavy menses or within 1 week of expected menses (relative)
- Pregnancy
- Active cervicitis
- High-grade lesions with a noncompliant patient
- Invasive lesions

Equipment (Fig. 25.1)

- Nitrous oxide 20-lb tank
- Flexible tubing from the tank to the probe
- Probe tips either flat or slightly coned. Sizes include 19 and 25 mm
- Vaginal speculum

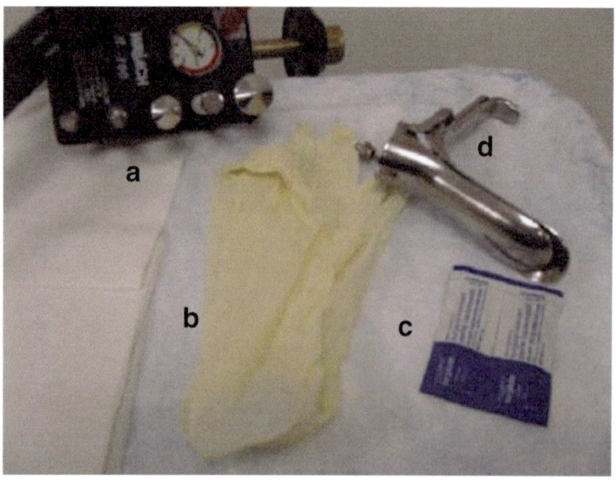

Fig. 25.1 Equipment tray for cervical cryotherapy: (**a**) Cryo tips with cryo tank and attachments (Wallach LL100 Cryosurgical System, Wallach Surgical Devices, Orange, CT); (**b**) gloves; (**c**) water-based lubricant Surgilube® (Fougera, Melville, NY); (**d**) speculum

- Water-soluble lubricant
- Colposcope (Some clinicians repeat the colposcopic exam at the time of the cryotherapy procedure.)
- 5% acetic acid

Optional Equipment

- Vaginal sidewall retractors
- Condom or glove finger for retraction of the vaginal wall

Procedure

1. Check urine pregnancy test prior to procedure.
2. Ensure the tank pressure is adequate and open the valve on the tank (Fig. 25.2). (The needle will be in the green zone on the pressure gauge.)
3. Place the patient in the dorsal lithotomy position.
4. Insert the speculum into the vagina.
5. Apply 5% acetic acid to identify the location and size of the lesion, with or without magnification from a colposcope.
6. Select the appropriate probe size.
7. Apply water-soluble lubricant to the tip of the probe to achieve an even freeze.
8. Apply the probe over the cervix, ensuring the entire lesion and transformation zone are completely covered.
9. Pull the trigger on the probe gun. The probe should adhere within a few seconds. Pull back slightly on the gun so the cervix is slightly forward, decreasing the likelihood of freezing the vaginal sidewalls (Fig. 25.3).
10. Continue freezing until a 7–10 mm ice ball is noted around the entire probe, with a minimum freeze time of 3 min.
11. Defrost the probe by releasing the trigger or pushing the defrost button, depending on your unit. The probe will detach shortly. *Do not pull on the probe until it is visibly defrosted to avoid pain and cervical laceration.*
12. Wait for the cervix to completely thaw, evidenced by a return of its pink color. A minimum of 5 minutes should be given.
13. Repeat the freeze–thaw cycle. Once the probe is disengaged the second time, the speculum can be removed.
14. Have the patient return to a sitting position slowly to avoid vasovagal symptoms.
15. Close the valve on the tank and discharge the remaining freezant.

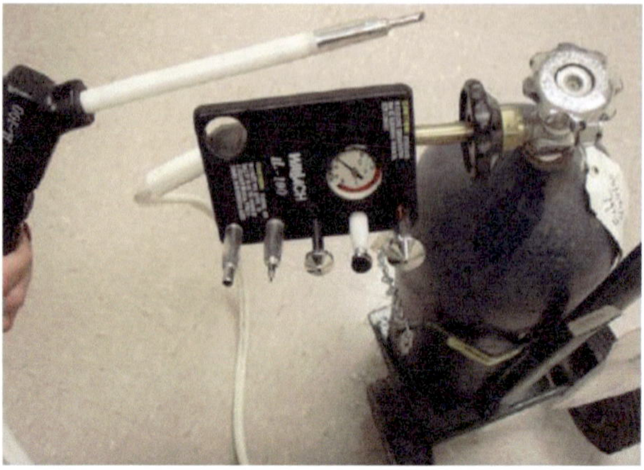

Fig. 25.2 Cryo tank with probe (Wallach LL100 Cryosurgical System, Wallach Surgical Devices, Orange, CT)

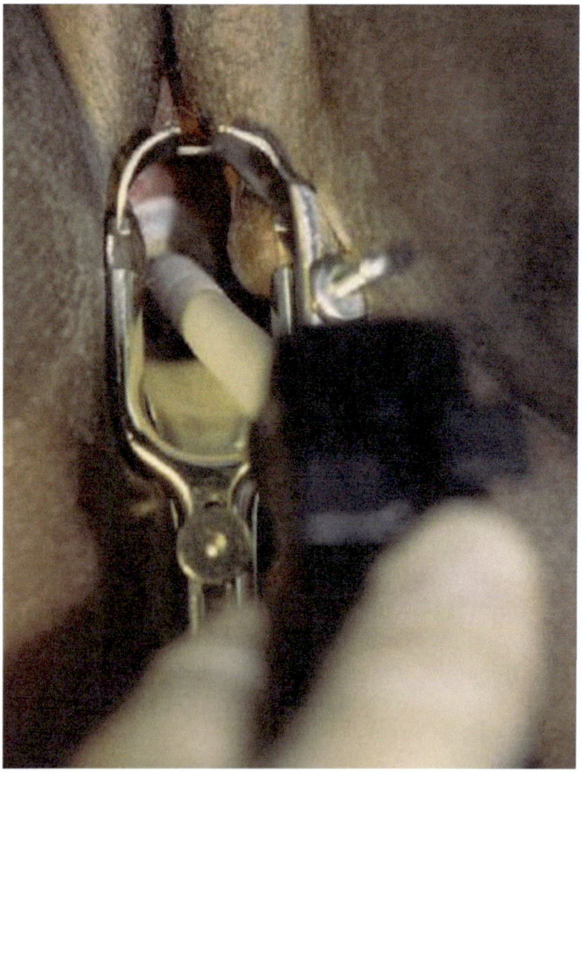

Fig. 25.3 Place probe onto the cervix after lubricant has been applied to the probe tip and pull trigger on the probe gun

Complications and Risks

- Treatment failure.
- Cervical stenosis.
- Difficulty with subsequent colposcopic exams as a result of the squamocolumnar junction retreating into the canal.
- Skip lesions (lesions further in the cervical canal behind the stenosis).
- Pelvic cramping typically lasts no more than a few days.
- Freezing of the vaginal wall.
- Profuse watery discharge which may contain a small amount of blood, often malodorous lasting 2–4 weeks.
- This occurs as a result of necrotic tissue and exudate being sloughed from the treatment site.
- Heavy bleeding and infection: very rare.

Tricks and Helpful Hints

- The optimal time to perform this procedure is 1 week after the start of the menstrual cycle. If a patient starts her cycle shortly after the procedure is performed, the subsequent edema of the cervix can cause stenosis of the os, retained menses, and significant pain and cramping. If this happens, the cervix can be probed with a cotton swab or cervical dilator, which will usually initiate the flow [2].
- Do not use "nipple-tipped" probes as they increase the rates of cervical stenosis and subsequent inadequate colposcopic exams.
- If vaginal side walls collapse into the canal and obscure full cervical visualization, the finger from a glove or a condom with the tip cut can be placed over the speculum blades, or vaginal sidewall retractors can be used to displace the redundant tissue and protect it from accidental freezing.
- Having the patient take 600 mg of ibuprofen 30–45 min prior to the procedure and every 6 hours (h) as needed over the next few days can reduce cramping.

Procedure Note

(Provider to fill in blanks/circle applicable choice when given multiple choices and to customize as needed.)

Date of Birth:_____________contraception_______________HCG________

G_________P_______A___Pap Smear History_______________

Reason for Cryotherapy:

____

___________________________*Smoking*_______________

Time Out completed.

(Final Verification of patient/procedure/site)

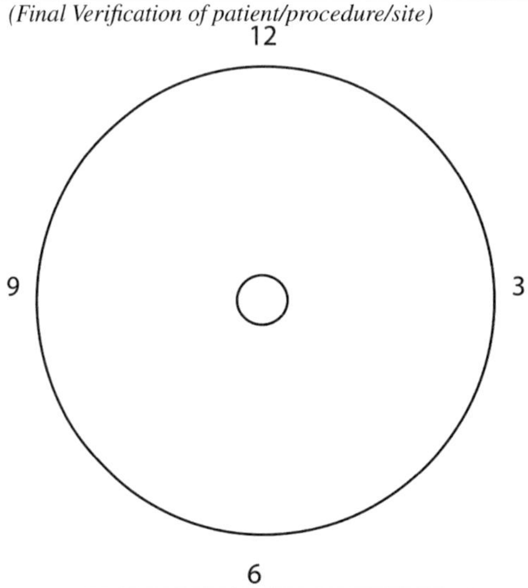

Colposcopy performed () yes () no

*Finding:*_______________________________

Cryotherapy:

A______cm flat/conical tipped probe was applied over the cervix with full coverage of the transformation zone and squamous lesion. The cervix was frozen yielding a ________mm ice ball. A full thaw was completed. The cervix was frozen a second time yielding a _____ mm ice ball. The speculum was removed, and the patient slowly returned to a sitting position.

*Complications:*____

*Impression:*____

*Suggest subsequent examination and/or follow-up:*____

____

Physician's Signature

Coding

CPT® Codes (Current Procedural Terminology, AMA, Chicago, IL)	
57511	Cryocautery of the cervix, initial, or repeat
ICD 10-CM-Diagnostic Codes (International Classification of Diseases, 10th Revision, Clinical Modification, Center for Disease Control and Prevention)	
N87.0	Mild cervical dysplasia (CIN 1)
N87.1	Moderate cervical dysplasia (CIN 2)
N87.9 D06	Dysplasia of the cervix uteri, unspecified Carcinoma in situ of the cervix uteri

Postprocedure Patient Instructions

The patient should be advised of the watery discharge that will ensue and persist for 2–4 weeks. Sloughing of the dead cervical tissue often causes malodorous discharge. Cramping is common and should be relieved with ibuprofen, 600 mg every 6 h. A small percentage will need stronger pain management. These patients should be reexamined to rule out an infection or retained menstrual flow prior to prescribing additional medication. The patient may have a small amount of spotting, but should not have significant bleeding. Infection is uncommon and can be greatly reduced by having nothing inserted in the vagina for 3 weeks following the procedure. Patients should call for any fevers, shaking chills, or pain unrelieved by nonsteroidals. Follow-up is essential after cryotherapy as failure of treatment does happen.

Follow-up testing after cervical cryotherapy is essential to ensure adequate treatment. It is important to refer to the ASCCP guidelines for follow-up recommendations as these are updated often based on the most current evidence. Currently, the recommendation for follow-up posttreatment of CIN 2 or 3 is HPV or co-testing at 6 months. If abnormal, colposcopy is repeated. If normal, then repeat HPV or co-testing should be performed annually until 3 consecutive negative results occur. Routine screening for these patients will be co-testing every 3 years for at least 25 years posttreatment. For patients with CIN 1, recommended follow-up is annual co-testing until 2 consecutive negative results occur, then return to routine age-based screening. Any abnormal result warrants repeat colposcopy [4].

Case Study Outcome

The patient had cervical cryotherapy performed without complications. Co-testing with Pap and HPV was done at 12 and 24 months; results were both negative. She resumed regular testing consistent with her age and risk group thereafter.

Patient Handout (Provider to Customize as Needed)

Cryotherapy is a method of treatment for cervical dysplasia (abnormal cells on your cervix that are precancerous) that involves destroying abnormal tissue in the cervix by freezing it. This is performed right in our office. The best time to have the procedure done is the week after your period has started, and this can be done even if you are still having a small amount of spotting.

The procedure starts like a Pap smear, with you lying on your back and your feet on the footrests (stirrups). A speculum will be placed in the vagina to visualize the cervix. A metal probe is placed on your cervix and gets very cold, allowing for the freezing. It is normal to hear a hissing sound as the procedure begins, and then you may feel some cramping similar to menstrual cramps. There is generally no pain beyond the cramps. Taking three 200 mg ibuprofen tablets (total 600 mg) 30 min prior to the procedure will help minimize this. You may also feel a little warm and flushed. This goes away within a few minutes after the procedure ends.

Cryotherapy is generally very safe and effective. The possible complications include cramping, infection, and narrowing of the cervical canal, which can very rarely be significant enough to cause difficulties letting menstrual flow out. This can be repaired. Finally, while cryotherapy is 85–95% effective in treating cervical abnormalities, failures can and do occur. Therefore, it is very important to continue to get regular follow-up Pap smears as directed by your clinician.

After cryotherapy, you can expect a profuse watery vaginal discharge that may have an odor and can last for 2–4 weeks. To decrease the risk of infection, we recommend that nothing be placed in the vagina (douching, tampons, etc.) and that you abstain from intercourse for 3 weeks. Typically, cramping may last for 1–2 days and can be minimized with ibuprofen, up to three 200 mg tablets (total of 600 mg) taken every 6–8 h as needed with food.

Please call us if you have any fever, bleeding heavier than a period, or abdominal pain not relieved with ibuprofen.

References

1. Cochrane Database Syst Rev. 2017; 2017(11): CD012847. Accessed 2 2024.
2. Pfenninger J, Fowler G. Procedures for primary care. Elsevier; 2020.
3. World Health Organization. Use of cryotherapy for cervical intraepithelial neoplasia. 2011.
4. Perkins R, Guido R, Castle P, et al. 2019 ASCCP risk-based management consensus guidelines for abnormal cervical cancer screening tests and cancer precursors. J of Lower Tract Dis. 2020;24(2):102–31.
5. Apgar B, Kaufman A, Bettcher C, Parker-Featherstone E. Gynecologic procedures: colposcopy, treatment of cervical intraepithelial neoplasia, and endometrial assessment. Am Fam Phys. 2013;87(12):836–42.
6. Sienstra K, Brewer B, Franklin L. A comparison of flat and shallow conical tips for cervical cryotherapy. J Am Board Fam Pract. 1999;12(5):360–6.

Chapter 26
LEEP: Loop Electrosurgical Excision Procedure

Stephen D. Hoag

Introduction

Loop electrosurgical excision procedure (LEEP) uses alternating electrical current to remove abnormal cervical tissue, which provides a specimen for pathological review. Historically, physicians have used high-frequency current for lesion removal as early as the 1940s. The introduction of the large loop with an insulated cross bar in 1989 by Prendeville revolutionized the treatment of cervical dysplasia. Cryotherapy and laser vaporization destroy tissue, whereas LEEP confers the advantage over cryotherapy and laser by providing tissue for histopathological review, thus allowing for prediction of recurrence of disease [1].

LEEP and loop electrosurgery remain the most common terms for this procedure, although diathermy loop treatment, loop excision of the transformation zone (LETZ), and large loop excision of the transformation zone (LLETZ) are other terms noted in the literature.

LEEP uses low-voltage high-frequency alternating current to produce an uninterrupted sine wave. As the loop is introduced into the tissue, an arc of current occurs causing the tissue cells to be rapidly heated and to explode into steam. The steam envelope allows for a continuous arc, thus allowing for a clean cut through the tissue and producing minimal thermal artifact. Once the tissue has been removed, the coagulation mode can be used with a ball electrode to fulgurate the tissue and cause hemostasis. With the more modern units, the coagulation and cut modes can be combined into a blend mode that produces less bleeding while minimizing the thermal artifact. The current is dispersed through a grounding pad with a large surface area to prevent burns.

S. D. Hoag (✉)
St. Joseph's Family Medicine Residency, Syracuse, NY, USA
e-mail: Stephen.hoag@sjhsyr.org

S. M. Sulik, C. B. Heath (eds.), *Primary Care Procedures in Women's Health*,
https://doi.org/10.1007/978-3-032-07061-6_26

The type of generator used for the LEEP procedure (Fig. 26.1) is similar to any electrosurgical generator used in either urological or laparoscopic surgery. The alternating current output ranges from 100 to 4000 kHz and comes with a variety of features. These features may include isolated circuitry and return electrode monitoring (REM). Isolated circuitry helps prevent alternate site burns by automatically deactivating the electrical surgical generator if any current transmitted through the active electrode is not returned through the patient electrode. The REM emits a warning sound and/or light if the return circuit is interrupted. Most generators will allow for combining the cut and coagulation modes into a blend mode. Blend 1 provides 75% cut with 25% coagulation, which helps decrease bleeding during the procedure. Higher blend modes, while available, can increase the amount of thermal artifact in the tissue and make pathological diagnosis of the margins more difficult [2].

Most loops have an insulated crossbar and shaft to prevent thermal injuries. The ball electrodes (Fig. 26.2) range in size from 3 to 5 mm, and both the ball electrodes and the loops are connected to a probe with a monopolar output. (The grounding electrode is usually an adhesive gel pad, or a solid "antenna" may be used.) The grounding pad should be applied near the operative site, usually the upper thigh or

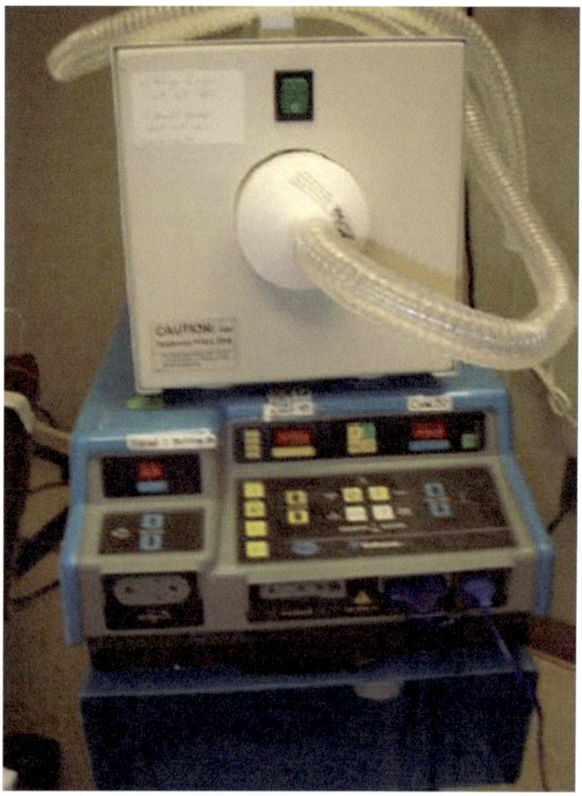

Fig. 26.1 Smoke evacuator and LEEP electrical generator

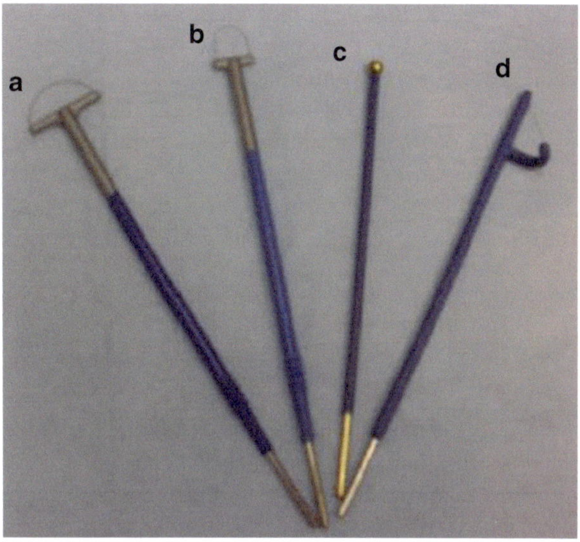

Fig. 26.2 Samples of loops and ball cautery tools. (**a**) 0.8 × 2.0 cm loop; (**b**) 1.0 × 1.0 cm loop; (**c**) ball electrode; (**d**) Fischer cone loop

buttocks. The pad wire should be connected to the generator and tested prior to the procedure to ensure the system is functioning properly.

A smoke evacuator is essential to remove the smoke plume during the procedure in order to provide adequate visualization. The smoke evacuator will filter any airborne particles and coexisting microorganisms into the plume and out of the air in the procedure room. Generally, the smoke evacuator is turned on prior to the generator and is a separate unit; however, there are a number of manufacturers that combine the smoke evacuator with the generator so that both turn on at the same time.

An insulated speculum is recommended for this procedure, and most have an attachment site for the smoke evacuator. This helps prevent secondary burns from the speculum to the vagina or vulvar areas. Special coated vaginal/lateral wall retractors are also available. Human papillomavirus has been isolated from laser plumes; thus, clinicians are encouraged to wear micropore or submicron surgical masks during the procedure.

Efficacy and patient acceptance of the LEEP procedure compare positively to other modes of treatment for cervical dysplasia. Studies indicate that LEEP is 91–98% effective in treating cervical intraepithelial lesions compared to 81–95% efficacy for cryotherapy and 83–94% efficacy for laser treatment of the cervix [1]. Most patients report the degree of discomfort with the procedure to be minor, with 85% of patients reporting no discomfort at all [3].

The morbidity associated with the LEEP is related to the volume of tissue removed and the depth of excision into the endocervical canal. This has direct implications in younger patients who have not completed childbearing. The overall rate of preterm delivery or spontaneous preterm premature rupture of membranes (pPROM) post-LEEP is directly related to the increased depth of the cervical tissue removed during LEEP. Patients who have more than 2.0 cm removed have a relative risk of pPROM at 4.91 compared to untreated women [4]. Women who have had LEEP are more likely to deliver preterm overall and to have more low birthweight babies; however, there are no differences in maternal or neonatal outcomes [5].

Posttreatment follow-up for the LEEP patient should include an office visit to discuss the pathology results and discuss a future surveillance plan per the ASCCP updated consensus guidelines. Patients with positive margins have a higher incidence of recurrent dysplasia usually within 2 years and a higher incidence of cervical carcinoma for at least 20 years posttreatment [6].

Case Study

A 39-year-old patient returns to your office after receiving a phone call from your nurse stating that you would like to discuss the abnormal Pap smear result. You inform the patient that the pathologist found a high-grade intraepithelial lesion (HSIL) on the Pap results and that you are recommending a further evaluation with a colposcopy. Colposcopy was performed, and biopsies were taken. The patient returns to your office for the results, which show severe dysplasia at the 4:00 and 6:00 biopsies with a negative endocervical curettage (ECC). You discuss the risks and benefits of the LEEP procedure for definitive treatment, and the patient elects to schedule the procedure.

Diagnosis

Severe dysplasia with negative ECC.

Indications (ASCCP Updated Consensus Guidelines) (Algorithm 26.1)

- Any biopsy-proven cervical intraepithelial neoplasia (CIN) lesion with adequate colposcopy.
- Diagnostic purposes for inadequate colposcopy.
- LEEP preferred over cryotherapy for the following:

  (a) High-grade lesions that encompass greater than 2 quadrants of the cervix.
  (b) Large lesions not covered by the cryoprobe.
  (c) Irregularly shaped cervix.
  (d) Recurrent CIN after previous therapy.
  (e) If "See and Treat" at a single visit is necessary (not the preferred method).

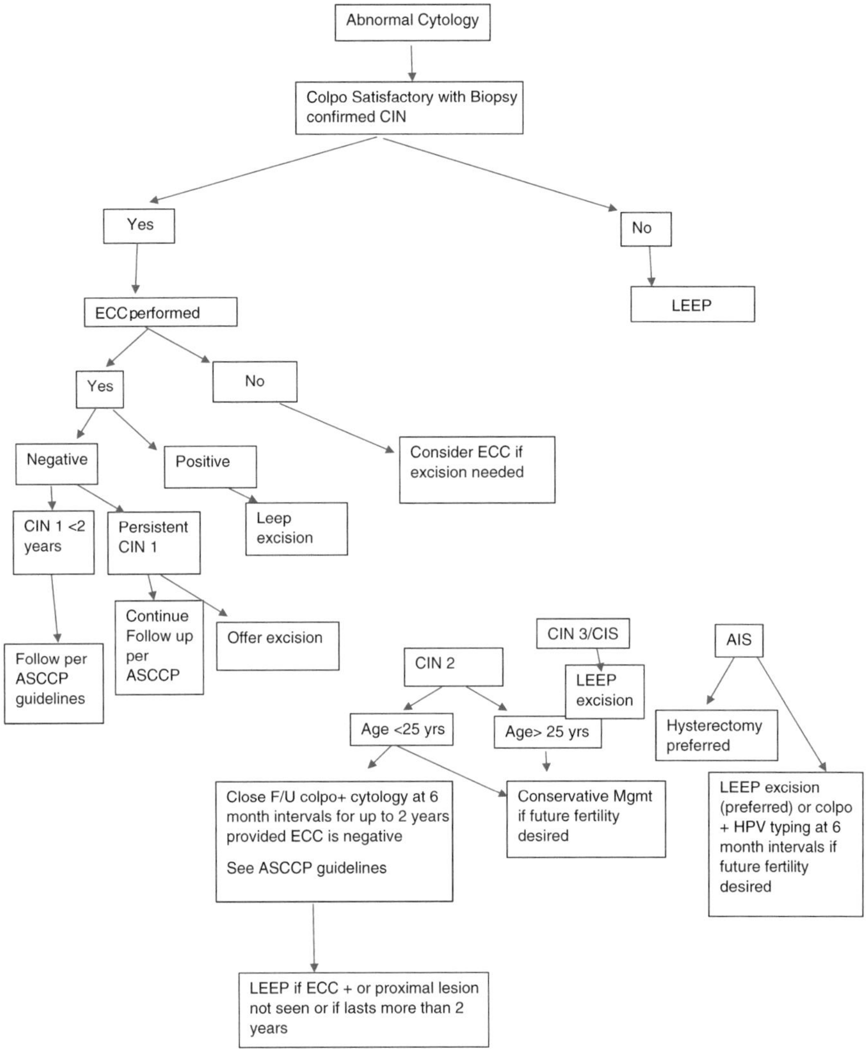

Algorithm 26.1 Flowchart for abnormal cytology and CIN workup leading to LEEP. CIN- Cervical intraepithelial neoplasia. ECC- Endocervical Curettage. CIS- Carcinoma in situ. AIS- Adenocarcinoma in situ

Contraindications

- Bleeding or coagulopathy.
- Less than 12 weeks postpartum.
- Clinically apparent invasive carcinoma of the cervix.
- Heavy menses (relative).
- Active/severe cervicitis (relative).

- Pregnancy (relative): should be performed only by an experienced specialist when carcinoma is suspected.

Advantages

- Allows for histologic audit of colposcopic diagnosis with histopathologic examination to rule out microinvasion.
- Allows for excision of the dysplastic lesion and transformation zone.
- Can treat lesions of all sizes involving all four quadrants of the cervix.
- Easily learned technique.
- Uses inexpensive readily available equipment with relatively low operating costs.
- Is office or outpatient procedure.
- Can be performed with initial colposcopy ("See and Treat," although this is not the preferred method of treatment).

Equipment (Fig. 26.3)

- Electrical generator.
- Smoke evacuator and tubing.
- Grounding pad.
- Insulated speculum.

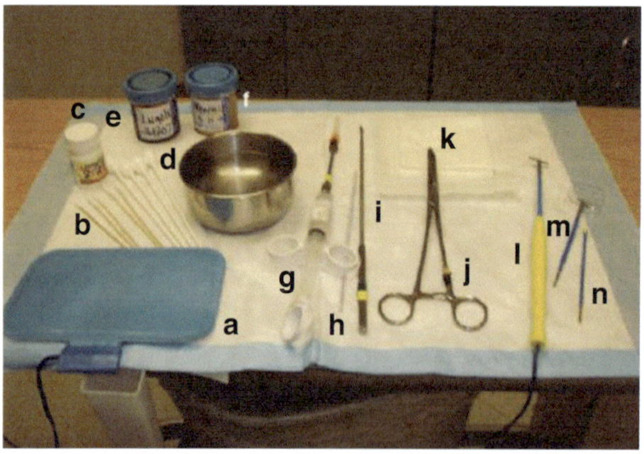

Fig. 26.3 Equipment setup for LEEP. (**a**) Grounding pad; (**b**) large and small cotton swabs; (**c**) Hurricaine® gel (Beutlich LP Pharmaceuticals, Waukegan, IL); (**d**) metal basin with acetic acid; (**e**) Lugol's solution; (**f**) Monsel's solution; (**g**) 10-cc syringe with 1% lidocaine with epinephrine with needle extender; (**h**) endocervical brush; (**i**) sterile endocervical curette; (**j**) sterile long Kelly forceps; (**k**) gauze; (**l**) monopolar probe with 0.8 × 2 cm loop attached; (**m**) 1.0 × 1.0 cm loop; (**n**) ball electrode

- Lateral wall spreaders: insulated (optional).
- Loops: range in sizes from 1.0 × 1.0 cm to 2.0 × 1.5 cm.
- Ball electrode: sizes range from 3 to 5 mm.
- 20% Benzocaine (Hurricaine® gel, Beutlich LP Pharmaceuticals, Waukegan, IL)
- 1% lidocaine with epinephrine: 5–10 cc
- Needle extender.
- 25- or 28-gauge needle
- Colposcope.
- Acetic acid.
- Lugol's solution.
- Monsel's solution.
- Specimen jar.
- Endocervical curette (ECC) (optional).
- Large cotton swabs (Scopettes®, Birchwood Laboratories Inc., Eden Prairie, MN).
- Small cotton swabs.
- Long Kelly or ring forceps.
- Face mask: micropore or submicron surgical face mask.

Optional Equipment

- Suture material: chromic or Vicryl 3.0 absorbable.
- Long-handled needle holder and scissors.
- Vasopressin for bleeding.

Procedure

1. Obtain informed consent and sign the permit including anesthesia.
2. Check a pregnancy test.
3. Place the patient in the lithotomy position; apply a grounding pad.
4. Check equipment to make sure all is functioning appropriately.
5. Insert an insulated speculum and visualize the cervix.
   (a) Adequate visualization of the entire cervix is key to a simple procedure.
   (b) Use the vaginal/lateral wall spreaders if necessary to provide adequate visualization.
6. Perform colposcopy and apply Lugol's solution.
7. Anesthetize the cervix.
   (a) Use 20% benzocaine (Hurricaine®) gel prior to lidocaine (Fig. 26.4).

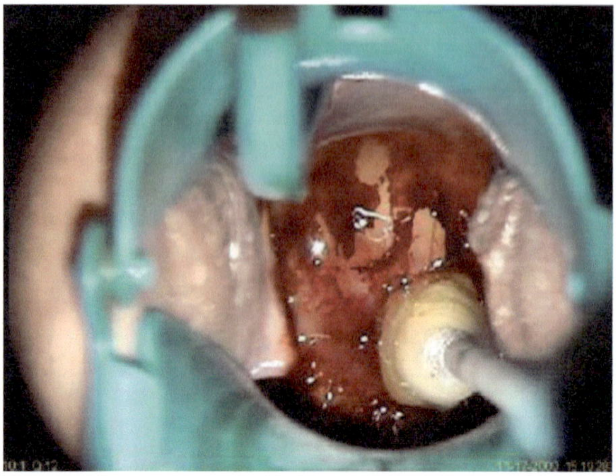

Fig. 26.4 Apply topical benzocaine to the cervix with a large swab prior to injecting the local anesthetic

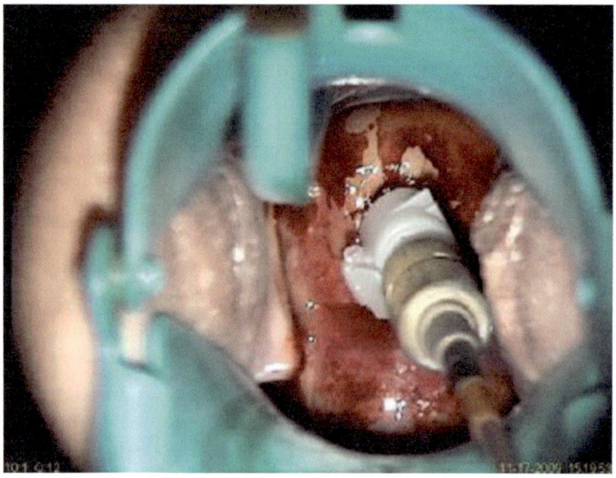

Fig. 26.5 Injection of lidocaine anesthetic at the 12:00 position on the cervix

(b) Inject at 12:00, 3:00, 6:00, and 9:00 positions around the cervix with up to 0.5–1 cc of lidocaine per site locally (Fig. 26.5). (Alternatively, you can inject at 2:00, 4:00, 8:00, and 10:00 positions.)
(c) Use depth of 1–2 mm only (submucosal).
(d) Allow several minutes to pass, and check to see if the area is anesthetized.

8. Choose an appropriate loop, and attach to the monopolar probe.
   (a) Check settings to ensure appropriate for the chosen loop.
   (b) Smaller loops require less current (i.e., 1.0 × 1.0 set at approximately 40 MHz, varies machine to machine).
   (c) Check to make sure the setting is on Blend 1.
9. Make a dummy pass over the cervix with a generator on stand-by to ensure adequate removal of the lesion.

10. Turn on the smoke evacuator and generator, and recheck settings.
11. Pass the loop into the tissue, and remove the entire transformation zone around the lesion (Fig. 26.6).
    (a) If necessary, make additional passes with a loop to remove the entire lesion.
    (b) Start the flow of current either by using the index finger to press the cut button on the handheld tool or by using the foot pedal.
    (c) Start excision approximately 5 mm lateral to the lesion, and place the loop just at but not touching the cervix. Start the flow of current prior to touching the cervix.
    (d) The cut should be made with a continuous flow of current, passing the loop to a depth of at least 8 mm—maximal crypt involvement of CIN reaches a depth of 5 mm. Stopping the flow of current can increase thermal artifact and may damage the loop.
    (e) Push the loop into the tissue and slowly draw the loop across the transformation zone with equal pressure until 5 mm past the lesion edge, and then remove the loop from the tissue perpendicularly (Fig. 26.7).
12. Remove specimen (Fig. 26.8) with long Kelly, after the generator is placed on stand-by.
13. Perform ECC if not done during colposcopy or if desired.
14. Use a ball electrode to fulgurate the base of the tissue crater and achieve hemostasis. Press the coagulation button on the handheld tool or with the foot pedal. *Do not fulgurate the cervical os* (Fig. 26.9).
15. Apply Monsel's solution to the crater.
16. Remove the speculum and grounding pad.
17. Mark the specimen as per your pathology department's recommendations and place it in a sterile container (Fig. 26.10).
18. LEEP Cone Procedure: looks like a reverse "cowboy hat" when completed.
    (a) Can be used when the lesion extends into the cervical canal.

Fig. 26.6 Pass the loop through the tissue in a perpendicular fashion

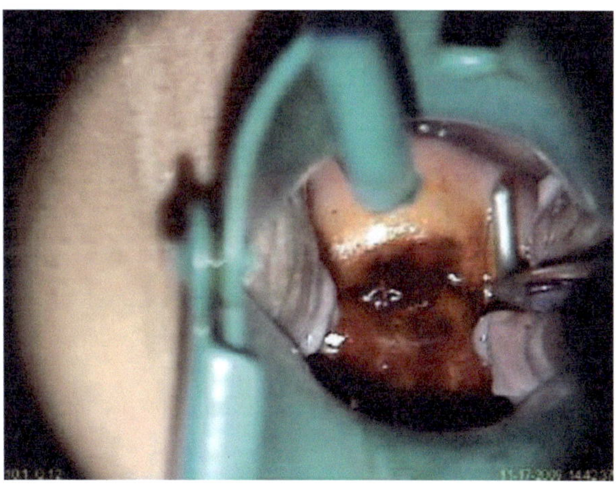

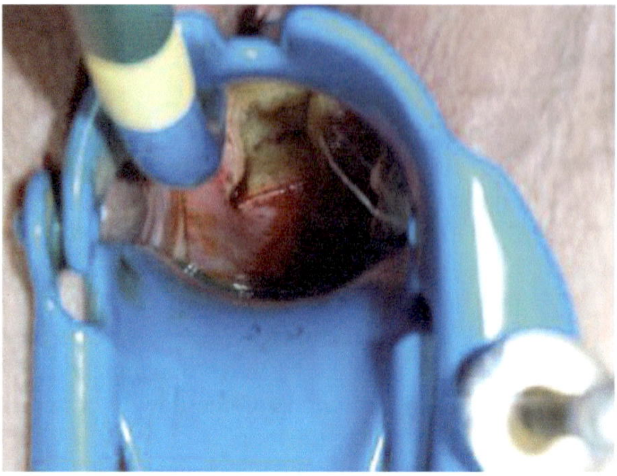

Fig. 26.7 Cervix with excision completed prior to hemostasis with ball cautery

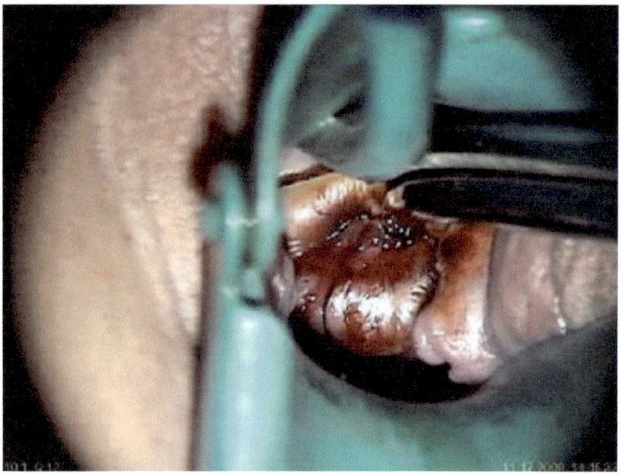

Fig. 26.8 Remove the cut specimen with a long Kelly

(b) Anesthetize the cervix in the same fashion, but use an additional 0.5–2 cc of lidocaine into the cervix to a depth of 1 cm at the 12 and 6:00 positions.
(c) Use a 1.0 × 1.0 or a square loop to excise a 9–10 mm portion of the endocervical canal. If doing this first, the specimen does not need to be marked, but if performing after the LEEP on the ectocervix, mark the endocervical edge of the specimen so that the pathologist can assess if the margins are negative for disease.
(d) The remaining transformation zone is excised in the usual manner as described previously.

19. Have the patient sit up slowly after the procedure to ensure vasovagal response does not occur.
20. Observe the patient for 15–20 min postprocedure before discharging to home.

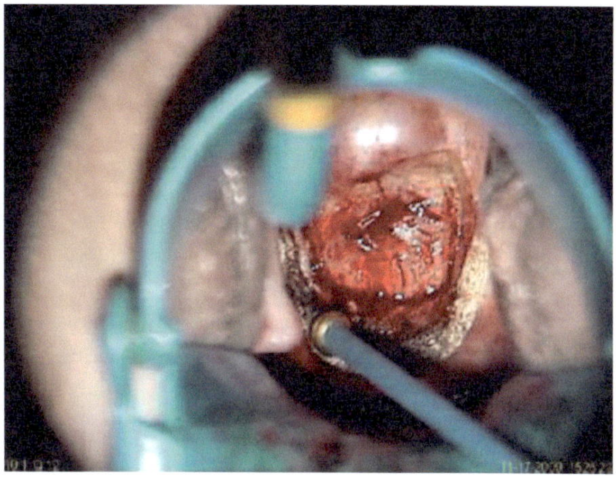

Fig. 26.9 Use the ball electrode to fulgurate the base of the excised cervix to achieve hemostasis

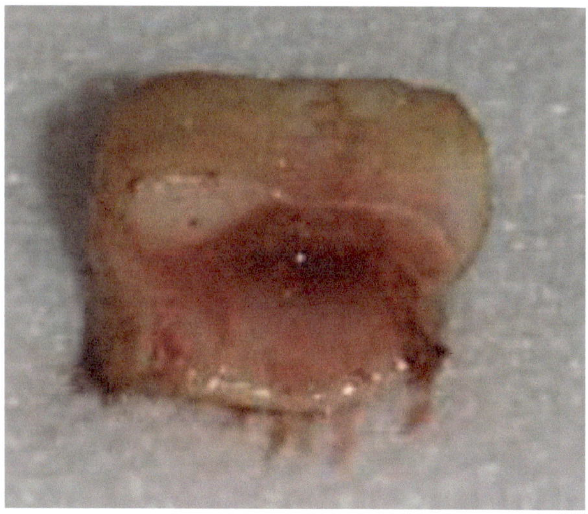

Fig. 26.10 LEEP tissue sample to be sent to pathology

Complications and Risks

- Burns to vaginal walls, usually due to poor visualization or operator inexperience.
- Bleeding: immediate bleeding 0.5–1%, late bleeding 1–8.5%. Perioperative bleeding is uncommon with the use of the blend-mode fulguration and Monsel's. Excessive bleeding can be controlled by the use of vasopressin. Rarely, a figure-of-eight suture is necessary to control the bleeding.
- Posttreatment cervical stenosis: more common with postmenopausal women, women on Depo-Provera® (Pfizer, New York, NY) or Implanon® (Schering Corporation, Kenilworth, NJ), or in breastfeeding women postpartum.
- Consider treatment with estrogen vaginal cream for several weeks post-LEEP.
- Infection: rare.

- Cervical incompetence.
- Positive margins or recurrent disease.

Tricks and Helpful Hints

- When using the lateral wall spreaders, a larger speculum is usually necessary: use a Graves or a long Graves.
- A cartridge system (Campion syringe or dental syringe) can be used for anesthesia. A thumb syringe with a dental extender, a spinal needle, or a Potochy Needle® (CooperSurgical, Trumbull, CT) can also be used.
- Consider adding 8.3% sodium bicarbonate solution 1:1 or 1:4 to decrease pain with the injection.
- Excessive bleeding can be controlled with the use of vasopressin:
  - Draw up 1 cc of vasopressin (20 units/cc).
  - Withdraw 40 cc of saline from the 100-cc mini bag and inject 1 cc vasopressin into mini bag. Draw up 10 cc of solution and inject directly into the cervix into the area of bleeding.
- Cone LEEP can also be done using a Fischer cone loop.

Interpretation of Results (See ASCCP Website)

- Review the pathology report to determine if the entire lesion is removed. Assess margins.
- If margins are positive, a closer follow-up is usually necessary.
- If margins are negative, follow up per ASCCP guidelines [7].

Procedure Note

(Provider to customize as needed.)

The permit was signed, and the pregnancy test was performed and is negative. The patient was placed in the lithotomy position, and the speculum was inserted. The cervix was visualized, and colposcopy was performed. The cervix was anesthetized with ___ cc of 1% lidocaine with epinephrine in the 3:00, 6:00, 9:00, and 12:00 positions infused locally. One pass with the 0.8 × 2.0 cm loop was made to remove the transformation zone in its entirety. Hemostasis with the ball cautery and Monsel's was done. The specimen was marked with suture at the _____ position and sent to pathology. The patient tolerated the procedure well and will follow up in 2 weeks for results.

Coding

CPT® Codes (Current Procedural Terminology, AMA, Chicago, IL)	
57,460	Colposcopy with loop electrosurgical excision or LEEP excision of the cervix
57,500	Cervical biopsy
57,520	Cervical conization with or without fulguration
57,522	Cervical conization using the loop technique
57,505	Endocervical curettage
99,070	Supplies and materials for kits and electrodes: A surgical tray charge is generally allowed for an office LEEP
ICD 10-CM-Diagnostic Codes(International Classification of Diseases, 9th Revision, Clinical Modification, Center for Disease Control and Prevention)	
180.9	Cervical cancer
N87.0	CIN 1 (mild dysplasia)
N87.1	CIN 2 (moderate dysplasia)
D06.9	CIN 3 (severe dysplasia)

Postprocedure Patient Instructions

- Instruct the patient to refrain from intercourse, tampons, or douching for 2–4 weeks post procedure, until all bleeding has stopped.
- Discharge is common for 2–3 weeks but may last up to 6 weeks.
- The patient should report any excessive bleeding (heavier than a normal period, or soaking a pad per hour) or any malodorous discharge.
- Instruct the patient to make a follow-up appointment to review pathology results within 2–4 weeks.
- Follow-up surveillance as per current ASCCP guidelines.

Case Study Outcome

The patient returned to your office for the LEEP, which was done without complications. The patient returns today for the pathology results which show severe dysplasia with negative margins. You instruct the patient to follow up in 12 months for a repeat Pap smear and high-risk HPV typing.

Postprocedure Patient Handout

You have just had a LEEP (loop electrosurgical excision procedure). This involves removing small pieces of abnormal cervical tissue that are then sent for pathologic evaluation. Most patients tolerate LEEP well, as the procedure generally causes little bleeding. However, in order to make sure that you heal well, we ask that you avoid putting anything in your vagina for the next 2–4 weeks until the bleeding has stopped. This means:

- No douching.
- No tampon use.
- No vaginal sex.

You should call your provider if any of the following occur:

- Increase in bleeding or heavy bleeding (more than a pad per hour).
- Fever, above 101 °F.
- Pelvic pain.
- Smelly discharge.

Discharge, even dark brown discharge, is common after LEEP.

Please make a follow-up appointment to discuss your results in 2–4 weeks. You will also need to discuss the frequency of Pap smears and follow-up plans at this appointment.

References

1. Martin-Hirsch PL, Paraskevaidis E, Kitchener H. Surgery for cervical intraepithelial neoplasia. Cochrane Database Syst Rev. 2013;6:CD001318.
2. Apgar BS, Kaufman AJ, Bettcher C, Parker-Featherstone E. Gynecologic procedures: colposcopy, treatment of cervical intraepithelial neoplasia, and endometrial assessment. Am Fam Physician. 2013;87(12):836–43.
3. Sadler L, Saftlas A, Wang W, Exeter M, Whittaker J, McCowan L. Treatment for cervical intraepithelial neoplasia and risk of preterm delivery. JAMA. 2004;291(17):2100–6.
4. Kyrgiou M, Athanasiou A, Kalliala IEJ, et al. Obstetric outcomes after conservative treatment for cervical intraepithelial lesions and early invasive disease. Cochrane Database Syst Rev. 2017;11:CD012847.
5. Wright TC, Massad LS, Dunton CJ, Spitzer M, Wilkinson EJ, Solomon D. 2006 consensus guidelines for the management of women with cervical intraepithelial neoplasia or adenocarcinoma in-situ. Am J Obstet Gynecol. 2007;197:340–5.
6. Alonso I, Torné A, Puig-Tintoré LM, Esteve R, Quinto L, Campo E, Pahisa J, Ordi J. Pre and postconization high-risk HPV testing predicts residual/recurrent disease in patients treated for CIN 2-3. Gynecol Oncol. 2006;103(2):631–6. Epub 2006 Jun 14
7. Massad S, Einstein M, Huh W, Katki H, Kinney W, Schiffman M, Solomon D, Wentzensen N, Lawson H. 2012 updated consensus guidelines for the management of abnormal cervical cancer screening tests and cancer precursors. J Low Genit Tract Dis. 2013;17(5):s1–s27.

Additional Resource

Article

Wright TC, Massad LS, Dunton CJ, Spitzer M, Wilkinson EJ, Solomon D. 2006 consensus guidelines for the management of women with abnormal cervical cancer screening tests. Am J Obstet Gynecol. 2007;197:346–55.

Website

www.asccp.org.

Chapter 27
Hysterosalpingography/ Hysterosalpingogram (HSG)

Sandra M. Sulik

Introduction

Hysterosalpingography (HSG) is a dye-based radiologic evaluation of the uterus and fallopian tubes. It is used primarily for the workup of infertility. Other indications include the evaluation of women with a history of recurrent spontaneous abortions, postoperative evaluations for women who have undergone reversal of tubal ligation, and assessment of women prior to undergoing myomectomy. The primary role of the procedure is to evaluate the patency of the fallopian tubes [1]. The optimal time for the study to be performed is day 7–12 of the menstrual cycle. This ensures that there is no pregnancy present and allows for optimal visualization of the endometrium in the proliferative phase. While the HSG is used to assess the tube patency, it has been known that some women will conceive within months of the test suggesting tubal flushing might play a role in improving fertility. Either oil-based contrast or water-soluble contrast material can be used to perform the test. Several randomized controlled trials have been done comparing the two types of contrast material and infertility rates with some suggesting that the use of the oil-based contrast might have a higher rate of pregnancy success [2]. Magnetic resonance hysterosalpingography (MR-HSG) with injection of gadolinium is also available in some areas. The diagnostic performance of MR-HSG for the analysis of tubal patency and intracavity abnormalities is similar. There is a significant decrease in pain associated with the MR-HSG as compared to the conventional HSG [3]. A recent systematic review of EMLA cream (Lidocaine 2.5%/Prilocaine 2.5%) prior to HSG showed a significant reduction in pain perception of cervical instrumentation with tenaculum and insertion of the HSG catheter [4].

S. M. Sulik (✉)
St. Joseph's Health; Professor Emeritus, Upstate Medical Center, Syracuse, NY, USA
e-mail: Sandra.Sulik@sjhsyr.org

S. M. Sulik, C. B. Heath (eds.), *Primary Care Procedures in Women's Health*,
https://doi.org/10.1007/978-3-032-07061-6_27

Case Study

A 34-year-old woman presents to your office with the concern that she is unable to get pregnant. She and her husband have been trying for the past year without success. She has had no other pregnancies, denies history of any sexually transmitted infections, and has regular menses. Her husband has a child from a previous marriage. You discuss the infertility workup and suggest an evaluation with a hysterosalpingogram.

Diagnosis (Algorithm 27.1)

Infertility investigation

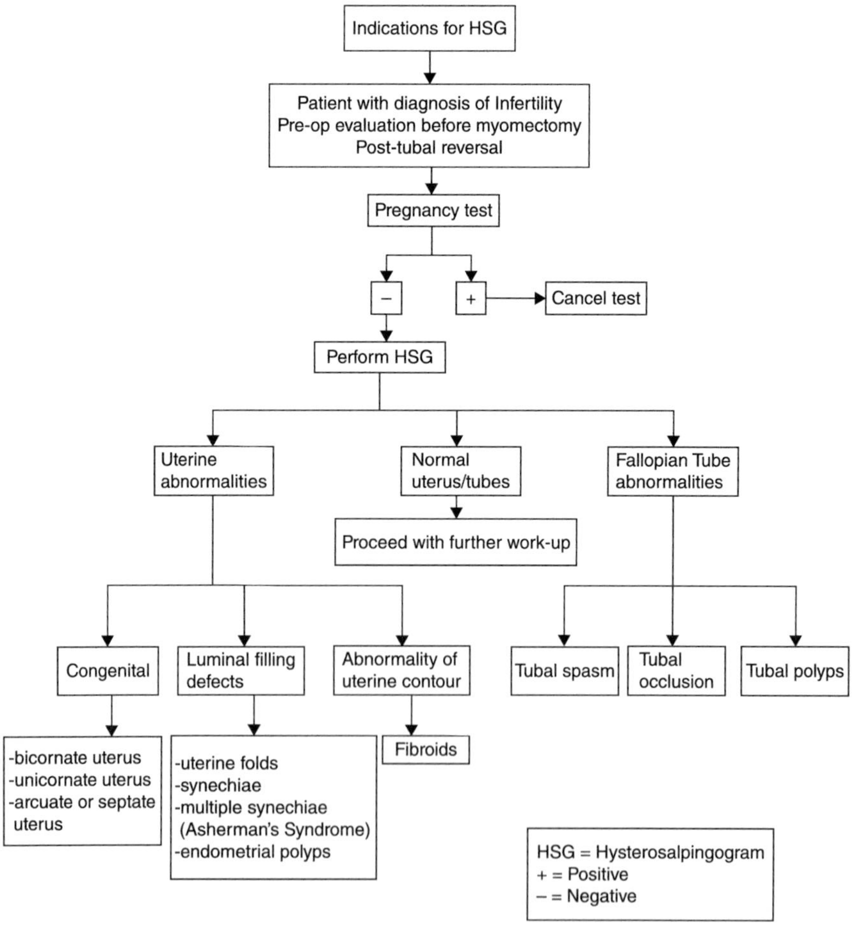

Algorithm 27.1 Indications and interpretations of HSG

Indications (Algorithm 27.1)

- Infertility
- Recurrent spontaneous abortions
- Preoperative evaluation prior to myomectomy
- Postoperative evaluation following tubal ligation reversal

Contraindications [1] (Algorithm 27.1)

- Pregnancy
- Active pelvic infection
- Active vaginal bleeding
- Allergy to contrast dye

Equipment (Fig. 27.1)

- Radiologic shields for the provider, radiologist, and technician
- Sterile tray with the following:
  - Sterile gloves
  - Sterile speculum
  - Small cup for antiseptic solution
  - Antiseptic solution
  - 3-cc syringe to test the catheter balloon
  - 10-cc syringe to inject dye
  - HSG catheter
  - Tenaculum
  - Contrast medium
  - Menstrual pad

Procedure

1. Perform a pregnancy test.
   - The patient should be instructed to abstain from unprotected intercourse from the onset of the menses until after the procedure is completed.

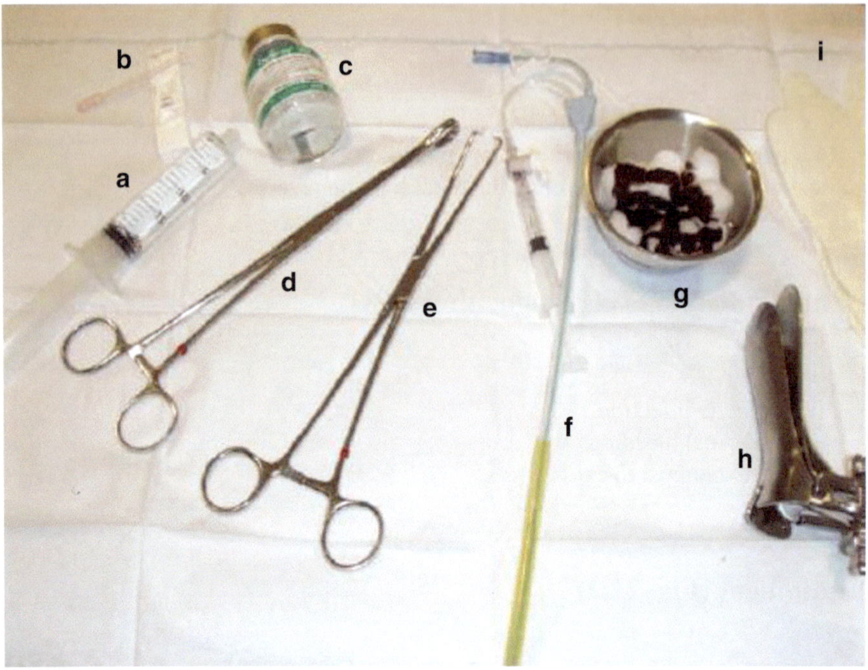

Fig. 27.1 Sterile tray set up for HSG: (**a**) 20-cc syringe filled with contrast dye; (**b**) pregnancy test; (**c**) contrast dye (e.g., Optiray®, Mallinckrodt Inc., St. Louis, MO); (**d**) ring forceps; (**e**) tenaculum; (**f**) hysterosalpingogram catheter, with 3-cc syringe attached; (**g**) metal basin with cotton balls soaked in iodine; (**h**) Graves speculum; (**i**) sterile gloves

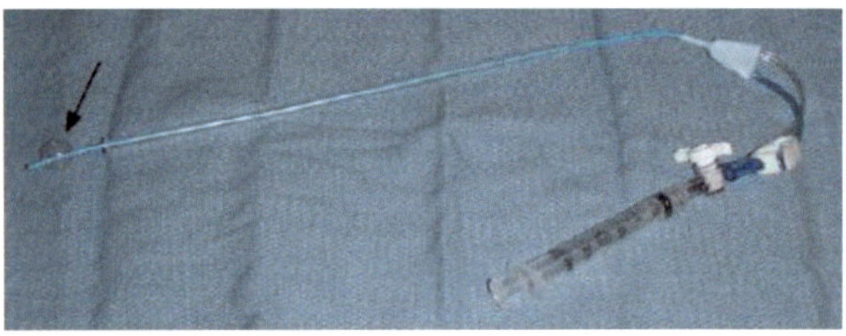

Fig. 27.2 Hysterosalpingogram catheter: check the catheter balloon prior to the start of the procedure

2. Patient is placed in the lithotomy position, supine on the fluoroscopy table. If using ELMA, place 3 ml of the cream into a cervical cup and apply to the cervix at least 30 minutes prior to cervical instrumentation [5].
3. Check the HSG catheter, and flush the catheter with contrast material prior to insertion (Fig. 27.2).
4. Insert the speculum, visualize the cervix, and clean with an antiseptic solution.

   - Insert the HSG catheter through the cervix into the endometrial cavity, and inflate the balloon using 3 cc of air. If necessary, use the tenaculum to help stabilize the cervix to insert the catheter.

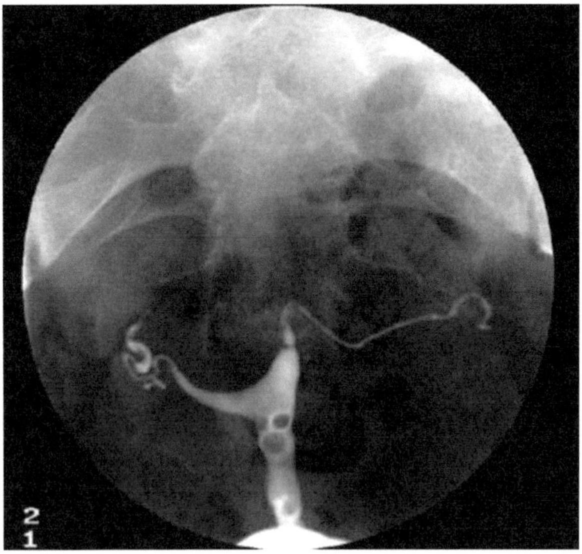

Fig. 27.3 Hysterosalpingogram with contrast spilling from both tubes

5. Turn the stopcock to keep the balloon inflated.
6. Obtain a scout radiograph to check the position of the catheter.
7. Inject contrast material slowly into the uterine cavity, until adequate fluoroscopic images are obtained.

   - Watch for spill of contrast medium into the fallopian tubes and then into the intraperitoneal area (Fig. 27.3).
   - Observe for filling defects and contour abnormalities as early filling occurs.
   - The shape of the uterus is best evaluated as the uterus is fully distended (Fig. 27.4).
   - Additional spot radiographs may be obtained to evaluate any abnormality that is seen.
   - Oblique views of the fallopian tubes may be needed and are obtained by having the patient roll from side to side (Fig. 27.5).
   - A radiograph can be obtained once the balloon is deflated to evaluate the lower uterine segment.

8. Once the radiographs are obtained, deflate the balloon and remove the catheter.

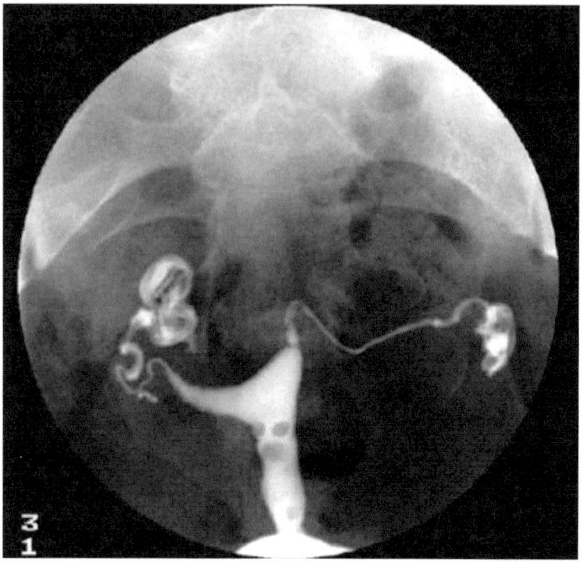

Fig. 27.4 The shape of the uterus is best visualized when fully distended

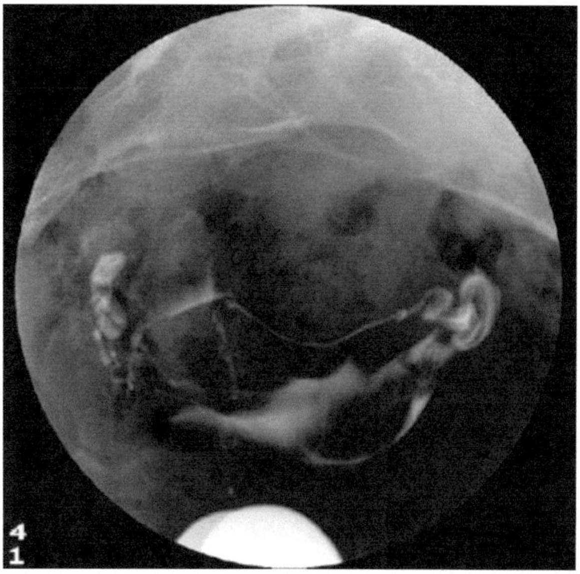

Fig. 27.5 Oblique views obtained by having the patient rotate side to side to assess for spill from both tubes

Complications and Risks

Spotting or pain

Rare Complications

- Heavy vaginal bleeding
- Infection
- Reaction to contrast medium
- Perforation of the uterus or fallopian tube
- Potential for irradiation of an early, unsuspected pregnancy
- Severe cramping causing need to terminate the study before completion

Tricks and Helpful Hints

- Use an inverted bedpan or a pillow, or have the patient place her hands under her hips, in order to raise the pelvis; this will facilitate insertion of the speculum and better visualization of the cervix.
- If unable to easily pass the catheter, use the tenaculum to straighten the cervical canal.
- Have the patient pretreat with a non-steroidal anti-inflammatory drug (NSAID) prior to the procedure.
- If cervical stenosis is present, use a small dilator to open the cervical os prior to insertion of the HSG catheter.
- Removing the speculum prior to the dye injection allows for better visualization of the lower uterine segment.
- Excessive injection of dye prevents proper evaluation of the uterine cavity [6].
- Use of intrauterine lidocaine is not effective in reducing pain during the HSG [7].

Interpretation of Results [1, 2, 6, 8] (Algorithm 27.1)

Uterus

- Should look like an inverted triangle with well-defined smooth contours.
- Uterine anomalies—three types:

1. Congenital abnormalities of shape:
   (a) Unicornuate uterus.
   (b) Bicornuate uterus: demonstrates a cleft in the outer contour of the fundus.
   (c) Arcuate or septate: shows a depression of the uterine fundus but a normal outer uterine contour.
2. Luminal filling defects (common):
   (a) Uterine folds: normal variants, parallel to the long axis of the uterus and can extend into the uterine horns
   (b) Synechiae (intrauterine adhesions) due to scarring/infection are seen as irregular filling defects; usually linear arising from one of the uterine walls.
   (c) Multiple synechiae—Asherman syndrome.
   (d) Endometrial polyps: well-defined filling defects best seen during the early filling stage. Sonohysterography is the preferred method of imaging endometrial polyps.
3. Abnormalities of uterine contour:
   (a) Leiomyomas most common, well-defined filling defects; only seen if submucosa. Seen best during early contrast filling of the uterus.
   (b) Large myomas can distort the size of the uterus.

Fallopian Tubes

- Tubes should appear as thin, smooth lines that widen in the ampullary portion.
- Vary in length (approx. 10–12 cm) and tortuosity.
- There should be free spillage of contrast material into the peritoneal cavity.
- Tubal spasm can occur rarely and is difficult to distinguish from tubal occlusion.
- Tubal polyps: Rare; appear as smooth rounded filling defects without tube dilatation or occlusion; less than 1 cm in diameter and can be unilateral or bilateral.

Procedure Note (Provider to Customize as Needed)

Informed consent was obtained. Pregnancy test was done and is negative. The patient was placed in the lithotomy position on the fluoroscopy table, and the speculum was inserted. The cervix was visualized and cleaned with iodine solution. The HSG catheter was gently inserted through the cervix, and the balloon was filled with air. Position of the catheter was confirmed with fluoroscopy. The radiologist was called and, when ready, the dye was instilled via *the catheter into the uterus. Spillage from both tubes was noted; no uterine abnormalities were seen. The study was completed, and the catheter was easily removed. The patient tolerated the procedure well.*

Coding

CPT® Codes (Current Procedural Terminology, AMA, Chicago, IL)
58340 Hysterosalpingography
74740 Hysterosalpingography, radiologic supervision, and interpretation
99070 Supplies and materials

ICD-10-CM Diagnostic Codes (International Classification of Diseases, 10th Revision, Clinical Modification, Centers for Disease Control and Prevention)
Q513 Bicornate uterus
N97.1 Infertility, female (626.2 of tubal origin) Infertility, female due to tubal occlusion N88.3 Incompetence of cervix Incompetence of cervix uteri

Patient Instructions

- The patient should call the provider when her menses are due so that the test can be scheduled at the end of the menstrual cycle, ideally days 7–12 of the cycle.
- She should be instructed to abstain from unprotected intercourse from the start of her menses until the procedure is completed.
- The patient should be instructed to take an NSAID, i.e., ibuprofen 800 mg, three times daily for 1–2 days prior to the procedure and the morning of the procedure (at least 30 min prior).
- The patient should be told to expect some cramping and flushing with the installation of the dye as well as with the insertion of the catheter. Some cramping can continue postprocedure but usually subsides shortly after the procedure is completed.
- The patient should expect sticky vaginal discharge after the procedure for several hours. Some spotting is also normal, but she should report any heavy vaginal bleeding or foul-smelling discharge.

Case Study Outcome

HSG was performed without difficulty, both tubes were patent, and the uterus appeared normal in contour. Results were reviewed with the patient and her husband, and the infertility workup was continued.

Patient Handout (Provider to Customize as Needed)

Your provider has ordered a hysterosalpingogram. This is an X-ray test done to look at the shape, size, and location of your uterus, fallopian tubes, and ovaries. Usually, this test is done to determine if the fallopian tubes are open and will allow an egg from your ovary to pass through the tube. This test is done as part of the workup for infertility.

Before this test, your provider will perform a pregnancy test. A radiology technician or nurse will assist your provider and radiologist with the procedure. They will ask you for the dates of your last menstrual period and if you have any allergies. Before the test is done, you will be asked to empty your bladder and put on a hospital gown.

Once ready, you will lie down on the X-ray table, and an X-ray of your pelvis will be taken. The speculum will be inserted into your vagina, and your cervix will be cleaned with an antiseptic solution. The catheter will then be threaded through your cervix into your uterus, and a small balloon will be filled with air. This will keep the catheter in the proper position for the test. Once the catheter is in place, the radiologist will be called in, the dye will be injected through the catheter, and the X-ray pictures will be taken. You may be asked to turn onto one or both sides in order to see both fallopian tubes. When the dye is injected, you may experience a warm flush and some cramping.

When the test is completed, the catheter and the speculum will be removed. You will be given a menstrual pad to wear. You may have some spotting and a sticky discharge for the rest of the day of the test. If you have cramps, you can take ibuprofen.

The radiologist will review the X-rays and will send a report to your provider. Your provider will schedule a follow-up appointment with you to review the test results and discuss a treatment plan.

References

1. Simpson WL, Beitia LG, Mester J. Hysterosalpingography: a reemerging study. Radiographics. 2006;26:419–31.
2. Fang F, Vai Y, Zhang Y, Faramand A. Oil-based versus water-based contrast for hysterosalpingography in infertile women: a systematic review and meta-analysis of randomized controlled trials. FertnStert. 2018;110:153–60. https://doi.org/10.1016/j.fernstert.2018.03.021.
3. Volondat M, Fontas E, Delotte J, Fatfouta I, Chevallier P, Chassang M. Magnetic resonance hysterosalpingography in diagnostic work-up of female infertility – comparison with conventional hysterosalpingography: a randomized study. Eru Radiol. 2018;29:501. https://doi.org/10.1007/s00330-018-5572-2.
4. Abu-Zaid A, Baradwan S, Abuzaid M, AlSghan OA, Salem H, et al. EMLA (lidocaine-prilocaine) cream for pain relief during hysterosalpingography: a systematic review and meta-analysis of randomised placebo-controlled trials. Hum Fertil Camb. 2023;26(5):978–86. https://doi.org/10.1080/14647273.2002.2040748.

5. Liberty G, Gal M, Halevy-Shalem T, Michaelson-Cohen R, Galoyan N, Hyman J, Eldar-Geva T, Vatashsky E, Margalioth E. Lidocaine–Prilocaine (EMLA) cream as analgesia for hysterosalpingography: a prospective randomized controlled double blinded study Human Reproduction 2007;22(5):1335–9. https://doi.org/10.1093/humrep/del517.
6. Lindheim ST, Sprague C, Winter IIITC. Hysterosalpingography and sonohysterography: lessons in technique. AJR Am J Roentgenol. 2006;186:24–9. https://doi.org/10.2214/AJR.05.0836.
7. Frishman GN, Spencer PK, Weitzen S, Plosker S, Shafi F. The use of intrauterine lidocaine to minimize pain during hysterosalpingography: a randomized trial. Obstet Gynecol. 2004;103(6):1261–6. https://doi.org/10.1097/01.AOG.0000127370.66704.f5.
8. Baramki TA. Hysterosalpingography. Fertil Steril. 2005;83(6):1595–606. https://doi.org/10.1016/jfertnstert2004.12.050.

Additional Resource

Article

Eng CW, Tang PH, Ong CL. Hysterosalpingography: current applications. Singap Med J. 2007;48(4):368–74.

Chapter 28
Breast Cyst Aspiration

Cathryn B. Heath

Introduction

A breast mass is a common presenting symptom in a primary care office setting, at times accompanied by symptoms of pain and tenderness. Patients may detect an asymptomatic mass during self-examination, or a clinician may discover during a clinical examination. Most breast masses are caused by fibrocystic changes of the breast, but these must be differentiated from breast cancer. Over half of the women in the United States will have fibrocystic changes sometime during their reproductive life; these changes are most common between the ages of 30 and 50 [1]. Fibrocystic breasts typically present in a patient starting in their 30 s, increase in their 40 s, and often resolve by menopause [2]. Fibrocystic changes consist of two different forms: fibroadenomas, which are solid, and cysts, which are liquid-filled sacs. Most fibrocystic changes fluctuate with hormonal cycles, worsening just prior to menses and improving after the initiation of menses. No matter when the mass is noted within the hormonal cycle or if it occurs postmenopausal, a diagnostic mammogram and sonogram should be ordered. If the breast cyst is complex and shows a thickened cyst wall, intramural tumor, multiple septae or is eccentric on ultrasound, it has a higher likelihood of being malignant [3] and should be referred for biopsy and/or excision. If the palpable mass is solid on ultrasound or mammogram, then the patient should be referred for evaluation and definitive biopsy. A breast mass must be evaluated even if the mammogram is read as normal, as breast cancer can present in a similar fashion.

It is unnecessary to aspirate a simple unilocular breast cyst unless the patient prefers to have it done due to pain or discomfort. Breast cysts are often

C. B. Heath (✉)
Rutgers University Student Health, New Brunswick, NJ, USA
e-mail: heathcb@scarletmail.rutgers.edu

S. M. Sulik, C. B. Heath (eds.), *Primary Care Procedures in Women's Health*,
https://doi.org/10.1007/978-3-032-07061-6_28

uncomfortable and can cause either cyclical or noncyclical pain. Breast cysts on ultrasound are typically oval and thin walled.

Breast cyst aspiration is a very easy office procedure that can be performed with minimal risks or complications. If the mass is not completely resolved with aspiration, referral to a breast surgeon or interventional radiologist for further evaluation is recommended. Follow-up in 2 weeks is recommended, as many breast cysts recur. Fluid that is gray-green in color is not usually sent for cytology, as it is considered benign [3, 4]..

Case Study

A 42-year-old patient presents to the office for left-sided breast pain for two months. She has a past medical history of fibrocystic breast changes. During the examination, a 3 × 2 cm mass is palpated in the upper outer quadrant of the left breast which is tender to touch. The mammogram shows a mass, and the ultrasound shows it is a unilocular (simple) cyst. She is uncomfortable due to its size and is requesting an aspiration.

Diagnosis (Algorithm 28.1)

Unilocular breast cyst.

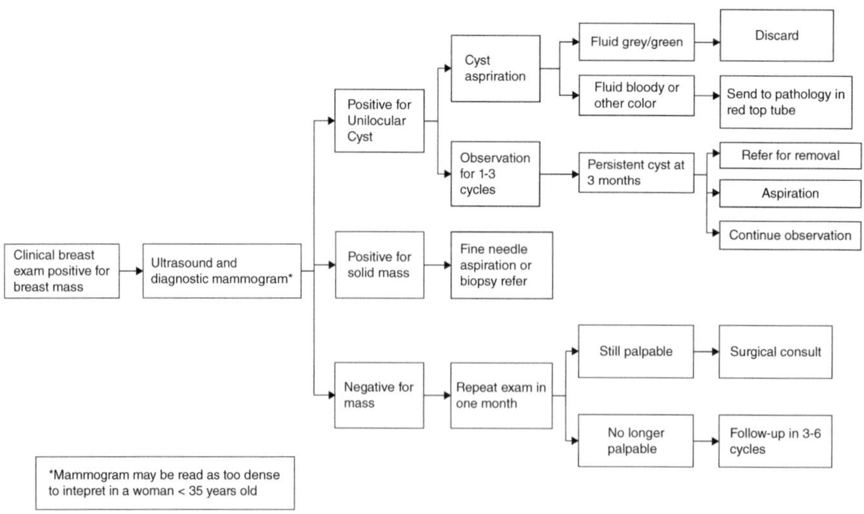

Algorithm 28.1 Decision tree for breast mass aspiration

Indications (Algorithm 28.1)

Uncomfortable breast mass documented to be an unilocular breast cyst by ultrasound.

Contraindications

- Previous history of breast cancer.
- Mass lying too close to the chest wall.
- Ultrasound shows non non-cystic lesion, a complex cyst, or a fibroadenoma.
- Uncertain diagnosis.

Equipment (Fig. 28.1)

- A 5–10-cc syringe (Fig. 28.2a) or butterfly needle with tubing attached to a syringe (Fig. 28.2b).
- 23- or 25-Gauge needle or butterfly with tubing (Fig. 28.2a, b)
- Hemostat.
- Antiseptic solution, such as povidone-iodine swab sticks.
- Ultrasound, if available.
- Surface anesthetic cream or spray freezant (i.e., ethylene glycol).
- Bandage.
- 2 × 2 gauze pads (for use for pressure under bandage if needed)
- Gloves.

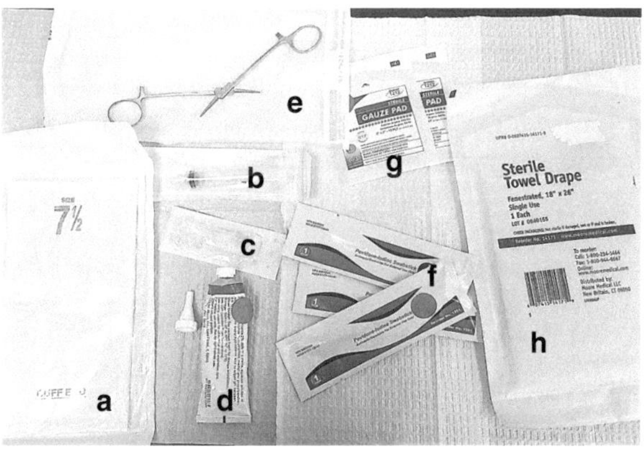

Fig. 28.1 Tray setup for breast cyst aspiration. (**a**) Sterile gloves; (**b**) 5-cc Luer lock syringe; (**c**) 23-gauge 1.5-in. needle; (**d**) topical anesthetic cream; (**e**) straight hemostat; (**f**) povidone-iodine swab sticks; (**g**) 2 × 2 in. gauze pads; (**h**) fenestrated sterile drape

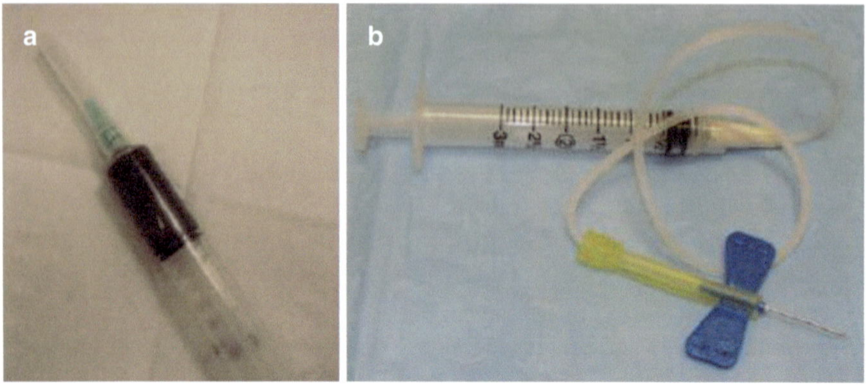

Fig. 28.2 (**a**) Syringe and needle, this one with gray-green fluid from a breast cyst. (**b**) Butterfly with tubing

Procedure

Breast Cyst Aspiration

1. Clean the area with an antiseptic solution three times in an outward circular fashion.
2. Spray ethylene chloride. Local anesthesia may be used instead but may distort architecture.
3. "Juice" the syringe (slide it back and forth a couple of times to ease aspiration later) and then leave 0.1–0.2 cc of air in the syringe prior to insertion. Put the needle on the end of the syringe.
4. Using gloves on both hands, grasp breast mass in the nondominant hand, cupping the mass within fingertips and applying some tension to remove it from the chest wall (Fig. 28.3). Alternatively, some clinicians capture the lesion between the second and third finger of the nondominant hand and pin the lesion above one of the patient's ribs (Fig. 28.4).
5. If ultrasound is available, ask an assistant to place the ultrasound lateral to the lesion, aiming toward the lesion.
6. Hold the syringe like a pencil during insertion, keeping the needle bevel up.
7. After insertion into the lesion, apply suction. This can be accomplished by placing the thumb under the plunger or inching one's fingers up the syringe to the plunger. Alternatively, you can have an associate withdraw the plunger to create the suction. With a pistol grip syringe holder, the syringe is held by the handle, with suction being applied after insertion by pulling back on the handle (Fig. 28.5).
8. Milk the mass (gently squeeze; Fig. 28.5) until it is totally gone. If there is too much fluid for the selected syringe, use the hemostat to twist the needle off the

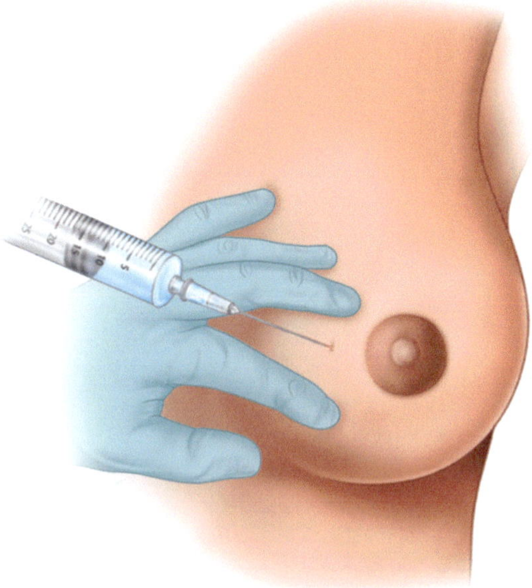

Fig. 28.3 Cupping cyst between the first and the second finger of the nondominant hand

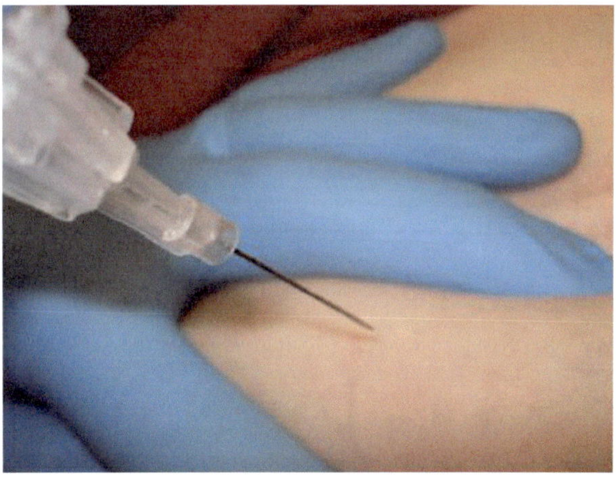

Fig. 28.4 Breast cyst localization with the nondominant hand

syringe, remove the fluid, and reinsert the syringe onto the needle again. It is not necessary to remove the needle from the patient.

9. When the mass is gone, stop applying suction and remove the needle. There is usually minimal bleeding involved. Apply pressure with the 2 × 2 gauze and then apply the bandage, if needed.
10. If the fluid is a clear, yellow, or grayish-green color (Fig. 28.2a), it is not necessary to send to the lab. If there is any blood or if the fluid is any other color, put the fluid into the dry red top tube for transport [3, 4]. Use as many red top tubes as necessary to send fluid.
11. If available, use ultrasound to document that the cyst is gone.

Fig. 28.5 Aspiration and "milking" of breast cyst

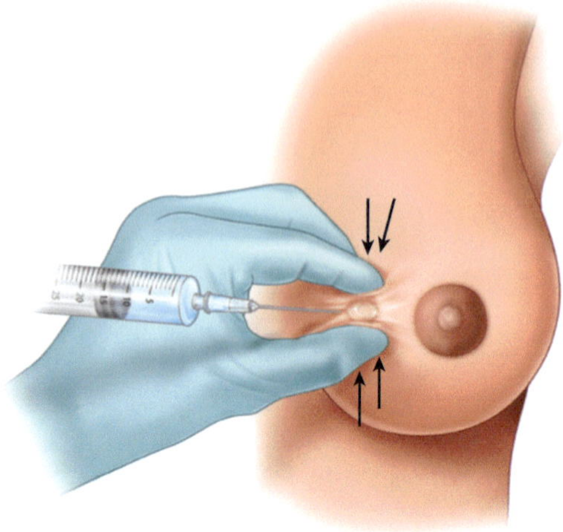

12. Document whether the mass is entirely resolved or still present. If still present, refer for further workup [4]

Complications and Risks

- Pneumothorax (rare).
- Bleeding (rare).
- Infection.
- Further workup if mass is not totally resolved with aspiration.

Tricks and Helpful Hints

- *Do not* let go of the mass or allow your associate to hold the mass while attempting to aspirate. This increases the likelihood of inadvertently causing a needle stick to yourself or your assistant.
- "Juice" the syringe by sliding the barrel up and down several times within the syringe prior to using on the patient. This facilitates easier withdrawal of the plunger during the aspiration.
- If possible, avoid the use of injectable anesthesia, as it distorts the skin above the mass and may make the mass more difficult to palpate. If necessary for patient comfort, consider using ethylene chloride or EMLA™. If applying EMLA™ topical cream, the patient should be instructed to apply it 60 min prior to having the procedure.

- Sebaceous cysts can also cause superficial breast lumps, so it is best practice to do an ultrasound prior to the aspiration.

Interpretation of Results (Algorithm 28.1)

- Gray-green fluid from a breast cyst is considered benign and can be discarded.
- Any bloody fluid should be sent to pathology for evaluation.

Procedure Note

(Provider to fill in blanks/circle applicable choice when given multiple choices and customize as needed.)

Breast Cyst Aspiration

Risks, benefits, and complications of breast mass evaluation discussed; alternative providers of the procedure discussed; consent signed. Patient placed in supine position, mass localized. Area prepped and draped in a sterile fashion. Topical anesthetic spray applied. Mass located and held with nondominant hand; breast mass aspirated with a 25-gauge needle on a 10-cc syringe. ________ccs of fluid obtained with complete resolution of breast cyst. Bandage applied. Patient tolerated the procedure well. Fluid noted to be gray-green in character and was discarded.

Coding

CPT® Codes(Current Procedural Terminology, AMA, Chicago, IL)	
88,170	Breast mass evaluation and recommendations for breast cancer screening
19,000	Aspiration and drainage of one breast cyst
19,001	Aspiration and drainage of breast cyst—each additional
ICD-10-CM-Diagnostic Codes (International Classification of Diseases, 10th Revision, Clinical Modification, Centers for Disease Control and Prevention)	
N60	Benign mammary dysplasia N60.0 solitary cyst of the breast N60.01 solitary cyst of the right breast N60.02 solitary cyst of the left breast

Case Study Outcome

Breast cyst was successfully aspirated in the office under local anesthesia. Gray-green fluid obtained, and mass completely resolved. No recurrence when reexamined in 1 month.

Patient Handout

(Provider to customize as needed.)

Breast cyst aspiration is an office procedure that involves putting a needle into the cyst and removing all the fluid. If you choose to have this done, plan on taking three 200 mg ibuprofen 1 hour before coming to the office. If you opted for topical anesthetic cream, apply it to the skin above the lump ~1 hour prior to the procedure. The area will be cleaned with an antibacterial disinfectant. The clinician will insert a needle to remove the fluid. After the procedure is done, a bandage will be applied. If the fluid is typical gray-green, it will not need to be analyzed. If it is otherwise, your clinician will send it for pathology.

Call your clinician's office if you are experiencing any warmth, swelling, bleeding, or shortness of breath after the procedure. Please make a follow-up appointment in 2 weeks to reevaluate your mass and discuss the results.

References

1. Calhoun BC, Grobmyer SR, Simpson JF. Benign, high-risk, and premalignant lesions of the breast. In: The breast: comprehensive management of benign and malignant diseases. 5th ed. Philadelphia: Elsevier; 2018.
2. Horton H, Abdo J, Tillman R, Seydel A. Management of cystic conditions. Surg Clin North Am. 2022;102(6):1089–102.
3. Sanders LM, Lacz NL, Lara J. 16 year experience with aspiration of noncomplex breast cysts: cytology results with focus on positive cases. Breast J. 2012;18(5):443–52.
4. Pearlman MD, Griffin JL. Benign breast disease. Obstet Gynecol. 2010;116:747–58. https://doi.org/10.1097/AOG.0b013e3181ee9fc7.

Equipment

Cameco pistol syringe holder syringe: http://www.belpro.ca/cameco.htm
Tao pencil grip syringe holder: http://www.taoaspirator.com/

Chapter 29
Management of Early Pregnancy Loss and Medication Abortion Using Mifepristone and Misoprostol

H Reeve Bright, Jennifer Amico, and Anna Sliwowska

Introduction

Half of all pregnancies in the United States are unintended, and half of these pregnancies end in elective termination [1]. At current abortion rates, one in four people capable of pregnancy will have an abortion by the age of 45 [2]. Despite the demand for abortion services, 90% of all counties in the United States have no abortion provider [3]. Furthermore, most patients seek abortion services at non-primary care sites, disrupting continuity of care for those who would prefer to access abortion services from their primary care provider. Over 90% of all abortions and pregnancy losses occur in the first trimester, when safe, simple, and highly effective services can be provided in the primary care setting [4]. If primary care clinicians were to offer abortion and medication-assisted early pregnancy loss care, they could greatly improve timely access to safe abortion and relevant reproductive health services, particularly in rural and underserved settings [5].

Offering medication abortion in the office setting does not require expensive equipment or specialized procedural training, thus facilitating its incorporation into primary care. Medication abortion offers an important alternative to procedure abortion from a patient perspective (see Table 31.1 in Chap. 31 on Manual Vacuum Aspiration Abortion). Patients' reasons for choosing a medication abortion include

H. R. Bright (✉)
Department of Family Medicine, Hoboken University Medical Center, CarePoint Health, Hoboken, NJ, USA
e-mail: henrietta.bright@carepointhealth.org

J. Amico · A. Sliwowska
Department of Family Medicine and Community Health, Rutgers Robert Wood Johnson Medical School, New Brunswick, NJ, USA
e-mail: jennifer.amico@rutgers.edu; anna.sliwowska@rutgers.edu

S. M. Sulik, C. B. Heath (eds.), *Primary Care Procedures in Women's Health*,
https://doi.org/10.1007/978-3-032-07061-6_29

a desire for privacy, a preference for a more "natural" method, and avoidance of an invasive procedure.

In September 2000, the U.S. Food and Drug Administration (FDA) approved mifepristone (also known as RU486 or Mifeprex®, Danco Laboratories, New York, NY) to be used with misoprostol (a prostaglandin) for medication abortion up to 49 days of gestational age. In March 2016, the FDA approved an updated protocol which endorsed the use of medication abortion up to 70 days of gestational age [6]. Since then, medication abortion has been proven to be safe and effective through 77 days of gestational age (off-label use) when given with two doses of 800 mcg misoprostol [7, 8]. This process first involves the administration of mifepristone (a progesterone antagonist), which effectively detaches the pregnancy from the endometrial lining and sensitizes the myometrium to prostaglandins. Misoprostol is administered approximately 24–48 hours(h) later, and stimulates uterine contractions, thus causing expulsion of the pregnancy tissue (Fig. 29.1).

While the FDA-approved 2016 regimen is widely utilized for medication abortion, other protocols utilize different timing or modes of administration of misoprostol. Though used less frequently, medication abortion can also be accomplished using methotrexate and misoprostol, or with misoprostol alone [9]. Advantages of using methotrexate include its relatively inexpensive cost and wide availability, and the fact that it can medically treat ectopic pregnancy under certain circumstances. However, given that methotrexate (used with misoprostol) can take a longer period for abortion completion (up to 4 weeks) and can only be used up to 9 weeks of

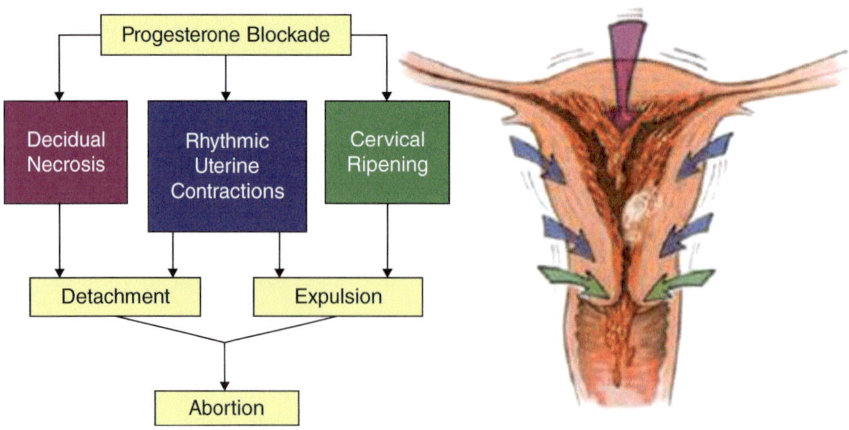

Fig. 29.1 Mifepristone and misoprostol mechanism of action. Mifepristone binds to progesterone receptors, causing decidual necrosis and detachment of the pregnancy from the endometrium. In addition, mifepristone induces uterine contractility and sensitizes the myometrium to prostaglandins. Misoprostol administration then promotes cervical ripening and further uterine contractions. The synergistic action of mifepristone and misoprostol ultimately causes pregnancy detachment and expulsion. (Reprinted with the permission of the National Abortion Federation. Early Options: A Provider's Guide to Medical Abortion. Medical Education Series. "Overview of Medical Abortion: Clinical and Practice Issues." 2005)

gestational age, it is not typically the regimen of choice for most US providers and patients [10].

After the Dobbs US Supreme Court decision in 2022, many states in the United States have outlawed abortion provision. Where abortion is legal, states may have laws regulating the provision of abortion services, including gestational age limits, mandatory waiting periods, parental consent for minors, physician-only laws, and/or mandatory health department reporting. Some states have also mandated that medication abortion follows only the FDA protocol, and the US Federal Court system is hearing a case arguing the legality of the 2016 protocol update as of the writing of this chapter. Clinicians should be familiar with state regulations prior to introducing medication abortion in their practice.

Medication abortion can be provided on a spectrum, from in-person care to telehealth visits to self-sourced abortion medications. Telehealth allows for a virtual office visit, and studies show it allows for earlier access to abortion care, has high rates of patient satisfaction, and no difference in the rates of abortion failure or complications. It is important for health providers to be aware that some patients will self-source their abortion medications outside of the clinical setting, purchasing mifepristone and misoprostol from an online platform or pharmacy [11]. These patients may come in seeking care after a self-sourced abortion and are not managed any differently than after an abortion provided via the healthcare system.

Case Study

A 23-year-old nulliparous patient presents to the office after missing her menses. Her last menstrual period was 6 weeks ago. She has regular menses and is sure of her last menstrual period. She and her partner experienced a condom break a couple of weeks ago, but she did not know about postcoital ("emergency") contraception. She is a young graduate student and does not feel ready to be a parent currently. She has no risk factors for ectopic pregnancy. After pregnancy options and abortion options counselling, she decides to proceed with a medication abortion.

Diagnosis (Algorithm 29.1)

- Six-week pregnancy with no risk factors for ectopic pregnancy.
- Desire for induced abortion.

Differential Diagnosis

- Normal, intrauterine pregnancy.
- Ectopic pregnancy.

- Heterotopic pregnancy: concomitant presence of an intrauterine and ectopic pregnancy.
- Early pregnancy failure: threatened, incomplete, or complete spontaneous abortion.

Indications (Algorithm 29.1)

- Induced abortion.
- May also be medically necessary for patients with comorbidities in which carrying pregnancy to term poses a threat to health and/or life.
- May be used for the completion of spontaneous early pregnancy loss (off-label use).

Contraindications (Algorithm 29.1)

- Confirmed or suspected ectopic pregnancy or undiagnosed adnexal mass.
- Intrauterine device in place (remove prior to treatment).
- Chronic adrenal failure (mifepristone contraindicated).
- Current long-term, systemic corticosteroid therapy (mifepristone contraindicated).
- Allergy to mifepristone, misoprostol, or other prostaglandins.
- Inherited porphyria.
- Hemorrhagic disorder or current anticoagulant therapy.

Special Considerations

- Patients with anemia (hemoglobin <10 mg/dl, hematocrit <30%) should be evaluated individually for symptoms and presence of current bleeding to determine the safest method of pregnancy termination.
- Any patient with chronic medical conditions (e.g., cardiac disease, hepatic disease, uncontrolled diabetes, uncontrolled seizure disorder, inflammatory bowel disease, renal disease, pulmonary disease) should be evaluated individually to determine the safest method of pregnancy termination.
- Breastfeeding patients: There is no evidence that mifepristone is harmful to breastfeeding infants. Patients should be warned that misoprostol can cause mild side effects such as diarrhea in infants, but they do not need to stop breastfeeding during this time.

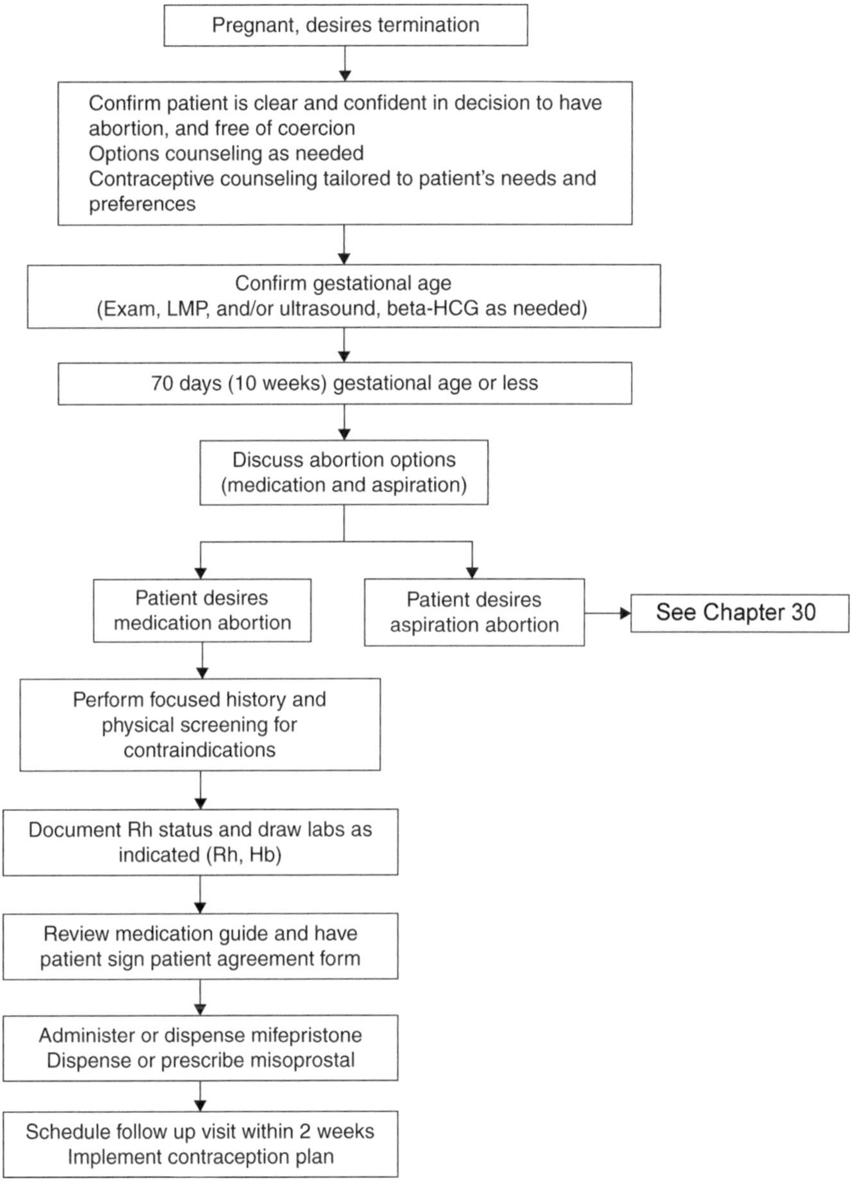

Algorithm 29.1 Decision tree for abortion options

Equipment (Fig. 29.2)

- Danco® Patient Agreement Form and the Mifeprex® Medication Guide (download from website www.earlyoptionpill.com).
- Patient Instructions for Medication Abortion Form (Fig. 29.2).
- Ultrasound—optional (not mandatory per FDA protocol).
- Ultrasound documentation form (if applicable).
- Mifepristone 200 mg pills (must be a registered provider with Danco®; http://www.earlyoptionpill.com).
- Misoprostol 200 mcg tablets (can order in bulk and dispense).
- Urine pregnancy test.
- Hemoglobin, if history of heavy menses.

Medication Abortion Instructions

Today you took mifepristone to end your pregnancy. You took 200 milligrams of mifepristone at ____am/pm. You may have some vaginal bleeding after taking this pill.

Any time from 24 to 48 hours after you took the first pill, _____am/pm, you must take another medicine, misoprostol (also called Cytotec). **Choose a time when you have had a good meal and plenty of rest.** Swallow one ibuprofen pill one hour before you take the misoprostol – this will help decrease your cramps. You must take the misoprostol even if you have started to bleed.

Each misoprostol pill is 200 micrograms. **Place 2 misoprostol pills in each cheek (4 pills total).** Leave them in your cheeks for 30 minutes. After 30 minutes, swallow the pills with water.

WHAT TO EXPECT

Cramping and Bleeding: Misoprostol causes cramping and bleeding, often with clots. The cramps and bleeding may be much more than you get with a period. The cramps usually start 2 to 4 hours after you take the pills, and may last for 3 to 5 hours. This heavy bleeding means that the treatment is working. The bleeding often lasts 1 to 2 weeks, and it may stop and start a few times.

You may have a lot of pain or cramps – if so, take pain medicine. You can take ibuprofen (Motrin or Advil) up to 800 milligrams every 8 hours and/or hydrocodone up to 2 pills every 4 to 6 hours. You can also use a heating pad to relieve the pain. You may have nausea, diarrhea, or chills. This should get better in a few hours.

Sadness or very emotional: You may feel very relieved when the abortion is over. You may also feel sad or moody. These feelings are partly from the changes in hormones, now that you are no longer pregnant. Feeling emotional at this time is normal. If you think your emotions are not what they should be, please talk to us.

When will your period come back? You can expect a period in 4 to 8 weeks. It is not the same for everyone.

You **should** call me if:
- Your bleeding soaks through more than 2 maxi pads per hour for 2 hours,
- You do **not** bleed within 24 hours after taking the misoprostol, OR
- You start to feel very ill after the heavy cramping and bleeding is over.

To reach me:
Call my 24-hour number: ________________________. If you have any questions or think something is going wrong, call this number and I will call you back. It may take me 10 to 15 minutes to return your call. No question is too small. **Please feel free to call me.**

Follow-up:
You will have a visit or phone call with me in 7-14 days to make sure that the abortion is complete.

Birth Control:
If you want to use birth control pills, patch, or ring, I have given you a prescription. You should start these on __________, even if you are still bleeding.

Fig. 29.2 Patient instructions for medication abortion. (Adapted from Reproductive Health Access Project http://www.reproductiveaccess.org/. Accessed January 23, 2024)

Procedure (Algorithm 29.1)

1. Confirm the patient is clear and confident about the decision to end the pregnancy and is free of coercion. If needed, perform pregnancy options counselling. Important points to consider for pregnancy options counselling:
   - Ask open-ended questions in a nonjudgmental manner (e.g., "How do you feel about being pregnant?").
   - Inquire about the patient's support network (partner, family, friends, etc.).
   - Discuss all options as necessary: continuing the pregnancy and becoming a parent; continuing the pregnancy and opting for an adoption; ending the pregnancy.
2. Confirm pregnancy diagnosis and gestational age:
   - Assess last menstrual period (LMP).
   - Obtain a urine pregnancy test or serum β-HCG, as indicated.
   - Obtain or perform a bimanual exam or an ultrasound, as indicated.

A Note About Ultrasound While ultrasonography is widely used for gestational age dating, it is not mandatory to perform an ultrasound for medication abortion per FDA protocol. According to the Mifeprex® Prescribing Information, "the duration of pregnancy may be determined from menstrual history and by clinical examination. Ultrasonographic scan should be used if the duration of pregnancy is uncertain, or if ectopic pregnancy is suspected" [6]. It has been shown that patients seeking abortions can accurately estimate their gestational age and that clinician assessment of gestational age (based on exam and LMP) had a high correlation with sonography [12]. Based upon this evidence, some providers have advocated for an "ultrasound as needed" protocol, such that an ultrasound is performed only under certain circumstances. This approach can greatly improve access to abortion services, particularly in sites where the cost of an ultrasound machine is prohibitive and/or there are no trained ultrasonographers.

Indications for ultrasonography prior to medication abortion:

- Discrepancy between gestational age as assessed by uterine size and LMP.
- Uncertain LMP or irregular menstrual cycles.
- Adnexal mass or pain.
- Recent use of hormonal contraception.
- Provider uncertainty with the exam.
- History of previous ectopic pregnancy.

At Mifepristone Visit

1. Confirm eligibility criteria and conduct other medical screening as indicated (e.g., Pap smear, testing for sexually transmitted infections). The performance of such screening tests in otherwise asymptomatic patients is not mandatory prior to providing medication abortion.
2. Help the patient choose a birth control method if desired. Discuss postcoital contraception and provide advance prescriptions if necessary.
3. Testing for hemoglobin or hematocrit is not mandatory per the Mifeprex® Medication Guide. Providers may choose to routinely screen for anemia depending on the local prevalence of anemia and/or by individual risk factors and clinical history [13, 14].
4. Review the *Mifeprex® Medication Guide* and have the patient review and sign the *Patient Agreement Form* (both required by Danco®, the manufacturer of mifepristone).
5. Counsel the patient on the procedure and expectations (Fig. 29.2).
6. The patient should pick a convenient time to administer the misoprostol, after mifepristone ingestion. Review *how and when* to administer the misoprostol, depending on which route has been chosen.
7. Advise on the use of pain and/or nausea medications prior to misoprostol administration (e.g., ibuprofen, promethazine).
8. Review when to call: if no bleeding occurs within 24 hours (h) of taking misoprostol, if soaking through two overnight pads an hour for two consecutive hours, or if sustained fever >100.4 °F.
9. Advise that cramping and bleeding will begin a couple of hours after taking the misoprostol, which may peak in 3–5 h. The cramping ranges from mild to intense. Approximately two-thirds of patients will complete the abortion process within 4 h. By 24 h, 90% of patients will have successfully completed the abortion.
10. The bleeding is like a heavy period with or without clots. The patient should be told that they will see blood and tissue and may recognize fetal parts starting at 9 weeks of gestation and above.
11. Either administer or dispense mifepristone. Document the time and date, as well as the lot number and expiration date of the mifepristone.
12. Prior to leaving, the patient should have the following:

    (a) Misoprostol tablets (record the lot number and expiration date) to self-administer at home.
    (b) Prescriptions for pain and/or nausea if desired.
    (c) Prescriptions for birth control and postcoital contraception, if desired.
    (d) The patient can start self-administered hormonal methods within 5 days of taking mifepristone, even if still bleeding.
    (e) A follow-up appointment in 2 weeks.
    (f) A 24-h provider contact number.
    (g) The Patient Instruction Form (Fig. 29.2).

A Note About Rh Testing Rhesus (Rh) factor testing is no longer indicated for abortions occurring at less than 12 weeks (84 days) of gestation according to the World Health Organization, the National Abortion Federation, and the Society of Family Planning [13, 14]. This includes both medication and manual vacuum aspiration abortions. The American College of Obstetrics and Gynecology still recommends it for all patients undergoing induced abortion or early pregnancy loss [15].

At Follow-Up Visit

1. Confirmation of pregnancy termination can be confirmed by the following:
   - Patient history (a description of cramping, bleeding, and passage of pregnancy tissue) with resolution of pregnancy symptoms.
   - Physical examination *or* ultrasound *or* documentation of declining serum β-HCG level (at least 80% decline from baseline over 5–10 days). Alternatively, patients can take a urine pregnancy test at home 4–5 weeks after the abortion if history is consistent with a successful abortion [16].
   - Postabortion indications for ultrasonography:
   - History not consistent with successful abortion.
   - Patient still feels pregnant.
   - Serum β-HCG not declining.
2. If the abortion is incomplete (persistent sac with or without evidence of ongoing pregnancy), the patient can be offered repeat medications or an aspiration procedure. An aspiration procedure may be required if the pregnancy has advanced beyond 77 days, if the patient has become anemic, or if the patient prefers faster resolution of symptoms.
3. Clinicians should inquire about the patient's experience with the abortion process and provide support and reassurance as appropriate.
4. Review the contraceptive plan and initiate the method that day, if desired and not yet initiated.

Complications and Risks [17]

Less than 1% of all US abortion patients experience a major complication. The risk of death associated with abortion in the United States is less than 0.6 per 100,000 procedures, which is less than one-tenth the risk associated with childbirth. Complications and risks are as follows:

- Significant bleeding requiring intervention: <1%.
- Infection: <0.5%.

- Sepsis: <0.01%.
- Incomplete abortion requiring a uterine aspiration procedure varies by gestational age:
    - 9w0d or less: <1%
    - 9w1d to 10w0d: 3.6% with a single 800 mcg dose of misoprostol, 0.4% with two 800 mcg doses
    - 10w1d to 11w0d: 8.7% with a single 800 mcg dose of misoprostol, 1.6% with two 800 mcg doses of misoprostol.

With medication abortion, the most common significant complication is the risk of ongoing pregnancy (1–3%) or retained tissue or sac (3–6%, varies by gestational age), so all patients should be counselled about the importance of the follow-up visit as well as the potential need for additional misoprostol dose or a uterine aspiration procedure at the time of medication abortion counselling.

A Note About Sepsis On July 15, 2005, the U.S. Food and Drug Administration (FDA) issued a public health advisory regarding four deaths in the United States (all in California) that occurred following vaginal administration of misoprostol after oral mifepristone for medication abortion. *Clostridium sordelli*, a virulent Gram-positive bacterium, was identified as the causative agent in all cases. Other cases of *Clostridium sordelli*-related deaths have involved cases of spontaneous abortion and childbirth. After an extensive investigation, the Centers for Disease Control and Prevention, the FDA, and the National Institute of Allergy and Infectious Diseases concluded that there is no definitive causal relationship between mifepristone and the deaths. Clinicians should be familiar with the signs and symptoms of sepsis and initiate prompt evaluation of patients who present with severe abdominal pain, prolonged heavy bleeding, syncope, or abdominal pain or general malaise, with or without fever, that occurs more than 24 h after taking misoprostol [17]. For more information on this topic, please visit the CDC website (https://www.cdc.gov/hai/organisms/csordellii.html.

Tricks and Helpful Hints

- Some patients who otherwise meet medical eligibility may not be appropriate candidates for medication abortion for psychosocial reasons.
- Clinicians should help patients identify possible barriers to seeking assistance during the medication abortion procedure including access to a phone, car, or childcare; distance from the office; and language barrier.

Procedure Note

See Fig. 29.3 for the Medication Abortion Charting Form.

(Provider to fill in blanks/circle applicable choice when given multiple choices and customize as needed.)

Chart Review Form
Medication Abortion

	Yes	No	N/A
Options counseling documented			
Adverse effects education documented			
Protocol explanation documented			
Informed consent form: signed, in chart			
Rh status documented Rhogam given, if indicated			
Contraindications ruled out No IUD in place No allergy to prostaglandins No chronic adrenal failure No long-term systemtic corticosteroid use No concurrent anticoagulant therapy No ectopic pregnancy No hemorrhagic disorder			
Iniital beta-HCG level obtained (if indicated)			
Ultrasound dating obtained (if indicated)			
Screening for anemia performed/documented (if indicated)			
Pain medication prescribed			
Follow up visit completed			
Assessment of abortion completed documented by History Beta-HCG level Ultrasound			
Contraception plan documented			

Fig. 29.3 Medication abortion procedure note/charting form. (Adapted from Reproductive Health Access Project http://www.reproductiveaccess.org/. Accessed January 23, 2024)

Coding

CPT® Codes (Current Procedural Terminology, AMA, Chicago, IL)		
For the visit	99204 or 99214	Level 4 new or established patient E/M visit
For the ultrasound	76817	Transvaginal ultrasound, pregnant uterus
	76815	Limited ultrasound, pregnant uterus
For medication(s)	J8499	Prescription drug, oral, nonchemo, not otherwise specified
	J3490	Unclassified drug
	90385	MICRhoGAM®, if given in the office (see *A note about Rh testing* above)
ICD 10-CM-Diagnostic Codes (International Classification of Diseases, 10th Revision, Clinical Modification, Center for Disease Control and Prevention) [non-comprehensive]		
Legally induced abortion, without mention of complication, complete		Z33.2

If J codes are not accepted by the insurance carrier, use 99,070 (a cost of materials CPT code) for Mifeprex® or S0190 for Mifeprex®. Note: Each insurance carrier may reimburse for Mifeprex® using a different code. The name of the drug (Mifeprex®), the dosage (200 mg), and the 11-digit National Drug Code (NDC) from the drug package must accompany this claim. In addition, submit a copy of the drug invoice to show the cost of the drug.

Patient Instructions

See Fig. 29.2.

(Provider to fill in blanks/circle applicable choice when given multiple choices and to customize as needed.)

Case Study Outcome

The patient took 200 mg of mifepristone the day of the office visit in the office. She took 800 μg of misoprostol buccally at home approximately 24 h later and experienced bleeding similar to a heavy period 1–2 h later, passing clots and tissue. She also had cramping that eventually subsided with ibuprofen and a heating pad. At her 1-month follow-up telehealth visit, she reported that her breast tenderness and nausea had resolved, and a home urine pregnancy test was negative. She continued to have intermittent, light bleeding without cramping and reported relief that the process was over. She started her birth control pills within 5 days of taking mifepristone, as you advised.

References

1. Finer LB, Zolna MR. Declines in unintended pregnancy in the United States, 2008–2011. N Engl J Med. 2016;374(9):843–52.
2. Jones RK. Population group abortion rates and lifetime incidence of abortion: United States, 2008–2014. Am J Public Health. 2017;107(12):1904–9.
3. Jones RK, Kirstein M, Philbin J. Abortion incidence and service availability in the United States, 2020. Perspect Sex Reprod Health. 2022;5449(41):1417–27.
4. Kortsmit K, Nguyen AT, Mandel MG, Clark E, Hollier LM, Rodenhizer J, Whiteman MK. Abortion surveillance—United States, 2020. MMWR Surveill Summ. 2022;71(10):1–27.
5. National Academies of Sciences, E. a. M. The safety and quality of abortion care in the United States. The National Academies Press. [Online]. 2018. Available at: https://doi.org/10.17226/24950. Accessed 2 Feb 2024.
6. Laboratories D. Mifiprex (package insert) prescribing information. New York City: Danco Laboratories; 2024.
7. Dzuba IG, Castillo PW, Bousiéguez M, Hernández EML, Vivar JJC, Smith PS. A repeat dose of misoprostol 800 mcg following mifepristone for outpatient medical abortion at 64–70 and 71–77 days of gestation: a retrospective chart review. [Online]. Contraception. 2020;102(2):104–8. Available at: PMID: 32474060. Accessed 02 Feb 2024
8. Kapp N, Eckersberger E, Lavelanet A, Rodriguez MI. Medical abortion in the late first trimester: a systematic review. Contraception. 2019;99(2):77–86.
9. Federation NA. Clinical policy guidelines for abortion care. [Online]. n.d.. Available at: ProChoice.org; 2020. Accessed 02 Feb 2024.
10. Wiebe E, Dunn S, Guilbert E, Jacot F, Lugtig L. Comparison of abortions induced by methotrexate or mifepristone followed by misoprostol. Obstet Gynecol. 2002;99(5 Pt 1):813–9. https://doi.org/10.1016/s0029-7844(02)01944-0.
11. Bearak J, Popinchalk A, Ganatra B, Moller A-B, Tunçalp Ö, Beavin C, Kwok L, Alkema L. Unintended pregnancy and abortion by income, region, and the legal status of abortion: estimates from a comprehensive model for 1990–2019. Lancet Glob Health. 2020;8:1152–61.
12. Raymond EG, et al. Early medical abortion without prior ultrasound. Contraception. 2015;92(3):212–4.
13. Horvath S, et al. Society of Family Planning committee consensus on Rh testing in early pregnancy. Contraception. 2022;114:1–5.
14. Mark A, et al. Foregoing Rh testing, and anti-D immunoglobulin for women presenting for early abortion: a recommendation from the National Abortion Federation's clinical policies committee. Contraception. 2019;99:265–6.
15. ACOG Practice Bulletin No. 225, 2020. Medication abortion up to 70 days of gestation. American College of Obstetricians and Gynecologists. Obstet Gynecol. 2020;136:e31–e47.
16. Iyengar K, et al. Self-assessment of the outcome of early medical abortion versus clinical follow-up in India: a randomized controlled on-inferiority trial. Lancet. 2015;2002(99):537–45.
17. Flemming M, et al. TEACH abortion training curriculum. s.l.:s.n. 2022

Additional Resources

Websites

For educational resources and a clinical curriculum regarding medication abortion, visit: (Dzuba IG, 2020). The National Abortion Federation: http://www.prochoice.org/education/resources/index.html. TEACH Abortion Training Curriculum: https://pressbooks.pub/workbook/

For information regarding abortion training in family medicine residencies, visit The Center for Reproductive Health Education in Family Medicine: www.rhedi.org

For information regarding state laws on abortion, visit The Center for Reproductive Rights: http://www.reproductiverights.org/ or the Guttmacher Institute: guttmacher.org

For patient and clinician resources regarding early abortion care (including the methotrexate/misoprostol regimen), visit The Reproductive Health Access Project: http://www.reproductiveaccess.org/

To obtain the Mifeprex® Medication Guide and Patient Agreement Form, visit: www.earlyoptionpill.com

Chapter 30
Manual Vacuum Aspiration (MVA) Abortion

H Reeve Bright, Anna Sliwowska, and Jennifer Amico

Introduction

Aspiration abortion is a safe procedure that can be performed in the office or in an ambulatory surgical center. It can be accomplished either by using a 60-cc handheld syringe (manual vacuum aspirator) or by using vacuum aspiration with an electric pump. These methods are commonly referred to as a "surgical abortion" and can be performed safely and effectively in an outpatient setting with local anesthesia alone or combined with light to moderate sedation [1]. Aspiration abortion is associated with lower rates of complications than sharp curettage (dilation and curettage), and along with medication-induced abortion is the preferred methodology of abortions whenever possible [2]. Aspiration abortion performed with a manual vacuum aspirator (MVA) is particularly adaptable for use in the primary care setting because of several features of the MVA: (1) low cost and ability to reuse the manual aspirator, (2) small size and portability of the manual aspirator, (3) its ability to aspirate tissue without extensive fragmentation, allowing for easier identification of early pregnancy tissue, and (4) its ability to work without an electrical source. The MVA is also a quieter device than the electric vacuum, which may reduce patient anxiety.

H. R. Bright (✉)
Department of Family Medicine, Hoboken University Medical Center, CarePoint Health, Hoboken, NJ, USA
e-mail: henrietta.bright@carepointhealth.org

A. Sliwowska · J. Amico
Department of Family Medicine and Community Health, Rutgers Robert Wood Johnson Medical School, New Brunswick, NJ, USA
e-mail: anna.sliwowska@rutgers.edu; jennifer.amico@rutgers.edu

S. M. Sulik, C. B. Heath (eds.), *Primary Care Procedures in Women's Health*,
https://doi.org/10.1007/978-3-032-07061-6_30

Use of the MVA is clinically indicated for induced abortion or completion of miscarriage up to 12 weeks by uterine size, ultrasound dating, or the last menstrual period (LMP). Beyond 12 weeks, an electric vacuum aspirator would be preferred. Other uses of the MVA technique include the treatment of incomplete abortion or miscarriage and endometrial biopsy.

After the United States (US) Food and Drug Administration's (FDA) approval of mifepristone for medication abortion in 2000, the number of medication abortions performed in the United States has steadily increased. Medication abortion offers an important alternative for patients seeking early abortion services (see Chap. 29). In order to provide comprehensive abortion options counseling, clinicians should be familiar with the advantages and disadvantages of medication abortion versus aspiration abortion from a patient perspective (see Table 30.1, patient handout).

Clinicians should be familiar with state regulations for first-trimester abortion provision prior to introducing MVA in their practice. Regulations may include gestational age limits, mandatory waiting periods, parental consent for minors, and/or mandatory health department reporting. Advanced practice clinicians (nurse practitioners, physician assistants) should specifically check if "physician-only" laws apply to abortion provision in their state.

Less than 1% of all US abortion patients experience a major complication [3]. The risk of death associated with a legally induced abortion in the United States is less than 0.65 per 100,000 of reported legal procedures, which is less than one-tenth the risk associated with childbirth [4]. The routine use of antibiotics just prior to or following induced abortions <16 weeks is associated with a 42% reduction in the incidence of postabortal upper genital tract infection, regardless of the patient's preprocedure risk status [5]. All patients undergoing a surgical abortion should receive prophylactic antibiotics using one of the following, single-dose regimens: doxycycline 200 mg by mouth once, azithromycin 500 mg by mouth once, or metronidazole 500 mg by mouth once. There is no known difference in effectiveness [6].

Table 30.1 Comparison of early abortion options: a patient resource

Abortion pill/medication abortion (mifepristone and misoprostol)	Aspiration abortion (suction or vacuum aspiration)
1. *How far along in the pregnancy can I be?*	
Up to 11 weeks from the first day of your last period.	Up to 12 weeks from the first day of your last period.
2. *What will happen?*	
The abortion happens at home.	The abortion happens in the office.
During your appointment, you will get the first abortion pill (mifepristone) which you will take during the visit or at a time that works best for you.	The actual abortion procedure takes 5–10 minutes.
You will likely feel fine after taking mifepristone. You may have some nausea or spotting.	Your healthcare provider puts instruments in your vagina and uterus to remove the pregnancy.
6–72 (ideally 24–48) hours later, you take four misoprostol pills.	You may have a return visit to your regular healthcare provider or to the office where you had the abortion 1–2 weeks later.
The cramping and bleeding start 1–4 hours after you take the misoprostol. You will have heavy bleeding and cramps for a few hours.	The abortion happens in the office.
3. *How painful is it?*	
You may have mild to very strong cramps off and on during the abortion. Your provider can assist with pain management options.	You may have mild to very strong cramps during the abortion. Your provider may have options for pain control available.
4. *How much will I bleed?*	
Expect heavy bleeding with clots during the abortion. After that, lighter bleeding may continue off and on for a few weeks.	You may have light bleeding for 1–7 days. Bleeding may continue off and on for a few weeks.
5. *How much does it cost?*	
For both types of abortion, the exact cost depends on where you go.	For both types of abortion, the exact cost depends on where you go.
6. *Can the abortion fail?*	
The pills work 98–99% of the time. If the pills fail, you may try the pills again or have an abortion procedure.	It works 99% of the time. If it fails, you must have a repeat abortion procedure.
7. *Can I still have children afterward?*	
Yes. Neither type of abortion lowers your chances of getting pregnant or staying pregnant in the future.	Yes. Neither type of abortion lowers your chances of getting pregnant or staying pregnant in the future.
8. *Is it safe?*	
Both pills have been used safely for over 20 years. Big problems are rare. Abortion is at least 10 times safer than continuing a pregnancy.	The suction abortion procedure has been done safely for over 50 years. Abortion in the first 12 weeks leads to very few problems. Abortion is at least 10 times safer than continuing a pregnancy.
9. *What are the advantages?*	

(continued)

Table 30.1 (continued)

Abortion pill/medication abortion (mifepristone and misoprostol)	Aspiration abortion (suction or vacuum aspiration)
You won't have shots, anesthesia, or instruments in your body.	It is over in a few minutes. It works 99% of the time.
It may feel more natural, like a miscarriage.	You see less bleeding than you would with a pill abortion.
Being at home instead of in an office may feel more private.	Medical staff members are with you during the abortion.
	It can be done later in the pregnancy than a pill abortion.
10. *What are the disadvantages?*	
It takes 1–2 days to complete the abortion.	A healthcare provider must insert instruments inside the uterus.
Bleeding can be very heavy and may last longer than with a suction abortion procedure.	Anesthetics and pain medicines may cause side effects.
Cramps can be severe and may last longer than with an abortion procedure.	You have less control over the abortion procedure. You may not be able to choose who is in the room with you.
It cannot be done as late in pregnancy as an aspiration abortion.	

Adapted from the Reproductive Health Access Project: www.reproductiveaccess.org with permission

Case Study

A 42-year-old G3P2002 female presents to your office with complaints of nausea. Her last menstrual period was 8 weeks ago. She stopped using birth control pills a year ago, citing that "I was too old to be on the pill." She and her husband already have two teenagers. She is shocked when her pregnancy test is positive and feels overwhelmed about the thought of having another child. After pregnancy options counseling, she goes home to talk with her husband. The couple returns the following week, having decided to proceed with an aspiration abortion. Her examination reveals an 8-week-sized, anteverted uterus. A transvaginal ultrasound reveals an intrauterine pregnancy approximately 8.6 weeks by crown-rump length.

Diagnosis (Algorithm 30.1)

- 8.6-week intrauterine pregnancy
- Desire for elective termination.

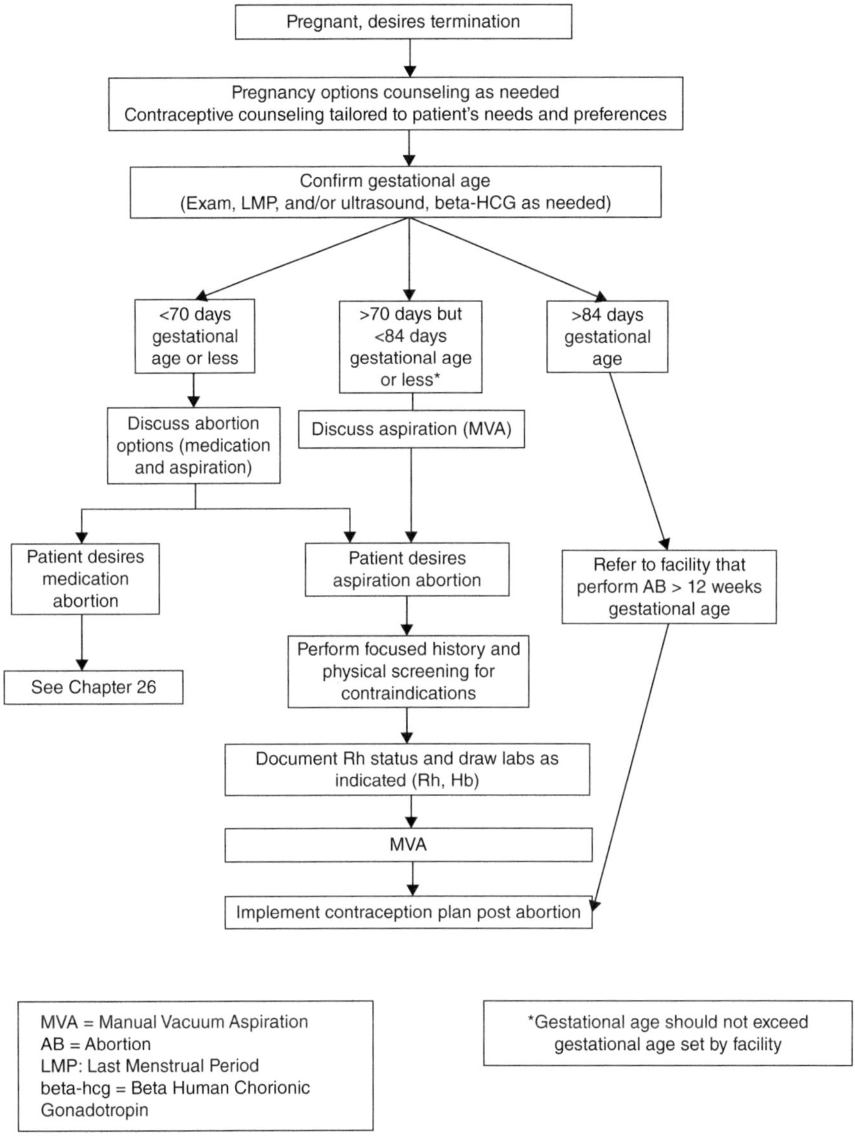

Algorithm 30.1 Decision tree for patients desiring elective termination

Differential Diagnosis

- Normal, intrauterine pregnancy.
- Ectopic pregnancy.
- Heterotopic pregnancy (concomitant presence of an intrauterine and ectopic pregnancy).
- Early pregnancy loss (threatened, incomplete, or complete spontaneous abortion).

Indications (Algorithm 30.1)

- Elective abortion up to 12 weeks.
- Treatment for early pregnancy loss up to 12 weeks.
- Medical necessity for patients with comorbidities in which carrying a pregnancy to term poses a threat to health and/or life.
- Endometrial biopsy (instead of using the endometrial pipelle).

Contraindications (Algorithm 30.1)

- Gestational age is greater than the limit set by the clinical site.
- Inability to tolerate MVA under local anesthesia and available analgesia.
- Known hydatidiform mole (should be referred to a tertiary care center for abortion).
- Hemodynamic instability (should be stabilized and referred to a tertiary care center).
- Severe medical illness (e.g., suspected diabetic ketoacidosis, uncontrolled seizure disorder, acute asthmatic attack) requiring hospitalization for management.

Special Considerations/Contraindications

- Active intrauterine infection: Clinicians should decide whether or not to proceed with the procedure depending on the patient's clinical status. Treatment should be initiated promptly per the Centers for Disease Control (CDC) Sexually Transmitted Diseases Treatment Guidelines [7].
- Mucopurulent cervicitis: The patient should be treated per CDC guidelines for presumptive gonorrhea and chlamydia cervicitis [7]. The patient can still undergo the procedure that day but should complete treatment postprocedure.
- Significant medical comorbidities: Examples include uncontrolled diabetes, cardiovascular or pulmonary disease, seizure disorder, and blood-clotting disorders.

Patients should be medically stable prior to the procedure and/or referred to a facility that is able to treat patients with such conditions.

- Cervical stenosis: May require cervical ripening agents, special dilation techniques.
- Severe anemia: Defined as hemoglobin <8 mg/dl, hematocrit <24%, and/or symptomatic anemia. Clinicians need to determine whether to proceed, delay the procedure, or refer to a facility with medications for postabortion hemorrhage or blood products.
- Suspected and/or known ectopic pregnancy: Evaluate, treat, and refer according to local protocol.

Equipment (Fig. 30.1)

Sterile instrument trays containing the following:
Procedure supplies:

- Specula (various sizes).
- Ringed forceps (sponge stick).
- Iodine cups.
- Tenaculums.
- Cervical dilators (e.g., Denniston or Pratt).

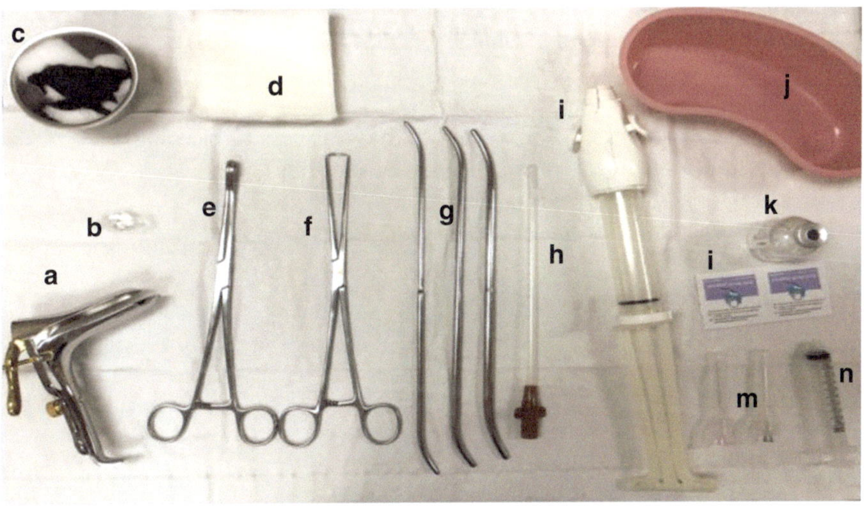

Fig. 30.1 Equipment setup for MVA. *Sterile*: (**a**) speculum; (**b**) surgical lubricant; (**c**) antiseptic-soaked cotton balls in basin; (**d**) sterile gauze sponges; (**e**) ring forceps; (**f**) single-tooth tenaculum; (**g**) cervical dilator set; (**h**) flexible cannula. *Not sterile*: (**i**) manual vacuum aspirator; (**j**) kidney-shaped basin; (**k**) lidocaine; (**l**) alcohol pads; (**m**) 18-gauge and 22-gauge 1.5-inch needles; (**n**) 10-cc syringe

- 60-cc aspiration syringe (e.g., IPAS MVA Plus®, IPAS, Chapel Hill, NC)
- Flexible cannulas in sizes 6–12 (e.g., IPAS Karman® [IPAS, Chapel Hill, NC], MedGyn® [Medgyn, Lombard, IL], Berkeley® [Berkeley Medevices, Richmond, CA]).

For viewing and processing products of conception (POC):

- Light box (available at a photography or craft store).
- Glass Pyrex dish (traditional pie size).
- Strainer (kitchen supply).
- Long forceps (to move and examine POC).
- Pathology specimen jars or disposal cups.

Additional supplies:

- Two 10–12-cc syringes.
- 22-gauge 1½-inch needles
- Sharps containers.
- Nonsterile gloves/sterile gloves.
- Sterile gauze.
- Betadine.
- Kidney basins.
- Autoclave and supplies for cleaning and wrapping equipment.

Medications:

- Lidocaine 1% (may dilute 50/50 with normal saline).
- Ibuprofen.
- Consider RhoGAM® (Ortho Clinical Diagnostics, Raritan, NJ).

For emergency use:

- Methergine® (Novartis, Basil, Switzerland) (for excessive bleeding).
- Misoprostol (for cervical ripening, excessive bleeding).
- Atropine (for sustained vasovagal reaction).
- IV tubing, IV fluid, IV catheters in various gauges, tape.
- Albuterol inhaler.
- Epinephrine 1:1000.

Ultrasound and supplies (if an ultrasound is on-site):

- Probe covers.
- Probe disinfectant.
- Ultrasound gel.
- Printer paper (if printer available).

Patient items:

- Drape.
- Gown.
- Sanitary napkins.

Documents:

- MVA Consent Form (Fig. 30.2).
- MVA Procedure Form (Fig. 30.3).
- MVA After-Care Instructions and Information (Fig. 30.4).
- Relevant birth control education.

Manual Vacuum Aspiration (MVA) Consent Form

____ I request a Manual Vacuum Aspiration (MVA), a procedure that will empty my uterus. This procedure may be used as a suction abortion or as treatment for a miscarriage, a failed medication abortion or for abnormal uterine bleeding.

____ I understand that if I am pregnant, my three options regarding this pregnancy are parenthood, adoption, and abortion. I understand that if I am pregnant, the MVA will end my pregnancy.

____ I understand that before the MVA, I may have blood tests done to check me for anemia and I will have to document my Rh type by history, blood donor card, prior blood test or a new blood test.
If I am Rh negative, I will be offered a shot of MicRhogam.

____ I understand that I might be offered medication before the MVA, ibuprofen to lessen the cramping. I will have local anesthesia with Lidocaine injected. To the best of my knowledge, I am not allergic to Ibuprofen or Lidocaine.

____ I understand that the possible complications from MVA include: incomplete emptying of my uterus, infection, bleeding, allergic reaction and perforation.

____ I have read this form and have had time to think about it. I have had all my questions answered.

____ I have been given an information sheet explaining how and when to get help should a question or problem arise after the procedure.

____ In the event of an unexpected complication during the MVA, I request and authorize the physician to do whatever is needed to protect my health and welfare.

____ I hereby consent that ______________________________ do the procedure “manual vacuum aspiration” for me.

____ If I had testing for sexually transmitted infections or blood type testing I will be available at this number to receive results:

My Phone: ________________________ May we leave a confidential message? ___yes ___no

Signature of patient: ____________________________**Date:**____________________

Witness: ______________________________________ **Date:** ____________________

Signature of Clinician:___________________________ **Date:** ____________________

Fig. 30.2 MVA consent form. (Adapted from Reproductive Health Access Project: http://www.reproductiveaccess.org/ with permission)

MVA PROCEDURE NOTE

Date:
Name:
DOB:

Physical Examination:
Uterus: Size in weeks (bimanual): ______ AV/Mid / RV Cervix: WNL / CMT, parous/nullip
Vagina: WNL / discharge noted:

Procedure:
- Cervix and vagina swabbed with Betadine.
- Lidocaine 1%, _________cc total injected.
- Tenaculum applied _________ o'clock.
- Cervix progressively dilated to: _________.
- Cannula inserted, size __________.
- Estimated blood loss: ________ cc.
- Additional comments:

Tissue Exam:
- Decidual tissue
- Villi
- Gestational sac
- Tissue appropriate for gestational age

Post-Op Ultrasound if done:
No IUP visualized
Other:

Assessment:
Patient stable, AB complete
- Pad checked for bleeding
  - o For complications, see progress notes
- Post-procedure vital signs: B/P____ P____

Plan:
- Expected symptoms discussed; post-procedure instructions given.
- Rhogam if needed:_______________
- Doxycycline 100 mg tabs 2 tab _______ Dispensed or ___ 1 gm Zithromax
- Contraception:____
- Follow up appointment recommended.

Clinician Signature:____

www.reproductiveaccess.org

Fig. 30.3 MVA procedure note and procedure note. (Adapted from Reproductive Health Access Project: http://www.reproductiveaccess.org/ with permission)

ABORTION PROCEDURE AFTER-CARE

Today you had an abortion procedure. You will probably feel fine when you go home. You can go back to your regular activities as soon as you want to. You can take a shower and wash your hair as soon as you want to. You can eat normally, although you may still feel nauseated for another few days.

Are there things you should not do? Yes. For one week, do not put anything in your vagina. Do not use tampons, do not douche, and do not have sex.

WHAT TO EXPECT Vaginal Bleeding: You can expect to have bleeding for up to 2 weeks. It is common for the bleeding to stop and start for several weeks after the abortion. Some people have no bleeding for 2 or 3 days and then begin to have bleeding like a period. Other people have only spotting for a few days and then no more bleeding at all. If you exercise or have a lot of activity, you may notice the bleeding increases; this is not dangerous.

Cramping: You may have cramps off and on during the week following an abortion. You can use pain medication like Tylenol, Ibuprofen (Motrin or Advil), or Naproxen (Aleve or Naprosyn). You can also use a heating pad, or drink some warm tea.

Sadness or very emotional: You may feel very relieved when the abortion is over. You may also feel sad or moody. These feelings are partly from the changes in hormones, now that you are no longer pregnant. Feeling emotional at this time is normal. If you think your emotions are not what they should be, please talk to us.

When will your period come back? You can expect a period in 4 to 8 weeks. Itis not the same for everyone.

You **should** call me if: Your bleeding soaks through more than 2 maxi pads per hour for more than 2 hours. Your cramps that are getting stronger and are not helped by pain medication. ! If your temperature is higher than 101 degrees (38.3 degrees Celcius).

To reach me:

Call my 24-hour number: ________________________. If you have any questions or think something is going wrong, call this number and I will call you back. It may take me 10 to 15 minutes to return your call. No question is too small. **Please feel free to call me.**

Follow-up visit: You have an appointment in 1 week, _______________ at ______am/pm.

Birth Control:

If you want to use birth control pills, patch, or ring, I have given you a prescription. You should start these on __________, even if you are still bleeding.

June 2016 / www.reproductiveaccess.org

reproductive health access project

Fig. 30.4 MVA patient instructions. (Adapted from: Reproductive Health Access Project: http://www.reproductiveaccess.org/ with permission)

Procedures

Preprocedure Steps

1. Perform pregnancy options counseling. Important points to consider.
   - Ask open-ended questions in a nonjudgmental manner, e.g., "How do you feel about being pregnant?"
   - Inquire about the patient's support network (partner, family, friends).
   - Discuss all options as necessary: (1) continuing the pregnancy and becoming a parent, (2) continuing the pregnancy and opting for adoption, or (3) ending the pregnancy.
   - Assess that the patient's decision, whatever it may be, has not been coerced.
2. Confirm pregnancy diagnosis and gestational age by assessing LMP, performing a bimanual examination, and obtaining an ultrasound. Obtain a urine pregnancy test or serum β-HCG, if indicated.
3. Confirm eligibility criteria and conduct other medical screening as indicated (e.g., Pap smear, STI testing). The performance of such screening tests in otherwise asymptomatic patients is not mandatory prior to performing MVA.
4. Help the patient select an appropriate birth control method, if desired. Discuss Emergency Contraception (EC) and provide advance prescriptions of EC if necessary.
5. Providers may choose to routinely screen for anemia depending on the local prevalence of anemia and/or by individual risk factors and clinical history [4].
6. Consider confirming Rh type (review blood donor cards, old prenatal labs, or send for testing), see note below.
7. Review the consent form and obtain the patient's signature (Fig. 30.2).
8. Provide a single dose of pre-procedure antibiotics [5].
9. Provide preprocedure analgesics with NSAIDs [8].

A Note About Rh Testing Rhesus (Rh) factor testing is no longer indicated for abortions occurring at less than 12 weeks (84 days) of gestation according to the World Health Organization, the National Abortion Federation, and the Society of Family Planning [2, 9, 10]. This includes both medication and manual vacuum aspiration abortions. The American College of Obstetrics and Gynecology still recommends it for all patients undergoing induced abortion or early pregnancy loss [11].

Performing MVA

Throughout the procedure, the "no-touch" technique should be followed such that instrument parts that enter the cervical os are never touched, thereby maintaining sterility.

Step 1: Prepare the Patient and Prep the Cervix (Fig. 30.5)

- Have the patient empty their bladder.
- Explain the procedure steps to the patient and answer all remaining questions.
- Help the patient into a dorsal lithotomy position on the table.
- Wash hands, put on appropriate barrier equipment; gloves can be sterile or nonsterile.
- Perform a bimanual examination, noting the size, shape, and position of the uterus.
- Insert the speculum so that the entire cervix is well visualized.
- Clean the cervix with an antiseptic-soaked sponge if desired; no proven effect on postabortion infection.

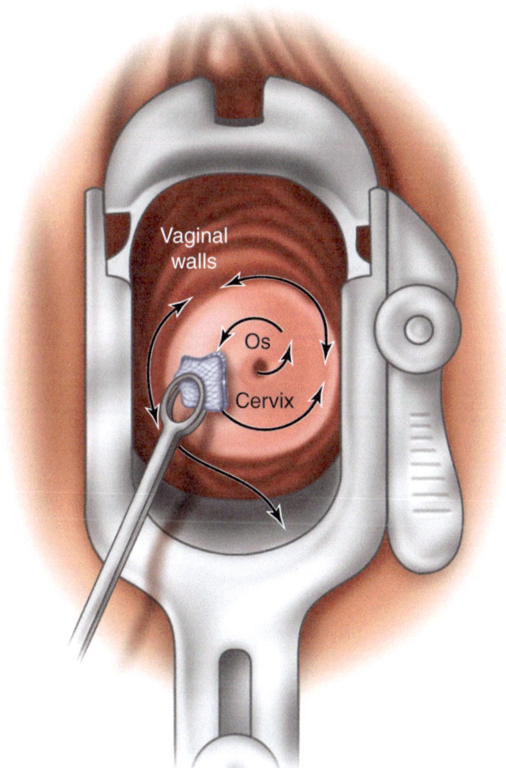

Fig. 30.5 Prepping the cervix . (With permission from IPAS, Stephen C. Edgerton, illustrator)

Step 2: Administer a Paracervical Block (Fig. 30.6)

- Inject 1–2 cc of local anesthetic at the planned tenaculum site (12:00 for an anteverted uterus, 6:00 for a retroverted uterus).
- Place the tenaculum at the anesthetized site by opening the tenaculum and closing it around a generous amount of cervical tissue, which allows gentle traction to be applied to straighten the uterus.
- Using the tenaculum, move the cervix to the side to visualize the "reflection," the site at which smooth cervical tissue meets vaginal tissue.
- Inject 5–10 cc of anesthetic into a depth of at least 1.5 cm at 2–4 points at the "reflection" (2 and 10 o'clock and/or 4 and 8 o'clock). Pull back on the plunger before injecting, to avoid administering into a blood vessel [12].

Step 3: Dilate the Cervix (Table 30.2)

Table 30.2 displays the recommended dilation and cannula size needed for the corresponding gestational age. During dilation, maintain gentle traction on the tenaculum to pull the uterine axis as straight as possible. Use a "no-touch" technique: only

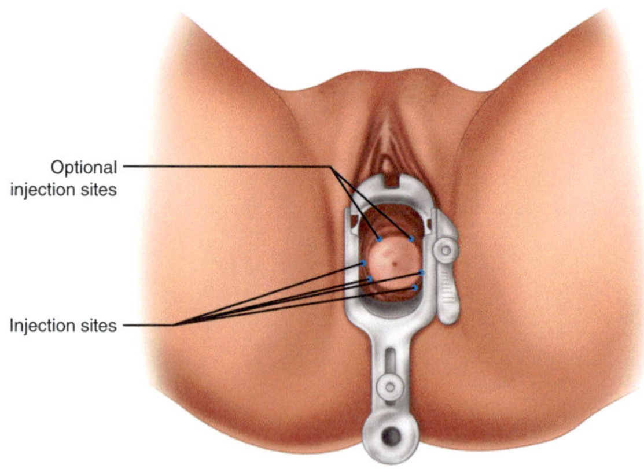

Fig. 30.6 Paracervical block sites. (With permission from IPAS, Stephen C. Edgerton, illustrator)

Table 30.2 Suggested dilation and cannula by gestational age

Gestational age (weeks) by ultrasound	Dilator size—measured in circumference (or in diameter; mm)	Cannula size (mm)
5.0–6.4	19 (6)	6
6.5–7.4	21 (7)	7
7.5–8.4	25 (8)	8
8.5–9.4	27 (9)	9
9.5–10.4	31 (10)	10
10.5–11.4	33 (11)	11
11.5–12.4	37 (12)	12

hold the instruments on parts that will not enter the uterine cavity, i.e., the middle of the dilators, the end of the cannula attached to the MVA.

1. Gently insert the first dilator into the cervix so that it is introduced just beyond the internal os. A slight “give” may be felt as the dilator slides from the wider external os past the internal os.
2. Take the dilator out and turn it over to dilate with the other side of the dilator (which is the next size up). Progressively dilate to the appropriate size.

Step 4: Insert the Cannula and Attach the Syringe (Fig. 30.7)

1. Insert the cannula into the cervix, past the cervical os and into the uterine cavity toward the fundus.
2. Attach a “primed” MVA syringe to the cannula, holding the tenaculum and the end of the cannula in one hand and the aspirator in the other.

Step 5: Evacuate the Uterus

- Release the valve buttons of the MVA syringe which will start the suction (Fig. 30.8).
- Gently and slowly rotate the syringe 360°, using an in-and-out motion at the same time. There should be a return of blood and tissue through the cannula and into the syringe (Fig. 30.9).

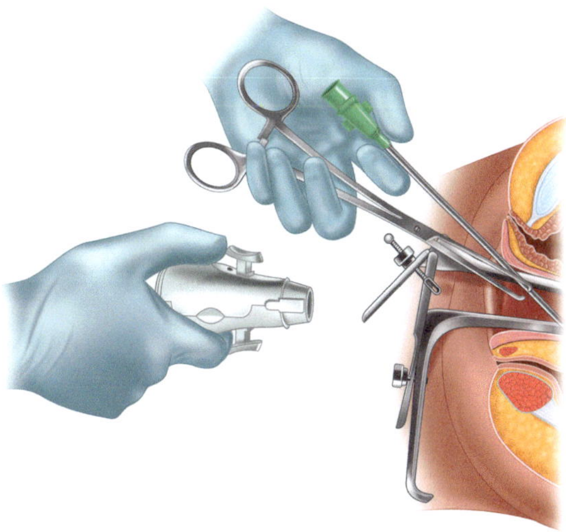

Fig. 30.7 Cannula inserted and attaching aspirator. (With permission from IPAS, Stephen C. Edgerton, illustrator)

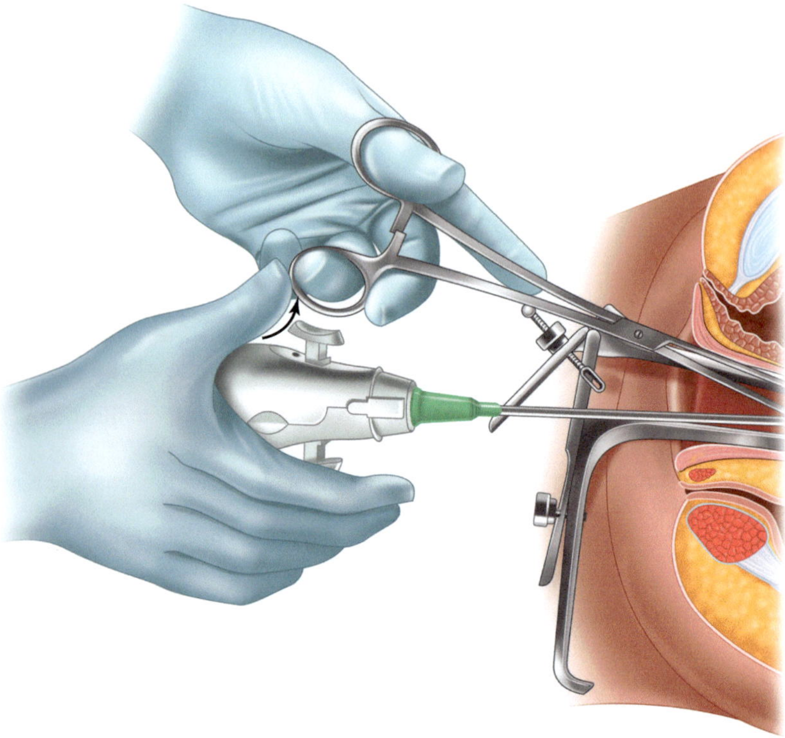

Fig. 30.8 Release the valve buttons of the MVA aspirator, which will start the suction. (With permission from IPAS, Stephen C. Edgerton, illustrator)

Fig. 30.9 Evacuating uterine contents. (With permission from IPAS, Stephen C. Edgerton, illustrator)

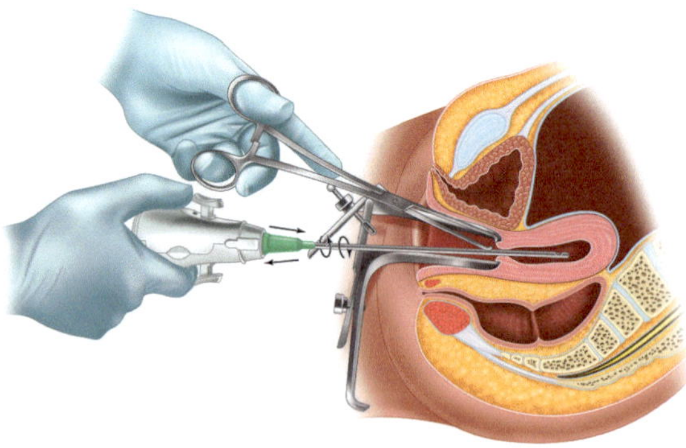

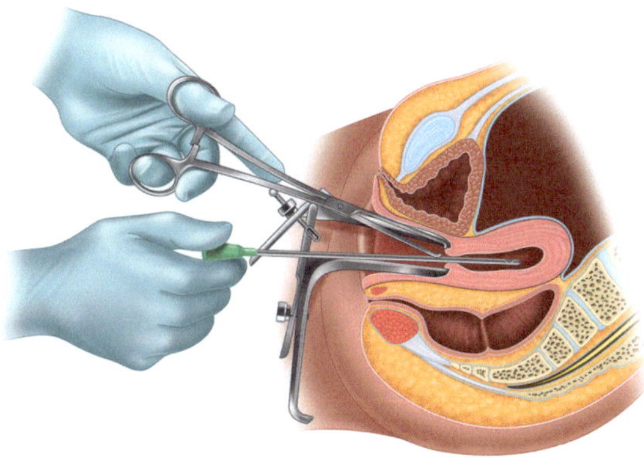

Fig. 30.10 Aspirator detached from cannula. (With permission from IPAS, Stephen C. Edgerton, illustrator)

- Once the aspirator is filled or once no further return of tissue occurs, withdraw the cannula beyond the cervical os until the vacuum is lost (a sound will be heard as the seal is broken).
- Reinsert the cannula just beyond the os at this time. Detach the aspirator from the cannula (Fig. 30.10). Empty the aspirator contents into a kidney basin.
- "Prime" the aspirator and attach it to the cannula. Repeat steps 4 and 5 until evacuation is complete.

Step 6: Assess for Complete Uterine Evacuation

The following signs indicate the uterus is completely evacuated:

- A "gritty" sensation is felt as the cannula passes over the uterine wall.
- The uterus "tightens" around the cannula.

Step 7: Complete the Procedure

- Take the cannula and aspirator out of the cervix.
- If an intrauterine device (IUD) is desired, it can be safely inserted at this time, although the expulsion rate may be higher when compared to delayed insertion [7].
- Take the tenaculum off. This can be facilitated by releasing the clamp and then gently rotating the entire tenaculum clockwise 180°, effectively lifting the "teeth" out of the cervical tissue.
- Use a sponge stick to gently swab any remaining blood out of the vaginal vault.
- Observe for any active bleeding, particularly from the tenaculum site and external os. Apply pressure to any sites of bleeding.
- Remove the speculum.

- Remove barriers and gloves, and wash hands.
- Help the patient into a comfortable position on the table.
- Offer contraception prior to leaving the office, long-acting contraception (LARC) preferred, Nexplanon can be inserted at the same visit if preferred over IUD. Start oral contraceptives or Depo Provera® on the day of the procedure.

Step 8: Inspect the Products of Conception (POC)

- The tissue should be rinsed in a strainer and placed in a clear, glass dish with water to help visualize the tissue.
- For best visualization, the dish should be placed on a light box.
- Identify villi, gestational sac, and decidual tissue (Fig. 30.11). As early as 8–9 weeks, fetal parts may be visible. Fetal parts must be positively identified in pregnancies at 10 weeks of gestation or greater.
- If no POC are visible or are less than expected for gestation age, an ultrasound and/or reaspiration should be considered, as well as re-evaluation of the diagnosis. The differential for absent POC or POC less than expected includes the following: (1) incomplete abortion, (2) spontaneous abortion that had already completed, (3) a uterine anomaly that precluded complete aspiration, (4) a failed abortion, or (5) ectopic pregnancy.
- After satisfactory inspection, the POC should be discarded per medical waste guidelines or sent to a pathology laboratory if required by institutional/state regulations.

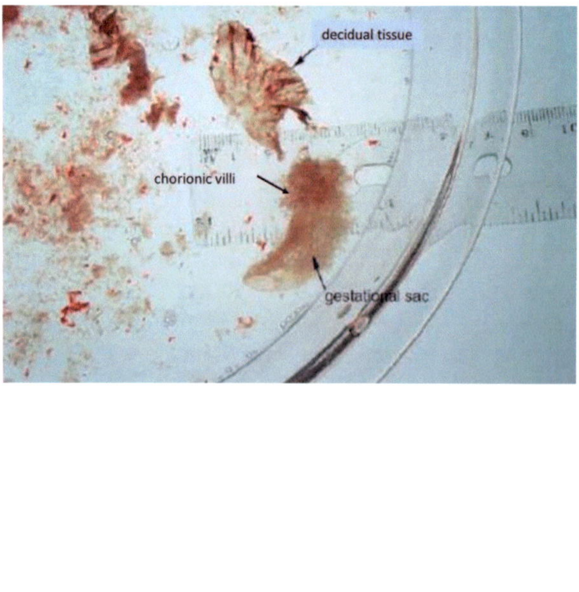

Fig. 30.11 Products of conception: villi/gestational sac and decidual tissue. (Courtesy of Deborah Oyer, MD, Seattle, WA)

Complications and Risks [3, 13–15]

- Significant bleeding (first-trimester rate): 0.07–0.4%.
- Infection: 0.01–0.4% (with the use of prophylactic antibiotics).
- Hematometra (accumulation of blood in uterus after procedure): 1.1%.
- Need to reaspirate (retained tissue or continuing pregnancy): 0.3%.
- Perforation: 0.02–0.07%.

Tricks and Helpful Hints

- Cervical preparation: Cervical priming with misoprostol (a prostaglandin agonist) for first-trimester abortion has been shown to increase initial cervical dilation, decrease blood loss, and require less dilation force [9]. The benefits of cervical priming must be weighed against the disadvantages of increased side effects, such as nausea, vomiting, diarrhea, bleeding, and cramping that can occur prior to the procedure. Common protocols for cervical priming include 400–600 μg (two to three tablets) of misoprostol taken 1–3 hours (h) prior to the procedure via buccal, sublingual, or vaginal administration [9]. Potential indications for preprocedure misoprostol cervical preparation may include the following:
  - Pregnancies over 11 weeks in nulliparous patients.
  - Any situation in which the risk of perforation is increased (e.g., stenotic os).
  - Pregnancies over 12 weeks.
- Performing the paracervical block: To reduce patient anxiety and pain, some clinicians like to ask the patient to cough just as the needle is inserted into the cervix. The cough serves to push the cervix forward toward the needle, and most importantly, it is a pain distracter. This technique can also be used when placing the tenaculum as well. Providers may opt to forego having the patient cough during times of high viral illness such as flu season or covid surges.
- Difficult dilation of an extremely anteverted or retroverted uterus: Changing to a shorter blade speculum (e.g., Klopfer, Weisman-Graves, Moore-Graves) allows the provider to bring the cervix closer. It also provides more anterior and posterior space to accommodate the dilators and cannula at a steeper angle to follow the uterine axis. The use of ultrasound to guide the path of the dilator may also be helpful.

Procedures

Coding

CPT® Codes (Current Procedural Terminology, AMA, Chicago, IL)	
For the visit	99,204 or 99,214 (level 4 new or established patient E/M visit)
For the ultrasound	76,817 (transvaginal ultrasound, pregnant uterus) or 76,815 (limited ultrasound, pregnant uterus)
For the procedure and medications:	
59,840	Induced abortion, by dilation and curettage
J2000	Lidocaine
64,450	Injection, nerve block
A4550	Surgical tray
99,000	Specimen handling
J2210	Methergine®
90,385	MICRhoGAM®
90,782	Therapeutic injection
ICD-10-CM-Diagnostic Codes (International Classification of Diseases, Tenth Revision, Clinical Modification, Center for Disease Control and Prevention)	
Z33.2	Legally induced abortion, without mention of complication, complete

Postprocedure Patient Instructions

- The patient may prefer to rest and recover for 15 minutes prior to leaving the visit.
- Continue to monitor symptoms and consider repeating vital signs after the procedure. Uterine cramping and bleeding should continue to subside. Prolonged cramping and excessive bleeding are not normal.
- The following items should be reviewed carefully with the patient (Fig. 30.4):
- Postprocedure self-care.
- Signs and symptoms requiring medical attention.
- How and when to start the desired contraceptive, review correct use, and possible side effects.
- The patient should be discharged home with the following:
- A follow-up appointment in 1–2 weeks (optional).
- Prescriptions or supplies for ibuprofen or analgesic of choice.
- Prescriptions or supplies of birth control to start as soon as possible.
- Prescriptions or supplies of a postabortion antibiotic dose if not administered prior to the procedure.
- A 24-h provider contact number.
- The Patient After-Care Instructions and Information Form (Fig. 30.4).

(Provider to fill in blanks/circle applicable choice when given multiple choices.)

Case Study Outcome

The patient underwent an uncomplicated MVA in the office. She had a copper intrauterine device placed immediately after the procedure. The products of conception were consistent with an 8–9-week pregnancy. She was discharged home in good condition.

Patient Handout

Preprocedure Handout Table 30.1
Postprocedure Handout Fig. 30.4

References

1. Westfall JM, Sophocles A, Burggraf H, Ellis S. Manual vacuum aspiration for first trimester abortion. Arch Fam Med. 1998;7(6):559–62.
2. World Health Organization (WHO). Abortion care guideline. Geneva: WHO; 2022.
3. National Academies of Sciences, Engineering, and Medicine. The safety and quality of abortion care in the United States. Washington, DC; 2018. p. 2018.
4. Henshaw SK. Unintended pregnancy and abortion in the USA: epidemiology and public health impact. In: Paul M, Lichtenberg ES, Borgatta L, Grimes DA, Stubblefield PG, Creinin MD, editors. Management of unintended and abnormal pregnancy. Comprehensive abortion care. Hoboken: Wiley-Blackwell; 2009.
5. Meckstroth K, Paul M. First-trimester aspiration abortion. In: Paul M, Lichtenberg ES, Borgatta L, Grimes DA, Stubblefield PG, Creinin MD, editors. Management of unintended and abnormal pregnancy. Comprehensive abortion care. Hoboken: Wiley-Blackwell; 2009.
6. Low N, Mueller M, Van Vliet HA, Kapp N. Perioperative antibiotics to prevent infection after first-trimester abortion. Cochrane Database Syst Rev. 2012;3:CD005217.
7. Centers for Disease Control and Prevention. Sexually transmitted diseases treatment guidelines. MMWR Recomm Rep. 2015;64(RR-3):51–82. Bednarek PH, Creinin MD, Reeves MF, Cwiak C, Espey E, Jensen JT. Immediate versus delayed IUD insertion after uterine aspiration. N Engl J Med. 2011;364:2208–17
8. Moayedi G, Tschann M. Pain management for first-trimester uterine aspiration. Obstet Gynecol Surv. 2018;73(3):174–81.
9. Mark A, Foster A, Grossman D, Prager S, Reeves M, Velasquez C, Winikoff B. Foregoing Rh testing and anti-D immunoglobulin for women presenting for early abortion: a recommendation from the National Abortion Federation's Clinical Policies Committee. Contraception. 2019;99:265–6.
10. Horvath S, Goyal V, Traxler S, Prager S. Society of Family Planning committee consensus on Rh testing in early pregnancy. Contraception. 2022;114:1–5.
11. American College of Obstetricians and Gynecologists (ACOG). Bulletin 225: medication abortion up to 70 days of gestation. Washington, D.C.; 2023.
12. Renner RM, Edelman AB, Nichols MD, Jensen JT, Lim JY, Bednarek PH. Refining paracervical block techniques for pain control in first trimester surgical abortion: a randomized controlled noninferiority trial. Contraception. 2016;94(5):461–6.

13. Flemming M, Shih G, Goodman S. TEACH abortion training curriculum. 2022. 7th ed.
14. White K, Carroll E, Grossman D. Complications from first trimester aspiration abortion: a systematic review of the literature. Contraception. 2015;92(5):422–38.
15. Upadhyay UD, Desai S, Zlidar V, Weitz TA, Grossman D, Anderson P, Taylor D. Incidence of emergency department visits and complications after abortion. Obstet Gynecol. 2015;125(1):175–83.

Additional Resources

Websites

For patient and clinician resources regarding early abortion care, visit The Reproductive Health Access Project: http://www.reproductiveaccess.org/

For information regarding abortion training in family medicine residencies, visit The Center for Reproductive Health Education in Family Medicine www.rhedi.org

For educational resources and a clinical curriculum regarding medication abortion, visit: (1) The National Abortion Federation: http://www.prochoice.org/education/resources/index.html. (2) TEACH Abortion Training Curriculum: https://pressbooks.pub/workbook/

For information regarding state laws on abortion, visit The Center for Reproductive Rights: http://www.reproductiverights.org/ or guttmacher.org

For information regarding MVA aspirators and supplies: www.ipas.org

Index

S. M. Sulik, C. B. Heath (eds.), *Primary Care Procedures in Women's Health*,
https://doi.org/10.1007/978-3-032-07061-6

L

M

MIX
Papier aus verantwortungsvollen Quellen
Paper from responsible sources
FSC® C105338

FSC
www.fsc.org

If you have any concerns about our products,
you can contact us on
ProductSafety@springernature.com

In case Publisher is established outside the EU,
the EU authorized representative is:
Springer Nature Customer Service Center GmbH
Europaplatz 3, 69115 Heidelberg, Germany

Printed by Libri Plureos GmbH
in Hamburg, Germany